Poverty and Health

This volume is published as part of a long-standing cooperative program between the Harvard University Press and the Commonwealth Fund, a philanthropic foundation, to encourage the publication of significant and scholarly books in medicine and health.

Poverty and Health
A Sociological Analysis

Edited by John Kosa

and Irving Kenneth Zola

Revised Edition

A Commonwealth Fund Book

Harvard University Press

Cambridge, Massachusetts

and London, England

Foreword

The reason for a second edition of *Poverty and Health* is eloquently stated by the late John Kosa in the first chapter. He comments on the fictional work of F. Scott Fitzgerald portraying the life of the wealthy, and Erskine Caldwell's writing about the poor, and states: "In this respect fiction illustrates a common characteristic of society: wealth is always noticed, but poverty is often overlooked, and not only by individuals, but also entire communities may be impervious to it."

There seems to be a need to rediscover the existence of poverty in our society. As a nation we have accepted equality of opportunity in principle and optimistically tend to think that the principle is universally applied. "Equal opportunity" implies that everyone has the chance to move upward in the social order if he works hard, saves, and plans ahead; "downward" mobility is the penalty for laziness, extravagance, and the desire for immediate gratification. Accordingly, poverty is essentially a self-determined condition, except for those handicapped by physical or mental defects.

This belief, firmly rooted in the Puritan ethic, and coupled with our commitment to a society which rejects the idea of a fixed class system, makes it difficult to deal in a realistic way with what Kosa terms "chronic poverty"— poverty which is lifelong and even multigenerational. Even our rediscovery of poverty in the 1960s and the well-publicized launching of the "war on poverty" have failed to make a lasting impact, and the greatest danger is that, as a nation, we will ignore the problem or at best think of it intermittently and in piecemeal terms.

This book reminds us that poverty continues to exist and documents once again the relationship between poverty and ill health. The evidence cited by each of the authors demonstrates over and over again that the poor fare less well than the affluent in almost every measure of health, both physical and mental, and they have far more difficulty in gaining access to adequate medical care.

A two-class system of medical care persists in this country, despite some blurring of the boundaries. By and large, the urban poor receive their ambulatory care in the emergency rooms and out-patient departments of large public and voluntary hospitals and, to a lesser extent, in community clinics. In-patient care for the urban poor is more likely to be on the "ward service" of the hospital than on the private service, and this is true whether or not the patient can pay via Medicaid or Medicare. The rural poor are less well provided for because physicians' services have all but disappeared from many poverty areas in rural America.

The liberal segment of our society, which is well represented in the Congress, feels that the two-class system of care should be eliminated and that as a matter of equity there should be one standard of care for all citizens. This position appears eminently reasonable, and yet differences in health between the poor and the non-poor cannot be reconciled so simply. Let us suppose, for example, that a sweeping new law were passed creating a national health insurance which would provide payment for all health services and that eligibility were universal with no differences between rich and poor, employed or unemployed. Would such legislation guarantee that the poor would be given the same quality of care as the affluent—even supposing that there were an equitable distribution of medical care resources? Not necessarily. Several of the authors of this volume note than an important characteristic of the poor is their sense of powerlessness, the feeling that they cannot influence institutions and that they are victimized by bureaucratic inertia.

It is quite possible that equal provision for payment by rich and poor alike would not result in equal care, because the poor are less able to insist on their rights than the affluent. The power structure of the medical profession, of hospital administration, and hospital governance is controlled by the middle class, and the poor have little opportunity to influence what the providers of care are willing to offer. There might be some refurbishing of hospital outpatient departments and renaming of ward services, but the poor might continue to receive care that is not very different from what they get now.

For the poor, one of the more attractive features of community clinics developed by OEO was community participation in governance. This gave rise to occasional conflict with the providers of care, and there were examples of waste, but for the first time the poor felt that they had some voice in the way a part of the health system operated. Yet, here was an example of care designed for the poor and not modeled on the customary private practice of medicine.

The provision of high-quality, comprehensive care for the poor will not automatically result from health legislation, no matter how liberally defined. The problem is more complex and is concerned with social and political factors rather than payment mechanisms. In other words, how do the poor learn to exercise sufficient power to be able to influence the health system so that it begins to serve their needs more adequately? There are signs that some elements of the urban poor have learned how to wield power within their communities, a development that should be applauded rather than feared by the middle class, for the exercise of power is a statement of group self-determination and the first step upward out of poverty.

A true health security bill would not solve the problems of health care for the poor, but it would be a beginning. Unfortunately, something less is likely to be legislated. The Congress may pass a national health insurance bill which contains provisions for co-insurance and deductibles. These are precisely the provisions which will hurt the poor most of all, but they may be legislated because the poor are not well represented in the halls of Congress.

Let us hope that this book will be read by those who can, by the force of their actions, influence the course of human affairs, There is much here to think about and, more important, to do something about.

Robert H. Ebert, M.D.
Dean, Harvard Medical School

Preface

The social sciences discovered illness in the 1950s, and rediscovered poverty almost a decade later. When the first edition of *Poverty and Health* was being planned, the three original editors (Kosa, Antonovsky, and Zola) were working on related issues in the Boston area. We debated whether to write a general treatise on the relationship between poverty and health or to assemble a collection of previously published articles. Finally, we decided to edit a book of original but collected essays, placing each author's contribution into a planned structure.

We prepared detailed outlines for every chapter and submitted them to the authors. To our gratification, this step did not give offense. The authors seemed to feel that the outlines enabled them to take off more freely, to divest themselves of the need to touch on every angle of the problem, and to write in the knowledge that they were writing for a book. These were the organizing principles of the first edition, published in 1969, and of this new edition. Two chapters and a technical appendix have been eliminated; one new chapter, on medical education, has been added. All the material has been revised and updated.

The idea for both the original and the new edition was John Kosa's. We became full partners as we worked through the detailed design and reworked and edited the various chapters. Kosa undertook the organizational work, greatly helped during the preparation of the first edition by the encouragement of Dr. Charles Janeway and the generous cooperation of Dr. Joel J. Alpert. For the second edition, we had the indispensable editorial assistance of Mrs. Judith

Auerbach. Without her, this book would never have been completed, for in mid-1972, John Kosa died. At the time of his death he was Director of the Medical Care Research Unit, Harvard Medical School, and Associate Professor in Sociology in the Department of Pediatrics, Harvard Medical School. This book testifies to his organizational ability, and although it would be naive to say that every subsequent decision was made with Kosa in mind, the intellectual give and take of our earlier decision-making was maintained.

I most particularly want to thank Aaron Antonovsky for his detailed and substantive criticisms of the manuscript.

Irving Kenneth Zola
Professor of Sociology, Brandeis University, and
Consultant Sociologist, Medical Division,
Massachusetts General Hospital

Waltham, Massachusetts
January 1975

Contents

Foreword by Robert H. Ebert, M.D.   v

Preface   ix

I.   The Nature of Poverty   1
    John Kosa

II.   The Social Aspects of Health and Illness   40
    John Kosa and Leon S. Robertson

III.   Social Differences in Physical Health   80
    Monroe Lerner

IV.   Social Differences in Mental Health   135
    Marc Fried

V.   Prevention of Illness and Maintenance
    of Health   193
    Irwin M. Rosenstock

VI.   The Help-Seeking Behavior of the Poor   224
    John B. McKinlay

VII.   The Treatment of the Sick   274
    Julius A. Roth

VIII.   Readjustment and Rehabilitation of Patients   303
    Marvin B. Sussman

IX.   Patient Care, the Poor, and Medical Education   335
      Raymond S. Duff

X.   The Reorganization of Practice in the   351
      Community
      John D. Stoeckle

      Notes   399

      Index   445

Tables

I-1.   Geographical factors in poverty   17

I-2.   Social factors in poverty   20

III-1.   Specific aspects of life-styles most relevant to the achievement of health among the three major socioeconomic strata   87

III-2.   Selected measures of overall mortality and infant mortality by residence and race   108

III-3.   Infant mortality by cause, 1962, in ten largest cities   120

III-4.   Days of disability per person per year by type of disability and family income   123

III-5.   Days of disability per person per year by type of disability, age group, and family income   124

III-6.   Percent distribution of persons by chronic condition and mobility limitation status   126

VII-1.   Relationship between income and having a physician   276

VII-2.   Repeated utilization of a pediatric emergency clinic   279

VIII-1. New career status and rehabilitation career interest   311

VIII-2. Tuberculosis patients with reduced rehabilitation potentials   315

VIII-3. Rehabilitation patients failing to participate in follow-up observations   318

VIII-4. Economic dependence and deterioration of activities among patients with fracture of the hip   320

VIII-5. Economic dependence and deterioration of activities among patients with first stroke   320

VIII-6. Length of hospital stay for patients discharged from a rehabilitation hospital, by source of funding   326

VIII-7. Costs of hospitalization in 1960 for 177 patients with completed rehabilitation   329

X-1. Out-of-hospital treatment organizations   354

Charts

II-1. The schema of the morbid episode   66

II-2. The place of morbid episodes in the social interaction pattern   76

VI-1.   Predominant service orientations and the typical utilization patterns of two social categories   265

X-1.   Treatment organizations and their use (estimated annual visits)   358

Poverty and Health

I. The Nature of Poverty

John Kosa

The biblical saying, "the poor always ye have with you" (John 12:8), hardly needs confirmation. Every epoch of history and every country on the map has had its share of the poor, although this name was given to groups of widely varying conditions. The slaves of the Roman Empire, the serfs of the Middle Ages, the peons of Latin America, the inmates of English poorhouses, or (in our country and time) the marginal farmers in Appalachia and the racial minorities in the urban ghettos were equally called poor, although they represented varying degrees of deprivation and different stages of forlornness. Small wonder that William Graham Sumner, a founder of American sociology and spokesman of laissez-faire philosophy, claimed that no definition of "a poor man" was possible. He deplored the use of the phrase because it seemed dangerously elastic and capable of covering a host of "social fallacies."[1] Yet, use of the word survived.

If a common adjective has been applied to so many groups with varying ways of life, this must have happened because the word "poor" denotes an ancient concept for expressing social differences between man and man, a concept coined long before the social sciences came up with their notion of social stratification. From time immemorial this ancient concept has clearly distinguished one segment

At the time of his death in 1972, John Kosa was Director, Medical Care Research Unit, Harvard Medical School, and Associate Professor in Sociology in the Department of Pediatrics, Harvard Medical School.

of the population from the rest and has gained general acceptance in our daily speech. Nowadays, for many good reasons, it cannot be replaced by more precise terms, such as the lower class or the blue-collar class, which—in spite of a considerable overlap—refer to a different system of classification and are not interchangeable with "the poor."[2] For example, the blue-collar class includes industrial workers above the poverty level, but excludes the poor of the farming areas; on the other hand, the lower class excludes many of the elderly who spent most of their lives outside the lower class and have become destitute as an unfortunate consequence of aging.

THE UNEQUAL DISTRIBUTION OF MEANS AND PRIVILEGES

As a more important difference, the word "poor" has an emotional appeal that the term "lower class" lacks. "Poor" is usually taken as a synonym of "needy," and whoever is in need can rightfully appeal for help to those who are more fortunate. Poverty calls for assistance, evokes our commiseration, moves our protective instinct, and claims our idealism. Quite in accordance with this emotional appeal, poverty is a relative term that reflects a judgment made on the basis of standards prevailing in the community. The standards change in time and place; what is judged poverty in one community might be regarded as wealth in another. Nevertheless, there is a reality behind the appeal to our nurturance, and the judgment is based on certain objective and even tangible criteria that are visible to the observer. Thus, the poor are those who, by the prevailing standards, are found to be deficient in means of subsistence and privileges of life.

In our economy the means of subsistence refers to money. Ours is a market economy in which money is the general medium for which the goods that people produce and the work that people perform are institutionally exchanged. Money is accessible to all, although in varying degrees; within the individual limitations of its availability, money buys everything that a person needs as well as many other things he does not need. In other communities of the past no market economy, or only an imperfect one, existed; money was not available to all, each household unit produced what it could for the preservation of its life and resorted to barter infrequently. Yet the material possessions, particularly the means of production such as land, work animals, and implements, were unequally distributed; the poor owned less, produced less, and subsisted on a precarious level.

The privileges of life can be described as intangible social and psychological possessions. They include a relationship to the social power, a participation in making decisions that affect the community, an ability to realize one's own decisions and plans, and a possession of knowledge; they include access to the pleasurable things of life and particularly to the services of others. In a primitive economy the services are rendered by servants whose main duty is to do heavy work and drudgery for the privileged ones; in our complex economy the most important services (medical care, education, police protection, and so on) are either institutionally marketed or dispensed by the government.

The privileges include access to health, wholesomeness, and all those services that promote a healthy way of living. It is by no means accidental that everyday language often compares health with material possessions and speaks of "poor" health and "needy" persons; its semantics are based on the facts of life. From the time of Hippocrates and into our own century the privileged classes have had at their disposal all the available health services, while the large unprivileged masses have had to content themselves with inferior services or no services at all.[3]

The means and privileges that are available in a community are interconnected, and the possession of one of them is likely to lead to the possession of another. In a primitive society, without an efficient market economy, the poor have fewer means of production, gather in a poorer harvest, and are more vulnerable to such natural disasters of life as famine and plague. In our society the doctor's son has a better chance than the tenant farmer's son to obtain a higher education, buy the pleasurable things, or take part in community decisions. It follows that within any group of people that is sufficiently large and has advanced beyond a rudimentary cultural development the means and privileges are unequally distributed, and there is a class that possesses both and another class that is deficient in both. Thus, when speaking of poor versus wealthy we apply a rather simple and unidimensional division to the community and overlook the more complex forms of stratification that can be discerned with finer analytical tools. It is this simplicity of outlook that recommends the concept of poverty and safeguards its currency, in spite of the objections of many scholars and even more non-scholarly representatives of conservatism. It is a concept that can be applied to almost any society and understood by anyone; it helps us to orient ourselves within any community because it makes one broad distinction between the wealthy and the poor.

The possession of means and privileges is visible and even conspicuous. The unequal distribution of worldly goods can be assessed and expressed without any special knowledge. A reasonably adequate judgment of the other person can often be formed without a personal acquaintance, and those who are familiar with their community can safely place their fellow citizens along the wealth. poverty line.[4] In fact, the designation of a person by his possession of worldly goods is a usual part of his full characterization, and writers of fiction seldom omit this trait when describing their fictional heroes. Compare F. Scott Fitzgerald with his fine differentiation among the wealthy and Erskine Caldwell with his compassionate rendering of the various shades of the poor; one gets the impression that while Caldwell urges us to help those in need, Fitzgerald does not seem to notice their existence. In this respect fiction illustrates a common characteristic of society: wealth is almost always noticed, but poverty is often overlooked, and not only individuals but also entire communities may be impervious to it.

ATTITUDES TOWARD POVERTY

As a part of our social life we tend to judge our fellow beings by their worldly goods; we perceive some of them as poor and set them apart from the rest of us. This is a motivated judgment that bolsters the judge's social position by defining others as being inferior to him in worldly possessions. It is a social judgment based on common standards and the consensus of the community. Hence, within the community the individual judgments follow a common pattern and end up in a consensual evaluation; but the communities greatly differ among themselves in the perception of poverty and in their response to its emotional appeal.

Some communities regard poverty as part of a permanent social order established by nature, divinity, or a mythical hero. The social order is codified in unwritten customs or written laws that in a statutory way deprive one broad group of people of means and privileges, relegate them to poverty, and enforce their deprivation. They establish slavery, serfdom, peonage, or any other of those disadvantaged statuses that exist in hierarchically structured feudal societies. Within the formally established social structure the status of the individual is often inherited, but it is, in any case, firmly assigned to him so that he can change it only in rare instances. The poor owe permanent services to the privileged and, in return, are supposed to receive some kind of protection, which, however, does not protect them against perennial pauperism. Poverty is not perceived as a separate phenomenon but is regarded as a relevant constituting element of a natural order.

Two examples may illustrate how institutionalized poverty is established within the total social structure. When in 1619 the first Negroes were introduced into the colony of Virginia, they were regarded as indentured servants. For the next three or four decades Negroes whose period of service had expired received land assigned to them in much the same way as white servants. Then the colony enacted a series of statutes which gradually excluded the Negro from the privileges of the indentured servants, making him instead a chattel and his servitude perpetual. Very few of the statutes dealt with the means of subsistence, but this was hardly necessary since deprivation of privileges implied a commensurate deprivation of means also. By 1670 slavery as a legal institution was firmly established, and the statutes of Virginia became models followed by the neighboring colonies.[5]

Another case of interest is Latin America, where sharp social cleavages exist among the various segments of society, particularly between the more privileged classes with their Hispano-American culture and the mestizo and Indian population with their native culture. As health insurance and social security programs have been established in the various countries, mainly during the last few decades, the services have been designed chiefly for the benefit of the privileged groups such as the military, governmental employees, white-collar workers, and groups of blue-collar workers with political weight and power. At the same time the mestizos and Indians, in spite of their conspicuous needs, have been left out of these programs.[6] Generally speaking, the new privilege of insured health care has been allotted in proportion to the privileges previously enjoyed, and in many cases the system of health insurance and social security has accentuated rather than mitigated the long-existing inequality of social classes.

Other societies, and notably those which have eliminated the remnants of feudalism, regard poverty not as part of an immutable order but as a condition created essentially by men. They acknowledge the existence of several social classes, distinguished informally and without any legal barriers separating one from the other. The means and privileges, although unequally distributed, are legally available to all, but the legal freedom of acquisition does not imply that everybody is equally free to participate in the resulting competition. Free competition hardly ever exists in social groups because it is restricted by several ubiquitous conditions—primarily by the unequal distribution of means and privileges. The possession of any one of the means and privileges helps the acquisition of another; that is, wealth helps toward successful participation in competition; poverty, on the other hand, restricts it. Moreover, numerous customs and prejudices (many of the latter reflect customs surviving from feudal times) further limit the poor in any acquisition, and the case of the Negro in present-day America well illustrates the point.

Under such conditions poverty may or may not be perceived. In any case, the designation of being poor signals unofficially the recognition of a social distance separating the poor from the rest of society, but no definitive exclusion from the means and privileges. Actually, the elastic structure of a class society offers opportunities absent in feudalism; the poor may take part in competition and, if successful, move upward on the social ladder. The elasticity of the structure and the rate of social mobility determine the success of the poor in upgrading themselves. An inelastic structure and slow mobility may perpetuate poverty within one segment of the population, as has happened in the rural South of the United States and, notably, in its Negro community. On the other hand, an elastic structure and rapid mobility may cause a rotating poor class, with many people moving upward while others are moving simultaneously downward or replenishing the poor class in some other way. The northern cities of the country, and notably their slums populated with successive waves of old-stock and new-stock immigrants, Negroes, and Puerto Ricans, present an example of this rotation.

The emotional appeal inherent in poverty may elicit a social response directed not toward the individual poor but toward poverty in general. The response takes one of two forms: it may be further deprivation or exploitation of the poor, as the case of the early Negroes in Virginia illustrates, or it may take the form of help on some community-wide basis, but this happens only when the "poor" are equated with the "needy." Help to the poor is not a consistent response; it is present in some communities but conspicuously absent in others. Its presence or absence is dependent on a more general orientation of the community, namely, whether or not poverty is taken for granted. As a rule, feudalism takes poverty for granted as a stable and even immutable institution and, accordingly, does not consider any helpful response necessary. A class society does not have a uniform response pattern because it may or may not take poverty for granted. It tends to respond in accordance with its moral sentiments and general conditions; if it views pauperism as a human condition subject to change, it is likely to extend help. To put it in plain words, however, it happens rather seldom that the sight of poverty leads to social concern.

Perception and response determine the attitudes that communities take toward poverty. Their combination yields four possible attitudes: (1) poverty is taken for granted, and its existence is not perceived; (2) poverty is taken for granted, but its existence is perceived; (3) poverty is not taken for granted and its existence is perceived; and (4) poverty is not taken for granted, but its existence is not perceived. Let us examine these attitudes as they evolved during their historical development.

Poverty that is taken for granted and not perceived has been a generally pervasive attitude all through the ages—a simple attitude of agnosticism that required no response to the existing facts. Supported by the belief in an immutable social order, the existence of conspicuous poverty was silently accepted and tolerated, as much by the poor as by the rich, without any manifest discontent or protest. The rich had few reasons, save that of conscience, to voice protest; but one notes with some amazement the docility with which the masses of slaves and serfs tolerated their institutional deprivation for centuries, and perhaps millenia, without any serious effort to change it. Slavery in America produced some localized revolts, but these were usually activated by slaves who were better off than their nonrevolting brothers and were not infrequently led by white persons.[7] The remnants of this ancestral acquiescence could still be discovered among the poor whom investigators just a short time ago were prone to describe as fatalistic, accepting deprivation as a natural part of life and showing relatively little inclination to diagnose and change existing situations.[8] Small wonder that present-day organizers of the poor advocate militancy as the necessary strategy to break the oppressive traditions of the past.

Poverty that is taken for granted while its existence is perceived was another common attitude of the past. Poverty was to some extent reconciled with the given social order, and treated in a superficial way without changing the social order or the causes of destitution. One response of this kind was summed up in the saying of the Romans: "panem et circenses." It described a policy toward the numerous poor in the imperial city whose revolutionary discontent was placated by distributing bread among them and furnishing games for their entertainment.

Christianity formed a more sublimated response by positing charity toward the poor as one of the three theological virtues. It was a symbolic response given to selected charity cases but denied to the overwhelming majority of the poor, who were excluded from the benefits of individual charity. The saints and heroes practiced charity, and their deeds were commemorated in many moving legends. The poor became the objects of charity, and their presence was needed for the daily practice of Christian virtues. Small wonder indeed that the Middle Ages did less than nothing to liberate the serfs and abolish the arrogant prerogatives of feudal lords; from time to time during that period a bloody cruelty was displayed in putting down the peasant revolts.

THE DISCOVERY OF POVERTY

The third community attitude, which does not take poverty for granted and perceives its existence, implies that poverty is a man-made condition, the result of human mismanagement of social affairs. It leads to a discovery of poverty in all its realistic details and to a desire to better the plight, not of a few charity cases, but of the whole class of the poor. This response does not necessarily mean that the community advocates revolutionary changes in the social structure, or that it has the required means and the knowledge of social engineering to carry out recommended reforms. The desire for improvement might be expressed in mere planning and scheming, much of which may remain naive, impractical, and even pettifogging, as it was with many early communistic schemes. However, the planning, whether good or poor, signals the readiness of the community to deal with poverty as a social problem.[9]

The famous Poor Laws of England codified this attitude perhaps for the first time. They were intended not to abolish pauperism but to alleviate the plight of the poor uniformly across the country, and in a crude way they contributed much to that noble goal. True enough, other countries did not seem to follow the English example, and England herself failed to adjust the Poor Laws to changing social conditions. But the medieval notion that the existing social order was a part of a cosmic divine order still held sway over people's minds and silenced the expression of any desire for social reforms. A general process of secularization was needed to change this mental attitude; when it came, it rejected the sacral notions surrounding the social order and contended that social structure was a human construct, free to be changed when change was desirable.

The modern discovery of poverty began with Adam Smith's notion that the "wealth of nations" was not a divine gift but rather the product of human labor, which could be manipulated for the attainment of greater wealth. His book contained some sensible passages on the poor (such as "Poverty sometimes urges nations to inhuman customs") but it somewhat vaguely predicted, as a general maxim, that poverty would eventually disappear. His optimistic prophecy sounded like a pleasant appeal to inertia; nevertheless, it furnished food for thought to many who wanted to fulfill the vague prediction with concrete plans of their own making. Robert Owen declared that poverty must be eliminated and recommended the Villages of Cooperation for this purpose. Saint-Simon outlined his hazy design for an industrial society without pauperism, and Marx developed an elaborate theory of socialism. With the arrival of Marx, poverty became the central issue in European politics and social philosophy.

The fourth attitude mentioned earlier does not take poverty for granted nor does it perceive its existence. Such a combination of views appears to be logically absurd, yet the attitude (either in a real or in an imaginary form) has exerted a tremendous impact upon present-day America. The writers who drew public attention to the problem in the early 1960's claimed that poverty was not known, and was ignored or hidden as if the nation wanted to close its eyes before a sight so disturbing to its conscience. Michael Harrington entitled the first chapter of his book "The Invisible Land."[10] A reviewer of the book, addressing the social conscience of the readers of *The New Yorker,* summed up the point concisely: "For a long time now, almost everybody has assumed that, because of the New Deal's social legislation and—more important—the prosperity we have enjoyed since 1940, mass poverty no longer exists in this country."[11]

It might very well be that the claim of the writers referred to an imaginary attitude, but, in any case, the claim appealed to the conscience of many and moved them to respond to the fact of poverty in an unprecedented way. It helped to launch the great national enterprise of the 1960s, the war on poverty, and if any attitude of not perceiving poverty had existed before, it certainly disappeared forthwith. In an almost cathartic outburst of emotions the nation suddenly realized that large-scale, unattended poverty existed in the most affluent country in the world and set out with earnest dedication to resolve this "paradox."[12]

One may question whether it is really paradoxical that poverty should exist amidst wealth and whether it is normal that wealth should bring forth an equal distribution of means and privileges. But perhaps the paradox might be better understood if we examine the origin of America's wealth. This conspicuous feature of our country can be attributed to an interplay of economic and social conditions, and among the latter the absence of feudalism as a social structure and the effect of the Protestant ethic upon national development loom large. The Protestant ethic, as embodied in the early beliefs of American Puritanism, emphasized "a devotion to the calling of making money," regarded money as the appropriate reward of man's work and recommended the application of men's best efforts to the pursuit of such reward.[13] During the historical development of national growth, the originally non-Puritan segments of our society came to adopt this ethic as part of their assimilation. Although the Puritan tenets of the Massachusetts Bay Colony changed much in time, their remnants can still be clearly recognized in the life style of the "middle class" or the "suburbanites," with its emphasis upon personal achievement, individual acquisition of means and privileges, high standard of living, and conformist behavior in the market economy.[14]

The Calvinist ethic left its imprint even upon the early discoverers of poverty in America. Benjamin Franklin, the Philadelphia freethinker and contemporary of Adam Smith, praised the blessings of wealth for the New Englanders and taught them in witty sayings about thrift and happiness.

Robert M. Hartley, a contemporary of Robert Owen and chief mover of the New York Association for Improving the Condition of the Poor, invented ingenious ways of making poverty less disturbing to the middle-class conscience through the application of organized charity. And finally Henry George, the nearest American approximation to Karl Marx, presented in the idea of the single tax a simple recipe, free from any taint of socialism, for the elimination of poverty.[15] In fact, every generation of Americans has had to discover poverty for itself, and our experience of the 1960s has been only the latest in a long series, although more promising for the future than the earlier ones.

A continual rediscovery of poverty was indeed necessary, because the traditions of the Protestant ethic set general standards for judging the poor and these standards changed with the passing of time. The generation of Robert M. Hartley, for example, applied such standards as a means test combined with an inquiry into personal probity and respectability of character; accordingly, it divided the paupers into the "deserving" and "undeserving" poor; made charity available for the former and showed its charitable wrath to the latter. Yet, in all these devices for improving the conditions of the poor, Hartley's generation was dominated by a Puritan conscience, with its particular principle of social justice and its middle-class determination to elevate the poor through the practice of philanthropy. It established organized philanthropy as a characteristic feature of American society and offered some kind of social nurturance to those who were deprived of their fair share of family security. Nurturance, originating in deep-seated psychological motives, is essentially irrational; accordingly, philanthropy chose its recipients without any rational plan, selecting them at random from the local scene. This incidental and parochial character has greatly restricted the social effectiveness of our magnificent philanthropies, even of our highly bureaucratized state philanthropy, the welfare system—the most important social nurturance that we extend to the poor.

THE POVERTY-PRODUCING FACTORS

The social effectiveness of our philanthropy has been further limited by the fact that the Puritan conscience had firm standards of propriety but less firm definitions of poverty. This was perhaps not the fault of the Puritan conscience, but rather a consequence of the existing circumstances—the open class system and rapid social mobility in America. Such circumstances produced transitional poverty, mainly among the immigrant groups. Immigration, as it rose to its peak before World War I, brought an influx of the poor and destitute who in their new homes continued the life of poverty. They crowded into cheap tenements, worked in the least desirable jobs, and showed all the symptoms of social disorganization attendant on pauperism. Yet in their case this state of deprivation lasted only for a while. In time they made their way out of poverty, some in the first generation and others in the second. The descendants of poverty-stricken immigrants now make up an indistinguishable part of the suburbanite class.[16]

The rise of the immigrant groups into affluence represents an interesting chapter in the American rags-to-riches story and a spectacular example of our system of social mobility. But it was due to motives and conditions indigenous among ethnic groups and absent from other segments of American society. While the descendants of the immigrants succeeded, oftentimes conspicuously, other groups remained in their previous state of poverty or sank into pauperism from a previously higher level.

It might very well be that social mobility in America is like Alice's Wonderland, where one has to run in order to stay in one place. In any case, it is reasonable to describe the poor of present-day America as a residual group that for some reason or another has not been able to take part in the general social mobility and acquire the means and privileges that insure a life above the poverty level. They have fallen short in personal achievement and other requirements of the Protestant ethic, and have been excluded from the country's general affluence.

The obvious failure of the poor cannot be described without inquiring into its causes. What keeps some people from acquiring the means and privileges that many others manage to acquire? We may dismiss moralizing answers that try to fix the blame for the failure, citing either the personal faults of the poor or the injustices of our social system. Poverty as a national phenomenon cannot be accounted for by any one cause; rather it must be regarded as the product of a great many factors of diverse origin and impact. For the sake of convenience in discussion, we may classify the factors into three main categories, geographical, social, and psychological.

It is an old observation that poverty is concentrated in certain areas of the country which can be clearly delineated on the map. For this purpose a listing of the 113 poorest counties of the United States, that is, those with a median income of less than $2,000, seems suitable. The income data listed in Table I-1 refer to 1959-60 because similar information based on the 1970 census was not available at the time of this writing. Although the income of the nation has considerably increased since 1960, the site of national poverty appears to be relatively inflexible and unchanged for quite a few decades.[17]

Table I–1. Geographical factors in poverty:
counties of the United States with median income of less than $2,000

| State | Counties with median income of less than $2,000 in 1959–60 | | |
	Number of counties	Population	Population as percent of state's population
Alabama	8	133,063	4.1
Arkansas	10	124,234	7.0
Georgia	14	120,497	3.1
Kentucky	23	265,216	8.7
Louisiana	1	11,796	0.3
Mississippi	25	477,639	21.9
Missouri	1	9,096	0.2
North Carolina	5	52,204	1.1
Oklahoma	2	22,200	0.9
South Carolina	4	104,510	4.4
South Dakota	1	4,661	0.7
Tennessee	13	181,273	5.1
Texas	5	57,010	0.6
Virginia	1	25,824	0.7

Source: U. S. Department of Commerce, Bureau of the Census, *County and City Data Book, 1967* (Washington, D.C., 1967), Table 2.

Table I-1 indicates that (in addition to pockets of poverty situated as far apart as South Dakota and Texas) there are two massive sites of greatest poverty in America: the Deep South—mainly its old plantation land—and southern Appalachia, mainly Kentucky and Tennessee. The former has retained many feudal remnants of the old plantation system, a generally antiquated social and economic structure that militates against material progress and discriminates against the Black population. Southern Appalachia, a predominantly white area, has perpetuated poverty through its marginal farming and mining as well as its distinct local culture, a special obstacle to progress.[18]

As Table I-1 further indicates, the site of the greatest poverty is rural America. The existence of oppressive pauperism in the great urban centers of the country cannot be denied, but poverty is not uniform, and its rural and urban aspects greatly differ in both their etiology and symptoms.[19] Rural poverty is mainly due to the effects of the geographical isolation which keeps out industrialization, restricts employment opportunities, and limits the marketability of farm products. The geographical factors of poverty that operate in the rural areas refer not to the infertility of the land or its distance from the seaboard, but to a combination of localized social and economic conditions which man has created or failed to create and which block the usual roads of social mobility—education, aspiration, high-return work opportunities. The combination of local conditions tends to produce further aggravating factors such as the poor distribution of governmental services, civic improvements, and welfare benefits. The state and county governments with the proportionally greatest number of poor provide the least of those services that may alleviate poverty. For example, in June 1971 the average welfare recipient under Aid to Families with Dependent Children received $67.25 in Massachusetts but only $13.45 in Mississippi, and this ratio of 5:1 appeared to be a fairly stable difference between the two states for a decade or more.

Altogether, the poverty-producing factors work in association, creating a vicious circle. If one factor is permitted to operate unchecked for any length of time, it tends to introduce another factor into the same area. The end result is likely to be an endemic poverty which the local residents are hard put to eradicate without outside assistance. The person unfortunate enough to be born or come to live in a poverty area is likely to be condemned to poverty—unless he moves elsewhere.

Urban poverty is much more uniform across the country and equally visible in New York, Chicago, Detroit, and in the many smaller cities. Its essential features must be explained, not by local conditions, but by those general social factors affecting and even determining the individual's place within an acquisitive society. Sex, age, work status, family structure and race—social characteristics that a person cannot change or has a limited power to change—help or hinder the acquisition of means and privileges. Their specific role is illuminated by the data in Table I-2, which summarize the effect of a few social factors upon the incidence of poverty in the United States.[20]

Each factor defines a specific impediment to the acquisitive life and identifies specific categories of deprivation. Farming areas generally have lower incomes; hence, residence on a farm increases, for the country as a whole, the risk of poverty by 50 percent. As for employment status, the simple dichotomy between working and nonworking makes a great difference in acquisitive potential, but this difference is further affected by the circumstance that puts any person out of work as well as by such contingencies of the working career as occupation and age. The poverty of the unemployed fluctuates according to the ups and downs of business cycles, while the poverty of the unemployable (who make up the majority of those "not in the labor force") remains much the same even in times of greatest prosperity.

Age affects poverty through the life cycle of earning capacity. The middle years of life (25 to 64) represent the acquisitive skills at their height and show uniformly low rates of poverty. On the other hand, families with young heads (under 25) fall much more frequently below the poverty level, and aging often leads to poverty.

Family structure affects poverty in several ways. Women in our society are greatly restricted in the job market because the important money-making activities are pre-empted by males. Moreover, care of children and home (a usual part of the female role) prohibits full-time employ-

Table I-2. Social factors in poverty:
families with income below the poverty level[a]
by selected social characteristics and race, 1966

	Number in thousands			Percentage of poor[a]		
	Total	White	Non-white	Total	White	Non-white
Total, U.S.A.	48,922	44,017	4,905	12.4	9.9	34.9
Residence:						
nonfarm	46,225	41,525	4,700	12.1	9.7	33.5
farm	2,697	2,492	205	18.1	14.0	67.3
Employment status of head:						
employed	38,885	35,261	3,625	7.8	5.9	26.2
unemployed	904	733	171	27.4	20.5	57.3
not in labor force	9,132	8,022	1,109	30.8	26.9	59.8
Age of head:						
14–24	3,011	2,676	335	16.9	14.0	40.6
25–64	38,982	34,971	4,013	10.3	7.8	32.7
65 and over	6,929	6,371	558	22.2	20.0	46.8
Type of family:						
male head	43,751	40,007	3,744	9.8	8.2	27.0
female head	5,172	4,010	1,162	35.0	27.7	60.2

Table 1–2. Continued

	Number in thousands			Percentage of poor[a]		
	Total	White	Non-white	Total	White	Non-white
Number of persons in family:						
2	16,354	14,942	1,412	13.9	12.7	26.8
3–4	19,498	17,841	1,657	8.6	6.9	27.8
5–6	9,627	8,604	1,023	11.9	8.5	41.2
7 or more	3,443	2,630	813	28.6	20.3	55.4
Number of earners:						
none	4,073	3,593	480	48.6	44.2	81.0
1	20,451	18,721	1,730	12.8	10.3	40.1
2	17,992	16,039	1,953	6.2	4.3	21.6
3 or more	8,405	5,663	742	5.9	3.0	28.0

Source: Mollie Orshansky, "The Shape of Poverty in 1966," *Social Security Bulletin,* 31 (March 1968), Table 6.

[a] As defined by the Social Security Administration with incomes ranging from $1,110 (for one-member farm family with female head) to $5,440 (for a nonfarm family of 7 or more members with male head).

ment to many women. Thus, the family with female head is three and a half times as likely as the family with male head to fall into the category of the poor. As for family size, the risk of poverty is the greatest for the large family, while the number of earners in the family is inversely related to the same risk.

Having considered all the variables involved, one may safely conclude that the nuclear family with a planned number of children is the ideal acquisitive unit because it implies the optional state of a male breadwinner and the

optional ratio of breadwinners and dependents. Any deviation from this ideal model tends to increase the risk of
poverty. The absence of earner and the presence of many
children signal partial deviation from the ideal and increase
the risk in proportion to that deviation. The "unrelated
individual," being totally deprived of the economic advantages of the nuclear family, represents the greatest deviation
as well as the greatest risk: 39 percent of these individuals
were poor in 1966.

RACE AND MINORITY STATUS

As Table I-2 also shows, race describes the category of
greatest and most consistent deprivation. For the country as
a whole the poverty rate is three and a half times as high in
the nonwhite as in the white population, and each category
of the table shows a staggering difference between the two
populations. As one example, of the families with three or
more earners, only 3 percent are poor among the whites but
28 percent among the nonwhites.

At the time to which the data refer, Negroes constituted
more than 90 percent of the nonwhite poor and at least 80
percent of the nonwhite population above the poverty level.
In connection with poverty, however, one should not speak
of a simple racial classification contrasting whites and nonwhites. The great majority of Puerto Ricans, Spanish-Americans and French Canadians appear under the classification
of white, but their poverty shows characteristics very similar
to that of nonwhites.[21] Evidently, not race in itself, but
rather minority status must be identified as a category of
deprivation, functioning as an impediment to acquisition in
a very similar manner among Blacks, Puerto Ricans, and
Chicanos as well. What are, then, the conditions operating
among minority groups generally?

First, various historical trends—Negro slavery, the social and economic underdevelopment of Spanish America, the old poverty-producing culture of French Canada—are still with us, and their effect upon the life of minority groups can be strongly felt. As a second and more general condition, minority status usually implies the existence of discrimination, which sets apart the minority group from the other citizens of the community. To be sure, discrimination is an imprecise word that denotes attitudes and actions of varying kind and intensity; it is known to vary from one community to the next and from one minority group to another. As a general rule, however, discrimination means that the poverty of the minority group is taken for granted and viewed as a part of the normal social order and, whether this poverty is perceived or not, the community sees no pressing reason for changing the established order of things.

Such an attitude, once it takes hold at any given place, deeply affects both sides. The community, in its efforts to uphold the existing order, closes the avenues of social mobility to the members of minority groups—in other words, consciously or unconsciously tries to perpetuate their existing poverty. The minority group is likely to answer such a closure with acquiescence; it gives up its incentives to improve itself and break out of poverty. In many cases, somewhat paradoxically, it accepts the view of the majority and with its defeatism contributes to the preservation of the existing order.

Under these conditions it is more or less inevitable that a power structure acquires a vested interest in the existing order, in having, for example, a large reservoir of unskilled workers available or in having the ultimate power of decision making in the local community. Thus, it uses its power to maintain the status quo, including the patterns of discrimination against minority groups.[22] In this way the poverty of minority groups becomes embedded in the total social structure and becomes a matter far beyond the potentials of the community, let alone those of the minority group itself. Against such a background the psychological factors involved in poverty may operate freely.

PSYCHOLOGICAL FACTORS IN POVERTY

At this point it is necessary to return to the family environment and consider it from another point of view. In our market economy every person is supposed to learn the standard acquisitive skills, and the basic part of this learning experience takes place within the family during the socialization process of childhood. The middle-class family (the usual model of the good in our American way of thinking) places heavy emphasis upon imparting those skills and teaches them with fair success. To be sure, the social, financial, and emotional stability that characterizes the middle-class family is a help, because the closeness of the family, as well as the active participation of both father and mother in the socialization process, greatly contributes to its success.

In contrast, poverty as an environment does not favor—or prohibits outright—the acquisition of those personality characteristics which would be useful in breaking away from poverty; it perpetuates and reinforces the personality of the pauper. The poor family seems to have a pattern of socialization in which the earning skills do not have a steady place and cannot be easily transmitted to the children. As one study concluded, the "task of the lower-lower class person is to evolve a way of life that will reduce his insecurity and enhance his power in ways that do not depend on achievement in the universalistic sector and on command of a rich and sophisticated variety of perspectives." Another study, dealing mainly with female-centered families, pointed to such "focal concerns" in their socialization process as a preference for using one's wits rather than doing steady dull work, a dislike of formal intellectual and scholastic activities, and an admiration for card sharks, gamblers, and con-artists as popular heroes.[23]

Two essential elements of the socialization process will help to explain the background. The middle-class family, being achievement-oriented, aims to provide its children with all those ambitions and practical and psychological skills that may promote their social and economic achievements in future life. The poverty family, on the other hand, sets more restricted aims and tends to provide the children with such skills and aspirations as are needed for the maintenance and continuation of the existing life style. There is perhaps a realistic judgment involved in this procedure, because the poverty family lacks those means and privileges that insure the motivation for achievement through generations.[24]

As another essential element in the socialization process, the middle class tends to build up a disposition for putting off the immediate gratification of wants for the sake of those ulterior gratifications that can be obtained at a later time.[25] This delayed gratification pattern operates when rational planning for the future is possible, when actions and their contingent rewards can be assessed, and the ulterior reward is deemed to be attractive enough to prevail over the impulse of immediate gratification. Such planning, when applied to career, financial management, marriage, and family, helps to assure the acquisitive success of the middle class. For example, the pursuit of higher education implies that a young man and his family postpone immediate gratification for the ulterior reward of a higher income and a more prestigious job to be gained upon completing his education.

The poor family is seldom in a position to impose this pattern because its environment lacks the necessary favorable conditions. As was noted, the lower-class child "lives in a world of anxiety about the immediate provisions for his basic needs of food, clothing, and shelter" and learns to seek immediate gratification in all his actions.[26] Accordingly, he is likely to drop out of school and rationalize his behavior by referring to discrimination on the part of his teachers. While discrimination and mistreatment must not be entirely discounted, his behavior is just as much motivated by the fact that in his unstable environment he is unable to assess his actions and their contingent rewards; consequently, he regards the ulterior gratifications that higher education can give as too uncertain to renounce, for their sake, his immediate gratifications.[27]

An unwillingness to defer gratifications seems to be a common characteristic not only of the budgeting and spending habits but also of the sex behavior of the poor. It was found that males with college education show the lowest and males with grade-school education the highest incidence rates of premarital intercourse, while the incidence rates of masturbation are reversed among the educational groups. [28] Dating and engagement were found to be more prevalent among youths of higher socio-economic level than among those of lower level. In fact, dating and engagement were described as typically middle-class rituals designed to prolong the preparatory stage to marriage. They were contrasted to the corresponding behavior of young people of the lower class who tend to "drift" into marriage, often under indications of premarital pregnancy, at a comparatively early age. A corresponding deferment of marriage can be observed: college-educated people tend to marry at a later age and are more likely to stay single than people with less education.[29]

According to a popular belief, sexual irregularities are common in the poor class, and a best seller of our poverty-conscious decade seems to teach that the wages of sex are poverty.[30] While marriage brings a happy ending in novels, in the life of the poor it is often followed by marital instability, broken families, and sexual behavior that is contrary to middle-class standards. Those upsetting events, crises, and stresses which may threaten daily life in any class, appear to be accentuated in the poor family, which, at any rate, has its undue share of "troubles"—brushes with the representatives of authority, including law, school, and welfare administration, as well as a high rate of delinquency, serious mental illness, and other difficulties that sociologists like to call social problems.[31]

In view of the momentous social changes that have taken place during the last few years in America, one might ask whether the psychological differences between the middle class and the poverty class still prevail. Are those many young people of the middle class who drop out of college still oriented toward achievement? Do those young people of the poverty class who nowadays enter colleges and embark upon a presumably middle-class career really differ in their psychological make-up from their middle-class colleagues? Does a difference still exist in the sexual behavior of young people of various classes? At present one could give speculative answers only, but one fact must not be forgotten. The class differences in child-rearing and socialization has existed for a very long time and one may assume that it requires more than the lapse of a few years to eliminate their effects entirely.

Another question must also be raised. Should the social

problems, so frequently observed among the poor, be attributed mainly to their life of deprivation or to their imperfect observance of the inhibitory system? The agencies of social control adjudge and treat deviants with due regard to their social status and community power; law enforcement and medical care adjust their rules of operation to the practical requirements of community life. Accordingly, they treat the same act as an offense by a poor person but not as an offense by a respectable citizen and may label the same symptom as a psychosis in the former case but not in the latter. Drunkards in the city jail and patients in the state hospital are likely to be poor, and in all likelihood they have been adjudged by standards that do not wholly apply to their more fortunate fellow citizens. Hence, a comparison across class lines of rates of delinquency, mental illness, and many other social problems invariably turns out to be unfavorable to the poor.[32]

At the same time, however, one cannot entirely overlook the differences anchored in the personality structure. The inhibitory system that keeps people out of trouble and makes them conform to communal standards is closely linked to the socialization process, and it operates differently in different social classes. Some of the taboos observed by the middle class are not known in the poor class, and other taboos are less firmly internalized and less rigorously observed. In any case, the observance of the taboos is reinforced with far greater efficiency in the middle class, where observance brings higher rewards and infringement causes heavier punishments. A jail sentence for public drunkenness may bring inestimable social loss, perhaps ruinous effects upon career and success, in the middle class, but may hardly affect the prestige and earning power of a laborer.

In their total effect the factors of poverty add up to what can be best described as a stigma, imprinted upon every poor person as a visible sign of his state, that accompanies him all the time and every place, and unfavorably influences his personality, behavior, presentation of himself, and chances to achieve a change for the better. Since the factors determine a specific behavior for the poor, it can be expected that this behavior manifests itself in the field of health also. The role of poverty in health status and care will be examined in the following chapter, but as a point of departure it is safe to assume that the poverty-producing factors are bionegative in their nature and determine poor health conditions for the poor.

TYPES OF POVERTY

So far, we have been speaking of the poor as a homogeneous class of people, seemingly overlooking the fact that they are not equal in their poverty nor are they people of the same kind. Poverty-producing factors bring forth a variety of poor. For example, physical disability and age-connected unemployment are often of a progressive nature; the loss in the earning power that they cause at their onset may fall anywhere between "small" and "great" and increase with the passing of time; and their total impact is further modified by the person's financial status at the time of onset.[33] The combination of several factors (such as disability, race, and occupation) introduces even greater variations. Therefore, a definition of several types of poverty might be useful.

The old moralistic typology of the deserving and nondeserving poor, although it has survived for a remarkably long time, is obviously inadequate and meaningless. A phenomenological typology is more relevant for descriptive purposes because the degrees of deprivation mark meaningful differences among the poor. Thus, a distinction between "poverty level" and "low income" level of poverty (as established on the basis of income by the Social Security Administration) delineates two empirical categories that greatly differ in size and social characteristics, or the distinction made by John Kenneth Galbraith between insular poverty and case poverty clearly points out its environmental and personal causes.[34]

Within the theoretical framework of this book we propose a relatively simple typology: we shall distinguish on the basis of different deprivation processes between chronic and acute poverty. The first, exemplified by the Negro in the rural South and the northern slums as well, implies a long-established—lifelong or perhaps multigenerational—deprivation process; the second, exemplified by the elderly, implies deprivation following a period spent above the poverty level. In the first case the acquisitive abilities have been chronically restricted and poverty is regarded as the usual and familiar state of life, often as the normal or natural life, viewed without much realistic hope for changing it. The chronically poor person has no personal knowledge of how to live above the poverty level and, if given some unexpected aid by a chairty organization, cannot live up to the expectations; perhaps, as has been suggested, he has to be taught the rudiments of middle-class life and spending habits.

In the case of acute poverty there has been a loss of acquisitive power. The loss is not necessarily complete; in many cases it amounts to "reduced means" and the retention of some of the privileges that may present a decided contrast to the deprivation of the chronically poor. The memory of former days is much alive and stimulates an active desire and effort to restore the former state, and any help given in these efforts is likely to be acknowledged and utilized.

Chronic poverty is self-perpetuating and preserves all the negative traits of pauperism mentioned above. Its characteristic response to the existing state of affairs is (or perhaps has been) either acquiescence or periodic and essentially futile rebellion. Acute poverty is largely free of the negative traits so shocking to the middle class, and its usual response to the existing state of affairs is either resentment at being déclassé or a refusal to identify oneself as poor. The diffident person who does not apply for welfare benefits is a case in point.

The typology might be helpful in assessing the changes that take place among the country's poor and in answering the question whether the number of poor is generally increasing or whether we are simply witnessing a shift from one type of poverty to another. Two important social forces, cybernetics and the aging of the population, function in such a way as to lead continually new masses into poverty. Cybernetics, as a sophisticated form of increasing mechanization, eliminates many unskilled jobs in services and industrial production. It regularly dislocates a great number of laborers whose chances to find new jobs on a shrinking market are proportionate to their educational and industrial skills; the undereducated among them are likely to face chronic unemployment.

The general increase in the number of the aged, a common phenomenon in the industrial civilizations of the Western world, poses a similar problem. The chance of being able to provide for old age and keep oneself above the poverty level is proportionate to one's educational and acquisitive skills; the chance is not given to the chronically poor and hardly given to the many marginal people remaining near the poverty line.

At the same time, other social forces work in the opposite direction and help to reduce the number of poor. Social mobility is still conspicuous in our society, and its usual road, the learning of acquisitive skills through higher education, is open to young people whose parents did not have the same opportunity. General economic progress, rising incomes, extended welfare programs and related governmental services, the civil rights movement and other measures to ensure equality for minority groups help to reduce poverty. But, again, the benefits that anyone may derive from such social forces are proportionate to his status and skill, and the poorest can benefit the least. One cannot entirely dismiss the total impression that the social forces, as they naturally operate in our society, may help to reduce acute poverty but tend to increase, or at any rate perpetuate, chronic poverty.

This was the background about 1960 when a number of conditions never before present in American history were manifest. The country reached an unprecedented affluence, but chronic poverty seemed to grow. The Puritan conscience—or what remained of its traditions in public opinion—felt troubled by this paradox, and its shame was heightened by the conviction that our industrialized society possessed the financial means and social engineering skills to eliminate poverty. If any further stimulus were needed to make the conscience work, this was given by the first great successes of the civil rights movement. The stimuli coming from different directions reinforced one another and created a psychological readiness to do something of lasting impact about the seemingly eternal poverty.

THE WAR ON POVERTY

The intellectuals of the country expressed the general mood; they argued for the necessity of a new approach to the old problem, and produced many new ideas and concrete propositions as their personal contribution to a national enterprise. Economists of both liberal and conservative persuasion set out detailed plans about possible governmental services, and writers and social practitioners added practical as well as ideological suggestions.[35] Among the philosophers of activism Saul Alinsky proved to be the most practical with his emphasis on organizing the poor to exercise direct political power against the bureaucratic efforts of local governments. Michael Harrington's theory about the decline of the poor from their position as the major revolutionary force of the last century appealed to the romantic imagination, while the ideas of the civil rights movement (such as Martin Luther King's program of nonviolence and Stokely Carmichael's principle of Black Power) gave additional weight to activating the Negro masses.[36]

The intellectual ferment played a major part in mobilizing public opinion and gathered enough support to initiate governmental action. The transition from intellectual planning to governmental action did not take a long time but lasted long enough to go through the usual motions of American reform movements—the reconciliation of the independent and often contradictory ideas into a practical compromise in which the leadership of the various kinds of social and political practitioners could prevail. Under such leadership the new action program became essentially nonideological and pragmatic; in fact, the prevalence of activists over the more theoretically oriented planners has been a characteristic feature, and perhaps shortcoming, of the whole poverty program. Yet, at the same time it turned out to be a vigorously antitraditional program in treating the poor.

Pragmatic as it was, the action program recognized that the treatment of acute poverty is a relatively simple task because it deals with people who, on the whole, anxiously endeavor to shake off their poverty; such supportive measures as health insurance for the elderly or job training and placement services for dislocated laborers are greatly effective in keeping these people above the poverty line. Chronic poverty, however, needs more than supportive actions; it needs massive intervention programs that are activated by the power structure residing outside poverty and are designated to alter radically yet systematically the general conditions existing among the poor.

Now public opinion and government were ready to initiate supportive measures as well as direct intervention. The total program amounted to large-scale social manipulation aimed at changing a basic psychological need as well as the underlying objective situation. The involvement of the federal government in the direct handling of poverty followed a long line of development which saw the extension of the federal authority over many new areas—in the present case, over the social manipulation of broad masses of our society. The federal government made funds available for nationwide coordinated programs; it aroused the attention of the nation and obtained safeguards against the political vagaries of local governments; and, furthermore, it made possible the participation of formerly apathetic individuals and of newly formed organizations.

The charity organizations of the past and the welfare structure of recent vintage were limited in their ability to handle the specific tasks of the new program. Private and church charities, as well as welfare administrations, were too parochial in their interests and too static in their goals. They aimed at maintaining an existing situation, helping the deserving poor, fighting the chiselers, but stopping short of any radical action that might affect the poor as a group. Thus, when it came to implementing the plans, the program could resort to new and often ad hoc organizations (such as the various community action groups) willing to assume the new responsibilities and work under great pressure, with a lack of routine and experience and with the urgency of extemporization. By their structure new organizations were supposed to be independent from the local centers of power, free of bureaucracy and eager to experiment with new methods of solving the poverty problem.[37]

With the help of this organizational structure the intervention program took a characteristically American direction. It remained pragmatic rather than ideological and worked toward an indirect redistribution of the means and privileges by furnishing the poor with standard acquisitive skills. It undertook to teach those skills both to the adult generation and young people. It designed job training programs, and, as a longer-range but more promising project, compensatory educational programs that would enable the children of the poor to reach out for higher income and take their places in acquisitive life. It launched community action programs that would establish a participatory democracy, make the poor active partners in civic actions and, in their psychological implications, end their powerlessness, apathy, forlornness, and enable them to cope with the tension and anxieties of acquisitive society. It initiated health programs that would transmit to the poor the rational and planned ways of healthy living, including family planning, as important conditions of middle-class life.

The war on poverty (as this very peaceful activity came

to be called for reasons of publicity) began with sanguine hopes, and perhaps nowhere were the hopes flying higher than in the Johnson Administration. Wilbur J. Cohen, Secretary of Health, Education, and Welfare, surveyed at one point the progress made and noted that in 1960 there were 40,000,000 Americans living in poverty, while in 1967 the figure was reduced to 26,000,000. On this basis he confidently predicted that by 1971 the poverty group would be down to 15,000,000 and by 1976 it would entirely disappear from the country.[38]

This optimism was not generally shared. In fact, as any public issue of controversial nature is apt to do, the war on poverty brought forth a torrent of criticism in which the representatives of poverty and vested interest, politics and scholarship, radicalism and conservatism, participated with equal zeal; some of its comments must be considered. [39] This study cannot make a complete assessment of the achievements and shortcomings of the war on poverty. At this point, however, with the large-scale national intervention program more or less ended, only those questions must be raised that refer to the theoretical considerations of this book: Is this national intervention program able to counterbalance the poverty-producing geographical, social, and psychological factors? Is it capable of correcting the effect of those social forces that perpetuate chronic poverty?

SOCIAL STRUCTURE AND WAR ON POVERTY

It is evident that poverty, as well as wealth or affluence, is a man-made condition that human effort and planning can change. But any intervention affects each of the poverty-producing factors in a different way, coping efficiently with some of them but remaining ineffective against others. Geographical factors such as isolation and local remnants of feudalism are easily amenable to manipulation; they are now removed with relative ease through roadbuilding programs in Appalachia and voter registration in the South. On the other hand, some of the social factors are resistant to any action program; old age will probably always constitute a deprived category in acquisitive competition, and little change can be expected. The psychological factors present a different problem: they are closely tied to the socialization process that works through the cycle of generations and cannot be changed in a short time.

The psychological lag that is the concomitant of any intervention program helps to explain the persistence of the poor in their ways of life. The hard-to-reach or hard-core family has long been known in social work and medical practice for of its conspicuous reluctance to change its way of life under professional guidance.[40] Such resistance to reasonable change can be understood: to many poor people any· change may appear as a threat to that personal security they perceive within the existing familiar order. Small wonder that the poverty program repeatedly encountered such resistance; still, it had better success in overcoming this reluctance than the previous fragmented and individualistic actions.

Whether dealing with social factors or real people, the nation's poverty program has been greatly reduced in its capabilities by organizational problems. The community action groups and agencies—new, innovative, and extemporizing as they were—encountered two forces that seem to pervade large-scale organizations—bureaucratization and power politics. Both of them pose inescapable threats. Bureaucratization tends, among other effects, to slow down operations and water down projects, particularly those of any innovative and radical bent. Power politics centers upon the authority of making decisions and all too often implies the threat of the power structure taking over the new spontaneous organizations, and where power structure is present the vested interest cannot be too far away.

If we compare the poverty program to the country's welfare administration (another large organization servicing humanitarian aims that struggled with bureaucratization and power politics for four decades), the poverty program has, perhaps, done not too badly; but neither has it done too well. Altogether, any assessment of our large humanitarian enterprises should humbly acknowledge our general inadequacy in organizational know-how. One lesson that we can safely derive from the history of the war on poverty is that we do not seem to know how to avoid the pitfalls of organizational life and how to marshal our forces for organized pursuit of large and noble aims.

Finally, the long-range limitations of the poverty program are defined by its problems. An adjective restricts the meaning of its noun: compensatory education is less than education proper, and participatory democracy is less than democracy; qualified education and qualified democracy are actually substitutes for more basic entities. Compensatory education is designed as a substitute for the middle-class socialization process, and participatory democracy is a similar substitute for the civic activity and political interest generally shown by the middle class. It remains to be seen how effective a substitute will be: whether the subtle effect of the total family environment upon the child can be replaced by some kind of formal education given at a much later stage of life; whether the required participation in community action or the instituted compliance with health programs will work out among the poor in the same way as the spontaneous activities of similar nature do in the middle class.

Yet it should not be forgotten that participatory democracy is a tremendous step forward when compared to the patterns of previous welfare administration and charity management. It is a part of the often praised, and just as often criticized, feature of the poverty program—of not distributing money among the poor in the guise of welfare, but working toward more essential goals. The achievements of the program consist of moving toward those goals. The poor of the country have been placed on the road of social mobility and prompted to participate in acquisitive life; the children of the poor have been influenced, and even prepared, to aspire for means and privileges represented by the affluence of the middle class. These social efforts have been well supported by the related achievements of the civil rights movement in assuring equality to minorities and of the federal legislation extending minimal health care to every citizen.

Such achievements reach beyond the purely emotional goals of lessening misery, humiliation, and deprivation. They work toward that idealistic aim, a more equalitarian society, which gives fair opportunities to everybody for starting out in life. To be sure, no perfectly equalitarian society can be conceived, and equal chances at the start turn into unequal achievements later in life. It is perhaps a vain hope that in the more affluent society of tomorrow, poverty, measured by the relative standards prevailing at that time, will be viewed as a thing of the past; in all likelihood poverty will always be with us. But the present intervention program, or call it "war on poverty" if you like, has attempted a major restructuring of American society, the reduction of the conspicuous differences in means and privileges, and the building of an ideal structure which, without setting a ceiling upon anyone's affluence, fixes a limit below which no family can fall in its standard of living.

II. The Social Aspects of Health and Illness

by John Kosa and Leon S. Robertson

The practicing physician, a proverbially busy person, tends to regard health, illness, disability, and death in their concrete relevance. For him the problem is how to diagnose the specific complaint presented by the patient and how to apply the treatment that is appropriate under the given circumstances. His attention centers around such practical details as the heart murmur of a middle-aged man, the examination of a healthy child, or the emotional difficulties of a suburban housewife. Amid such preoccupations, definitions of health and illness appear to him as matters all too abstract and removed from the current problems.

When, however, we have to move beyond the clinical appearances of health and illness to a level where they cease to be unique events and become parts of a complex social situation or a national policy, their conceptual clarification becomes necessary. If a national health policy has to be considered or the relationship of health and poverty to be assessed, the unique clinical observations need to be synthesized into a general conceptual framework where health

Dr. Leon Robertson is on the staff of the Insurance Institute for Highway Safety, Washington, D.C.

and illness become social as well as medical phenomena. Accordingly, this chapter aims to present, first, a critical review of the existing models and definitions, and then, a theoretical framework for the interpretation of health and poverty.

THE MEDICAL VIEW

One definition, found in medical writings throughout the ages, is broadly utopian. Galen, writing *On Health Care* in the second century, described health as a "condition in which we neither suffer pain nor are hindered in the functions of daily life," that is, when we are able "to take part in government, bathe, drink, and eat, and do other things we want."[1] In our times, the World Health Organization placed the following definition in the preamble of its constitution: "Health is a state of complete physical, mental and social well-being and not merely the absence of disease or infirmity."[2] The striking similarity of the two statements indicates an old tradition in medicine; yet this tradition always had its disputants. One critic, reading the definition of the World Health Organization, exclaimed, "This sounds more like a coma than health."[3] To be sure, it is the definition of a policy incorporated in a constitution, which spells out the aims of an action-oriented organization. It is far too general to be useful in understanding the etiological, therapeutic, and behavioral aspects of health phenomena.

Physicians engaged in clinical work have always been greatly interested in the specific theories of illness that promised to explain their bedside observations and promote better methods of treatment. The fanciful theories of the prescientific age hardly need to be described here; it is sufficient to concentrate on the main ideas that have developed in modern medicine since the time of Louis Pasteur.

The germ theory of disease helped to vanquish many dreaded infectious diseases; the traditional epidemiological theory, which viewed illness as a battle of three interacting entities, the host, the agent, and the environment, helped to defeat the epidemics; the cellular concept of disease, emphasizing the changes within the cell as the basic components of disease, was associated with the rapid progress of the biological sciences in our century; and the mechanistic concept, which viewed disease as a defective part of the machine, reflected a similar progress in surgical procedures. All four theories were overwhelmingly specific, concerned with unraveling the mysteries of given pathological conditions and applying this knowledge to a clinical conquest of the pathology. In an era in which infectious diseases posed the major threat to mankind, the specific approach was indeed useful. But once society had moved beyond this state, a fully comprehensive theory, applicable to all groups of infirmities, became essential.

Two comprehensive, although simplistic, views have gained wide acceptance among medical authorities and lay people as well. One view regards as illness any state that has been diagnosed as such by a competent professional. It certainly reminds us of Occam's razor, but its simplicity is deceptive. Many illnesses and infirmities are never brought before professionals for diagnoses; in many other cases the professionals are by no means unanimous in their diagnoses.[4] Let us consider two hypothetical patients: one with high blood pressure and electrocardiographic evidence of left venticular strain who has not missed a day's work and insists that he feels great; and another whose father dropped dead at an early age and who ever since has led a life of restricted activities in spite of the negative findings of innumerable laboratory procedures. Both patients are likely

to receive contradictory diagnoses from different professionals who may disagree about which one of the patients is
ill.[5]

The other widely accepted view defined illness in the
patient's terms: whoever feels ill should be regarded as sick.
The importance of such a subjectively based concept should
not be underestimated because it calls attention to that
personal feeling that leads the patient to the doctor and
initiates medical action. However, the use of such a subjective criterion raises a problem of its own, that of distinguishing between a bionegative feeling and an objective state of
disease. The problem was well posed by the question
whether the experience of grief, which ordinarily follows
the loss of a loved person, a valued possession, or an ideal,
should be regarded as a disease.[6]

Psychologically oriented authorities have consistently rejected the specific explanations of diseases, and have preferred to view disease in its relationship to the whole person, regarding it as a situation that naturally arises in life; as
a phase of life that alternates with phases of health, as a part
of a continual adjustment to the momentary exigencies of
life; as a dynamic process taking place in an ever-changing
environment; or a natural course of changes resulting from
an accumulation of stress.[7] These views tend to emphasize
that disease is more than a symptom and prefers to speak of
sick people rather than of diseases.

Influenced by the advances of psychiatry, medical thinking has come to consider that a great many social and
psychological variables are involved in sickness. These variables could be well reconciled with the clinical concept of
sickness, so much so that an entire school of investigators
has pointed to certain combinations of organic and non-
organic factors as the real determinants of illness. Their

views appear to be prevalent in present-day medicine, but the variables named by them are too numerous to be adequately reviewed in this context. Therefore we select only those which refer to stress and hormone production and discuss them at some length. This discussion, we believe, will illustrate both the strengths and weaknesses of the multifactor theory of disease etiology.

THE DETERMINANTS OF ILLNESS

The traditional epidemiological model of illness focuses on those factors that result in a noxious agent coming in contact with a tissue and producing a change which is defined as morbid. Social variables such as occupation, family characteristics, and ethnic background have been shown to be important in this model with respect to a number of diseases. Graham has illustrated the value of such a model in research on scrotal and lung cancer, and has cited numerous other examples of relationships between social variables and various chronic diseases. However, the noxious agents involved in most of these diseases have not been specified. This may be a partial result of overemphasizing exogenous physical, chemical, and biological agents. As it was stated, "most diseases are the result of a pathologic environmental agent brought into contact with a host individual genetically susceptible to this agent."[8]

Only the broadest definition of "a pathologic environmental agent" allows its inclusion in the model of stress, the factor that increasingly is hypothesized as playing a major role in most chronic illnesses and perhaps in the onset of some acute infectious diseases as well. Some of the findings in recent research on stress and illness and basic research on stress suggest that an exogenous physical agent is often necessary but not sufficient for illness to occur. Indeed there are some diseases in which no such agent is present. In view of this, an alternative to the epidemiological model is offered by King.[9] The model focuses on the possible inter-action processes of genetic predispositions, exogenous and endogenous physical agents, and stress and coping mech-anisms which may result in the onset or avoidance of disease. The interaction processes that result in illness have not been specified. In this section we discuss one theory that is derived from knowledge of the behavioral and disease correlates of hormonal reaction during stress.[10]

Stress has been implicated in a remarkable variety of pathological conditions. However, all writers do not agree about what constitutes stress. Selye concentrates on phys-ical agents (heat, cold, infection) as stressors and uses stress to denote the conditions that result from these agents. Stress itself does not refer to a specific state such as nervous tension but is an abstraction "manifested by a specific syndrome which consists of all the nonspecifically induced changes within a biologic system." Included in the changes are fluctuations in endogenous elements such as the "anti-inflammatory hormones" (adrenocorticotropic hormone, cortisone, cortisol), the "proinflammatory hormones" (somatotrophic hormone, aldosterone, desoxycor-ticosterone), the adrenalines and thyroid hormone.[11]

Maladaptation occurs when the secretion of these hor-mones is out of balance with the requirements of the organism in adjusting to the stressor. This maladaptation, along with dietary, hereditary, and other factors, is posited as important in the development of the following diseases: high blood pressure, heart and blood vessel diseases, kidney diseases, eclampsia, rheumatoid arthritis, inflammatory dis-eases of the skin and eyes, infections, allergic and hypersensitivity diseases, nervous and mental diseases, sexual derangements, digestive diseases, metabolic diseases, cancer, and diseases of resistance.

Advocates of the psychogenic theory of illness accept the proposition that excessive or insufficient hormone production is a factor contributing to the onset of various illnesses, but they emphasize psychological rather than physical stress as the major source of changes in hormone secretion. Simmons argues that disease results from a "weakness of the adult personality structure," which is a function of "defective relationship patterns in childhood."[12] Stress, although not carefully defined, is said to be the result of an extreme and/or prolonged emotional reaction to a situation that is unusually meaningful for the person. A precise link between the personality structure and stress is not offered except for the statement that "emotional stress plays the role of catalyst." The disease-producing hormonal changes are thought to be consequences of the intensity and duration of emotional stress rather than a maladaptation of response to the stressors.

The weakest aspect of the psychogenic theory is the position of a weak personality structure as the central factor. Personality traits are often correlated with a higher incidence of certain illnesses. Eysenck cites a number of studies which show higher than usual extroversion on the part of persons with heart disease and cancer.[13] Extroversion is also high in heavy smokers, indicating the possibility that a more complex relationship than the simple smoking-cancer or smoking-heart disease relationships may be plausible. King, in a review of the literature on rheumatoid arthritis, points to studies that characterize arthritics as shy, feeling inadequate and inferior, self-sacrificing, overconscientious, unable to express anger overtly, obsessive, and compulsive.[14] However, the critical mind demands that the process whereby personality traits, stress and hormone over-abundance or inadequacy combine to produce or exacerbate illness be specified. To say that persons become ill because of weakness, approaches tautology.

The behavioral scientist must leave research on the hor-mone-illness relationship to medical and biological scien-tists. Nevertheless, the hypothesis that sustained overpro-duction or underproduction of hormones causes disease or lower resistance to infectious agents gives the behavioral scientist a task on which he can work. The most appropriate task would seem to be to specify the process by which personality traits, stress, and other possible factors result in sustained levels of hormone production.

Social situations must also be considered as possible fac-tors in disease. Indeed many of the factors that Simmons terms psychogenic might more appropriately be called soci-ogenic. Interpersonal relations, divorce, and financial re-verses are not exclusively psychological. The prevalence of such events preceding the onset of illness is striking. One study compared the two-week period before and the two-week period after the appearance of streptococcal infections and found that the incidence of crises (such as death of grandparents, change of residence, father's loss of job, unu-sual pressures on the infected person) were four times as frequent before the illness as after it.[15] Chronic family disorganization and the sharing of bedrooms by children also appear to be related to increased susceptibility. There is evidence that a concentration of social stresses exists before the onset of various illnesses.[16] Sanatorium employees who contracted tuberculosis were compared to a matched sample of healthy employees with respect to social stresses in a ten-year period, and the stresses of the ill group were found to be skewed significantly in the two years before illness. Similar studies of cardiac patients, persons with skin disease, inguinal hernia patients, and both married and unmarried pregnant females show the same results. Sophisticated scales of stressful life change events are being developed and show considerable promise in the prediction of onset and severity of a variety of types of illness.[17]

THE DEVELOPMENT OF STRESS-RELATED ILLNESSES

Basic research on stress also points to the importance of social factors in the mode of reaction to stress. Funkenstein and his associates show that college male subjects in an experiment designed to induce stress manifest cardiovascular responses much like those which occur when either epinephrine or norepinephrine (adrenal hormones) are injected in subjects not under stress. The subjects' verbalized emotional responses are related to physiological reactions. An angry response is more often accompanied by a norepinephrinelike response, while self-blame or anxiety are more frequent when the response is epinephrine-like. These reactions, as the psychogenic theory would predict, are also related to the subject's recall of childhood relations with parents. When the father is characterized as a stern and distant authority and the mother is warm and affectionate, blame of others is more frequent. Self-blame occurs more often when father is a mild and affectionate authority and mother is the primary source of affection. When the mother is both authority and source of affection, the response to stress more often is anxiety.

The psychogenic theory is not supported, however, when the reactions to two subsequent encounters with the stress are observed. The Funkenstein group classifies the reactions to the three stress situations in the following ways: (1) mastery, i.e., no severe anxiety in the first two encounters and performance anxiety or no emotion in the third encounger; (2) delayed mastery, i.e., severe anxiety in the first or second encounter and no emotion or performance anxiety in the third encounter; (3) unchanged reaction, i.e., the same reaction excluding severe anxiety in all three encounters; and (4) deteriorated reaction, i.e., severe anxiety in the third encounter regardless of the first two responses. There are no relationships between this classification and the above-mentioned initial reactions or the recall of relationships with parents. Mastery of stress in this context is found to be related to scales designed to measure the degree to which the subject's concept of himself differs from his view of his peer group's feelings about him. While the mastery group's view of self is congruent with their estimate of peers' impressions of them, the delayed mastery group indicates feelings of being overevaluated by peers, and the deteriorated group shows feelings of being under-evaluated.[18]

A number of studies demonstrate the physiological correlates of group characteristics and interpersonal relations. One of them reports differences in free fatty acid in plasma of subjects in groups with varying cohesion, conformity, and leadership.[19] Others find that the heart rates of patient and therapist in psychotherapeutic interviews are alike depending on the content of their interaction.[20] Another research project demonstrates a relationship between positive, neutral, and negative sociometric pair choice and degree of covariation in galvanic skin response during five discussion sessions.[21] Each of the physiological indicators in these studies is related to hormone output. These findings suggest that it is not a personality characteristic per se that determines the individual's mode of handling stress but perhaps the degree to which the personality is congruent with the social environment.

The emphasis in the theory of hormone nimiety or deficiency as a factor in illness is on the sustained nature of the hormone condition. Presumably, a pathological state develops only when hormone production is beyond certain limits for an extended period of time. One theory of mental illness, for example, suggests that hallucinogenic derivatives of hormones may be factors in producing the symptoms so labeled.[22] Funkenstein reports that patients diagnosed as paranoid manifest an excess of norepinephrine while those diagnosed as depressive show an overproduction of epinephrine. These physiologic reactions are sustained for the patients but are not so for the student subjects in the experiment discussed earlier. Whether or not the reactions would have become prolonged for those who did not master the stress in subsequent encounters is, of course, unknown.

Feedback is one of the possible processes that might result in a sustained level of stress with the noted physiological consequence. If some combinations of personality trait and social environment cause stress, reinforcing, in turn, the personality trait and/or social environment toward producing more stress, then the basis for a prolonged state of stress exists. Recent research on affiliation suggests the possibility of such a process.

Schachter's experiments show that the only and first-born children in a condition presumed to provoke fear (in this experiment the threat of electric shock in a forbidding environment) express a desire to wait with others (affiliation), while later-born subjects prefer to wait alone.[23] No significant birth order differences occur among subjects in the nonfear condition. Interpretation of the results is based on another finding that the only and first-born children have higher dependency needs than later-born children. [24] Affiliative behavior is highest among first-born children who react to a stressor in an epinephrinelike manner and whose parents are highly expressive. These conditions are hypothesized as precursors of dependency.[25]

Assuming that this is true, what happens if persons with such needs are socially isolated or, conversely, if nonaffiliative persons are in situations where social contact is inescapable? A partial answer to this question is provided by the Dohrenwends.[26] When subjects are isolated in a sensory deprivation experiment, the only and first-born children display higher symptoms of stress, while later-born children show lower stress symptoms than they displayed before the experiment. However, in a slum area with crowded living conditions, the later-born respondents report a significantly higher number of stress symptoms than do the only and first-born respondents. Similar findings are reported by MacDonald, who randomly placed subjects together or in social isolation while awaiting a test.[27] First-born subjects more often show reduced anxiety when forced to wait with others while later-born subjects show reduced anxiety more frequently when in social isolation.

These findings suggest that two types of persons will develop stress-related illness: (1) affiliative persons who are in isolation from which they cannot escape and (2) nonaffiliative persons in situations where social interaction is unavoidable. Further, it is hypothesized that a feedback process is operating in these two cases. Stress increases the need of the affiliative person for social interaction. If the interaction is not available, the person is again stressful, and the process continues until interaction becomes available or the sustained stress with its accompanying hormone state produces illness. The following analogous chain is hypothesized for the nonaffiliative person: stress—need for isolation—isolation not available—stress—need for isolation—and so on.

The conditions of poverty are major stressors. The correlations of poverty and various diseases, including the stress diseases, are discussed in subsequent chapters. These correlations suggest that the stress of poverty may have a direct, cumulative effect on the probability of disease. It is also likely, however, given the theory exposited here, that there are interaction effects between the personality and familial correlates of reaction to stress. Thus, the stresses of poverty may have differential effects on disease rates depending on personal and familial characteristics. The obvious example from the studies referred to is the greater number of stress symptoms noted in later-born children in crowded slum conditions when compared with first-born children in the same environment.

At present, however, the theory cannot answer certain important questions that its critics may justly raise. It cannot specify the types of illnesses that develop from stress-related processes because this specification may need, as a basis, the presently unavailable knowledge of genetic predispositions with respect to susceptibility to endogenous or exogenous agents. In addition, it may be necessary to know whether or not the hormonal predisposition is connected with specific emotions under stress and whether or not particular types of hormones are affected by given emotions. In spite of such deficencies in knowledge, it is likely that the riddle of disease etiology will be solved by exploring feedback or other processes involving social and personality variables rather than by relying on such vague concepts as a "weak personality structure."

A SOCIOLOGICAL VIEW OF ILLNESS

The behavioral sciences, not being directly involved in clinical work and not necessarily oriented toward an organic view of illness, have been mainly interested in a model for human behavior in health and illness—a model that fits the statistical requirements of empirical research. Statistics dissect any broad concept into measurable components that can be established on the basis of empirical observations and applied to a quantitative interpretation of the whole concept. Thus the National Health Survey, when studying the relationship of family income and health, selected for measurement three types of health characteristics: disability, hospitalization, and injury; it subdivided each characteristic and classified, for example, disability into four subcategories: restricted activities, bed rest, inability to work, and inability to attend school.[28] Such a treatment of the topic (just as the contemporary medical views of disease) suggests that health is a multidimensional variable. It is a concept so broad or abstract that in its totality it is not available for immediate observation; its clarification must depend upon a great many facets.

Psychology illuminates reasonably well the many-faceted nature of health, and its contribution to the topic leads us back to the definitions of Galen and the World Health Organization. Psychological studies have found that avowed happiness had three general correlates: youth, health, and good education. A low socio-economic status is associated with unhappiness, but materialistic luxury and good treatment, as implied by the wealth and education of one's parents, are not related to the avowed happiness. On the other hand, health has a stable relationship to happiness, even in populations that are, on the average, probably quite healthy.[29]

Sociology might be the useful discipline to deal with the many facets of health because it places illness and health in a social context in which not only the sick person but his whole environment, and particularly those significant persons who try to heal him, find their places. It regards the problems of health as parts of a dynamic interaction process, views illness in its relativity, and assumes that the extent and meaning of any illness can be understood only in relation to other healthy and sick people.

The great pioneer of medical sociology, Henry E. Sigerist, presented the concept of the "special position of the sick." As he reasoned, "To be ill means to suffer," and every culture defines its stand toward suffering. While many cultures of the past tended to view illness as a punishment of the wicked, modern civilization grants, as a general rule, a privileged position to the sick and manifests a systematic concern with the healing and welfare of sick people.[30]

Talcott Parsons elaborated this reasoning and placed it in the framework of a theory of social systems. In his conception, a person's illness needs to be legitimized by the authority of the medical profession, his intimates, or other people having influence over him. When the illness is legitimized, the person assumes a special sick role that replaces, or modifies, his usual occupational or familial roles. The sick role permits him to observe specific norms such as freedom from the usual obligations; at the same time it imposes specific norms on people near to him such as family members or attending physicians.[31]

This theory has gained wide popularity in sociology; however, empirical studies have found a limited usefulness for it. Role playing implies a relatively stable and lasting position that a person takes in the stream of social interrelationship. Occupational and family roles last for many years, and people usually wish to maintain their accepted roles; for example, many workers are unwilling to relinquish their occupational roles at the mandatory age of retirement. But illness is seldom lasting and even less seldom stable in its effects; as a rule, it is not associated with endeavors for its unrestricted prolongation. Because of such differences one may ask whether there is any state to which the term "sick role" can properly be applied; at any rate, its use needs to be restricted by sheer logic to the chronic illnesses in a more-or-less stationary state.[32]

More recent theories have attempted to fill this gap and offer a broader explanation of health-related phenomena. King emphasized the perceptual component of illness and described "one crucial variable" in any health-related action: the way in which man "sees or perceives the situation of disease and all of the social ramifications that accompany it."[33] Mechanic built on such a basis the concept of illness behavior, concerned with "the ways in which given symptoms may be differentially perceived, evaluated, and acted (or not acted) upon by different kinds of persons."[34]

Following a different chain of thought, Suchman presented a theory of stages of illness and medical care that discerns five stages "demarcating critical transition and decision-making points in medical care and behavior." The five stages are symptom experience, assumption of the sick role, medical care contact, dependent-patient role, and recovery or rehabilitation.[35] Finally, Kasl and Cobb distinguished health behavior, illness behavior, and sick-role behavior, reasoning that "the likelihood that an individual will engage in a particular kind of health, illness, or sick role behavior is a function of two variables: the perceived amount of threat and the attractiveness or value of the behavior."[36]

The last four theories agree on certain points. They relegate the stationary sick role to a restricted place, emphasize the dynamic nature of health-related episodes, and regard the alternations of good and ill health as a continuous process evolving within a social context. In the present discussion we are attempting to build upon their concepts, reconcile those concepts with the views commonly held by the medical profession, and formulate a sufficiently broad and flexible theory to explain the health-related phenomena. In this attempt it is necessary to re-examine the usual dichotomy between health and illness. This dichotomy was formulated long ago, when epidemics and other serious illnesses were common, when the generally inefficient medical care could offer hardly any effective help beyond a placebo, and when any illness was likely to last for a long time. Since then the advent of scientific medicine and the improvement of health care have basically changed all those conditions. They have vanquished many of the life-threatening diseases, made reasonable health care available to practically all people, and greatly reduced the duration of many common ailments. As a result, man in his life cycle now enjoys a long period of good health (roughly from the age of fifteen to forty-five and perhaps beyond) during which he survives for many years without presenting any serious illness to his physician. The health problems that he presents are, in all likelihood, not the serious organic damages of the past epochs, but illnesses with psychosomatic components, emotional and social complaints, or problems of a preventive nature.[37]

One is reminded of the stimulating idea of Thomas S. Szasz that the word *illness* should not be applied to *mental illness*.[38] It would not be quite proper to apply this idea to physical health. However, it is evident that the most common health-related actions and experiences of our times cannot be clearly labeled as *illness* or *health*. This dichotomy does not accommodate the preventive measures that are so common among healthy people and include such activities as daily physical exercise, a reducing diet, or a check-up with physicians. It does not accommodate the small incidents of life (abrasions, lacerations, common colds) that temporarily may upset the family but have no significant duration or consequences. It does not fit many common forms of disability that are compensated, rehabilitated, or corrected either naturally or with professional help by wearing eyeglasses, dentures, protheses, or tooth fillings. Finally, it excludes a whole set of complaints that stretches from the psychosomatic component of every illness to the nonincapacitating and not-treated but serious psychoneuroses.

THE CONCEPT OF MORBID EPISODE

As an appropriate concept that includes the measures, conditions, and disabilities mentioned above, as well as the traditional symptoms and illnesses, we present the term *morbid episode*. *Episode* refers to man's persistent view that such an act or condition must be an interruption of the normal or desired course of events because the normal or desired state is characterized by freedom from such episodes. One may argue that physiological normality does not exclude repeated occurrences of symptoms, illnesses, and disabilities, but (as will be presently discussed) the health behavior of people seems to be governed by the belief in a desired state of health rather than by the teaching of biological sciences.

All these episodes (including the preventive measures) have reference to morbidity. The extent of the morbidity present in any episode cannot escape attention; it is assessed crudely by the patient or other layman helping him and more exactly by professional health personnel. This assessment initiates a social-psychological process of handling the morbid episode. The process is an integral part of the usual pattern of social interactions in which the patient and other significant persons are involved. Its regular course can be broken down into four elementary parts: (1) the assessment of a disturbance in, or of a threat to, the usual functioning of physiological-psychological health; (2) the arousal of anxiety by the perception of such an incidence; (3) the application of one's general medical knowledge to the given disturbance; and (4) the performance of manipulative actions for removing the anxiety and the disturbance. Let us discuss each element separately.

The disturbance or threat is assessed by the patient or

somebody near to him such as a family member. What a "layman" perceives is a comparative difference between the present (acute) functioning of health and its previous or usual functioning. The felt difference is communicated in the relative terms of symptoms which furnish rather imperfect clues to the total disturbance and (with a few exceptions such as fever) cannot be quantified by the layman. Given the broad range and limited quantification of disturbances, the layman tends to use subjective criteria in judging whether an observed phenomenon should be assessed as a symptom, and these criteria vary according to the circumstances.

Any disturbance must reach a certain degree of seriousness or duration in order to be assessed as a symptom; below that degree a person may experience a cough, pain, a discomfort without perceiving them as symptoms (subliminal symptoms). This perceptual threshold changes with the circumstances: it is lower in summer when people do not expect illnesses and higher in winter when respiratory ailments and other illnesses are frequent; it is lower on work days and higher over the weekend when the pattern of recreational activities blocks the usual assessment of disturbances; it is lower for children and higher for adults. [39] Furthermore, one may expect that the perceptual threshold changes with social class and income level, and low-income groups differ in their assessment of a given disturbance as symptom.

Any threat to one's security and physical and psychological well-being evokes anxiety that, in case of health disturbances, is aggravated by the ultimate anxiety of death. Thus, any morbid episode appeals to the deepest fear of man, the fear of death, and sets more powerful psychological forces into motion than the word *episode* would indicate. On a psychological level, disturbance and threat are inseparable. The experience of fever and pain or the expectation of fever or pain evokes as its psychological response a specific anxiety that tends to be proportionate to the seriousness of the symptom or threat. The symptom is assessed by the measure of anxiety it arouses, and the anxiety introduces the many subjective variations in setting the perceptual thresholds.[40]

Any threat to a beloved person, such as a family member, evokes an essentially similar anxiety and causes the emotional involvement of several people in the morbid episode. Every disturbance of health originates a specific anxiety in the patient as well as in people near to him. Thus, an episode seldom remains the affair of only one individual, the patient; usually it involves other people also, initiates a chain of interactions between the patient and the others, and the extent of the interactions tends to be proportionate to the seriousness of the episode. At the same time, a threat releases general or floating anxiety, usually present in the psychological makeup of every person, and focuses it on the threatened person. This anxiety is pre-existent to, and independent from, the morbid episode; it is a function of psychological and social factors. In contemporary American families the child is the most likely focus of anxiety; the relative living in the household the least likely focus; while self and spouse are in between. Accordingly, when mothers were asked to report all symptoms experienced by family members within a month, children were most frequently mentioned as having had symptoms, relatives least frequently, with mothers and fathers falling in between. The more serious symptoms (those requiring two or more days of restricted activities), when separately examined, did not show a similar frequency distribution.[41]

RESPONSES TO ANXIETY

Evidently, any sickness is likely to direct the floating anxiety toward the sick person and allot to him the "special position" described by Sigerist. Threatening events, unrelated to health, may also release the floating anxiety, focus it upon one person, and affect the morbid episode. Such an extraneous event as the loss of the father's job may either focus anxiety on the child's illness and cause unreasonable concern about it, or may act just the other way, detract from the anxiety focusing upon the sick child and result in a neglect of his illness. Thus the degree of the floating anxiety does not necessarily correspond to the seriousness of the health disturbance. The total anxiety, present at the time of a morbid episode, is not a simple outcome of the perceived disturbance but a fusion of two independent anxieties; hence it is in its extent and manifestation always individualistic and subjective.

The natural response to a feeling of anxiety is the endeavor to remove or relieve whatever its cause might be. In daily life, however, the cause of anxiety can seldom be ascertained unambiguously. The feeling of anxiety and the response to it arc linked through a vague and uncertain causal relationship that is common in the realm of psychology. To any given anxiety people respond in many ways, and the relieving effect of any of the alternative responses depends on many individual circumstances. One frequent response is the one which often follows the dictates of the avoidance-escape mechanism. In case of health disturbances this kind of response means an attempt to forget about the matter and put it out of one's mind—a common enough response that can be observed in delaying health care, breaking appointments, and refusing to participate in reasonable health plans.[42] Another frequent form of response seeks the help of superhuman powers and uses magic or superstition in an attempt to remove the cause of anxiety.[43]

Very often such responses have a useful function in relieving anxiety; so it is in bereavement where forgetting is a common reaction. Health disturbances, however, present a special case. Here forgetting or denial may immediately alleviate the existing anxiety but lead in the long run to dangerous consequences—neglect of treating an acute and curable disease. The danger is great. Fortunately, there exist control systems that subject the responses to the censorship of higher-order psychological functions (learning, reasoning, judgment) and work to bring forth a reasonable response that is judged to be beneficial to health. Such control systems are, on one level, personal knowledge and, on another, the social organizations of the family and professional medicine.

Since morbid episodes occur regularly, their course can be observed and their treatment explored; thus, people acquire a general body of knowledge about health, illness, and therapy. This knowledge corresponds to the cultural level existing in the community, and it might be described as magic belief in one community, folk medicine in another, and medical science in a third.[44] On each level knowledge is likely to include some kind of classification of morbid episodes, evaluation of the nature and seriousness of the common illnesses, and predictions relating to the eventual outcome and possible handling of the symptoms. On every cultural level this body of knowledge is available in two forms—a popular one accessible to the average person and an esoteric form accessible to the professional healers. The popular form of knowledge depends on the professional one for its source and authority; in many instances it attempts to imitate the professional know-how existing in the community. Although popular, it is not an equally general knowledge; those persons who have the special duties of nurturance (mothers, older women) are its usual repositories.[45]

This lay knowledge, acquired to a great extent from past experiences, is applied to the perception of morbid episodes. It functions as a rational censorship of anxiety and prompts people to consider the whole situation in the light of their available knowledge. It influences them to make judicious decisions about taking actions for the removal of the cause of anxiety and the possible elimination of the health disturbance. The soundness of the decision depends on the medical knowledge available, but knowledge is never equally distributed among the social classes. Thus one may expect that low-income and other underprivileged groups handle health-related anxiety and decision-making differently from the privileged groups.

When this knowledge is applied to the state of good health, it tends to act in accordance with the floating anxiety and initiate preventive actions. For centuries, popular knowledge has recognized that disturbances in health can be prevented and has recommended preventive measures of the kind of "an apple a day keeps the doctor away." Furthermore it has prescribed a great number of harsh and even painful preventive treatments (purgation, bloodletting, circumcision), that can be hardly understood without considering the interplay of floating anxiety.

When the same knowledge is applied to a disturbance in health, it helps to assess the total situation, particularly, the level of seriousness and the necessity of taking actions. In many cases no action is taken, in others only a psychologically supportive response is given to the patient because it is believed that the episode will run its usual course and resolve itself without the necessity of any outside interference. In other cases, again, the disturbance is treated at home by the patient or by a member of his family, while the more serious cases are brought to the attention of professional healers.

The actions that people take are of manifold nature and effectiveness, but all of them have two characteristics in common: they take part within the framework of the usual interaction pattern, and aim at the satisfaction of a basic psychological need (such as relief from anxiety) by changing the underlying objective situation (the disturbance in health). Such complex goal-directed actions are best denoted as manipulations, and the name can be properly applied to the health-related actions, many of which do not have a rational relationship to genuine therapy.

THE MANIPULATIVE ACTIONS

Both lay persons and professional healers carry out manipulations. The former are likely to be family members and other intimates who are affected by the anxiety surrounding the health disturbance and are emotionally involved in the total episode; they have a high motivation to manipulate but no systematic knowledge of health and illness. The professionals (who are not necessarily physicians or approved by the medical profession) do not share the anxiety and emotional involvement and take up manipulation usually upon the formal request of the patient. On the other hand, they have a special knowledge, characteristic of their profession and the cultural level of the community.

Such a duality of manipulators implies that "simple" actions that do not require special knowledge are carried out by lay persons and complex actions by professionals; however, the duality does not coincide with the therapeutic or nontherapeutic nature of the action. Lay people often take therapeutically sound actions, particularly in case of common, simple episodes, while many medically non-approved practitioners manipulate the anxiety rather efficiently without proper therapy for the underlying disturbance.[46]

The authority of performing manipulative actions is, on the whole, ambiguously defined. Both personal involvement in the anxiety and special knowledge of health entitle people to take such actions, and the perceived seriousness of the episode designates the point where the authority of the lay person is supposed to yield to the authority of the professional healer. This general ambiguity leads to many dilemmas, particularly when it comes to selecting one out of several alternative manipulative actions; at the same time, it prompts the professional healers to impart a popularized form of their special knowledge upon the lay public.[47]

Manipulative actions aim at simultaneously removing both the health disturbance and anxiety. The achievement of this ideal goal is not always possible because disturbance and anxiety are to a certain extent independent in their origin as well as behavior, and the alleviation of one does not automatically alleviate the other. While the alleviation of a disturbance is likely to reduce the specific anxiety (although it may leave unaffected the floating anxiety), the alleviation of the anxiety, as a rule, does not reduce the underlying physiological disturbance. Other times anxiety may linger on after the apparent cessation of the disturbance, for example, in the form of a fear of its reoccurrence.

It is, therefore, practical to classify the manipulative actions according to their intended effectiveness in dealing with the health disturbance only. On such a basis we may distinguish between therapeutic and gratificatory actions. The therapeutic action aims at the removal or arrest of the disturbance, giving, at the same time, proper consideration to the anxiety surrounding it, in accordance with the standards set by the competent healing profession. It is likely to be the outcome of a reasoned judgment which establishes priorities among the possible aims and actions and proceeds consistently toward the desired end.

Gratificatory manipulation is essentially nonrational and has a main aim other than the professionally defined cure of the disturbance. It may aim at a relief of the anxiety without arresting the underlying disturbance, or at the gratification of wishes and needs not directly related to the morbid episode. Certain specific instances of it are particularly common, such as the escape-avoidance of painful or threatening therapy or the unwillingness to give up a pleasurable activity for the sake of health. The patient's desire for prolonging the sickness is frequent in mental and psychosomatic illnesses; for example, patients use hysteria for the gratificatory aim of dominating their family and, accordingly, to resist professional therapy.[48] Faith healers and cultists are likely to gratify various needs not related to the disturbance; the gratificatory nature of their manipulations helps to explain the popularity they enjoy with the public.

The manipulation of one symptom may include several actions; hence, therapeutic and gratificatory actions can be taken simultaneously. In the health care of the American middle class, manipulatory gratification has an adjunct role, secondary to the therapeutic one, and shows up, for example, in the usual pampering that patients give themselves or receive from others. In an adjunct role the medical profession also uses gratificatory manipulations (by "sweetening the pills," recommending bed rest or a "change of air") either as the signs of nurturance given by the healing professions or as psychologically effective means in the total therapeutic management.

To summarize the proceding discussion, Chart II-1 shows the schematic representation of the morbid episode as the patient's experience. From the patient's point of view, the four elements (perception, anxiety, knowledge, and manipu-

Health disturbance (threat)		Anxiety aroused		Pertaining knowledge	Manipulation		Preventive measures
Perception	Assessment	Floating	Specific		Gratification	Therapeutic	
Disturbance not perceived (subliminal symptoms)	Non-serious	Varying by extraneous factors	Little ⟷ Great	Lay knowledge	None		
Perceived symptoms	⟷ Serious				Requiring none		
					Requiring emotional manipulation of the anxiety only		
					Responding to lay manipulation (home treatment)		
				Professional knowledge	Requiring medical attention		

II-1. The schema of the morbid episode

lation) are interrelated; each of them affects all the others and, at the same time, is affected by them. Thus existing medical knowledge, while functioning as a rational censorship of anxiety, modifies the perception and manipulation; and, in turn, this knowledge is modified by the experience gained in each morbid episode.

It must be realized, however, that the patient, although the center of the episode, is seldom able to handle it by himself. He needs the assistance of persons in his immediate environment, particularly in his family. He finds further help in the more distant environment—in his community where professional health care is organized for giving support and nurturance in case of need. The resolution of the morbid episode requires interactions on the levels of his primary and secondary groups, represented by the family and the system of professional health care.

THE INTERACTION PATTERN OF
FAMILY AND MEDICINE

The family is the primary protective social organization that regularly dispenses nurturance.[49] In the pursuit of this main goal each family member has to perform a specific task—breadwinning, homemaking, preparation for adulthood. The systematic performance of such tasks establishes statuses within the family which, in turn, outline the channels for the flow of nurturance. The main channel leads from parents to children. The parents are the main dispensers of nurturance, but sex roles differentiate between their activities: the mother almost invariably is put in charge of health and nursing care, while the father is charged with certain supportive activities the extent of which greatly varies by social class and ethnic group. Among the children, age and order of birth differentiate in the form and amount of nurturance received.[50]

The floating anxiety, usually present in the family environment, is likely to move along the regular channels of dispensing nurturance and readily focuses upon the usual recipient of nurturance. Thus morbid episodes (even though essentially similar in nature) evoke varying degrees of anxiety depending on the family status of the receiver as well as the dispenser of anxiety; the greatest anxiety is likely to move from the mother toward her young child, while a usually "neglected" member of the family is just as likely to be neglected in his health needs also.

The systematic performance of specific tasks and the regular flow of nurturance establish a routine in family life with daily and weekly cycles of activities. The routine, although informal and flexible, serves as the framework of the family's daily life, supports the effective discharge of nurturance, and strengthens the cohesiveness of the family unit; its maintenance is a common concern of the family members. But the occurrence of a morbid episode disrupts the established routine. It demands a rearrangement in the usual flow of nurturance so that special care can be focused upon the afflicted member, and sometimes it demands a rearrangement of the usual tasks so that the family members can be free for the performance of manipulative tasks.

The family has to find ways to minimize the disruption and maintain the routine. This is achieved by varying the criteria which are used in judging the seriousness of symptoms and selecting manipulative actions. The systematic changes of those criteria mark weekly and seasonal cycles as well as variations by family status among morbid episodes.[51] In this way the family censors the experience of the patient and adjusts it to the necessary routine. While this is usually done with reasonable care, in its total effect it amounts to the family operating as an inhibitory system against the wishes and desires of the sick person. In particular, the family tends to enforce the primacy of the routine-like tasks over the immediate gratification of pleasurable needs, restricts the gratificatory manipulation of morbid episodes in favor of therapeutic ones and, more generally, aims to decrease the number and duration of morbid episodes.

Needless to say, certain types of families are more vulnerable to disruption by morbid episodes than others. In addition to the structure and size of the family, social class and income appear to mark important differences.[52] The question is not simply a matter of measures—whether the poverty family experiences more anxiety; after all, anxiety is highly subjective and often eludes the measurement techniques of research workers. But on a qualitative level there cannot be much doubt that the usual routine of the poverty family is more precarious and, on the other hand, the means and privileges of the well-to-do class represent great advantages in coping with anxiety and mastering stressful situations. The thesis and its consequences will be discussed in the following pages.

The secondary helper in morbid episodes is professional health care. It is an extremely complex system that provides care through a huge network of practitioners with special skill and knowledge and of institutions with trained manpower and special equipment. In accordance with the old professional ideology, each practitioner and each institution is supposed to be independent; many of them are, while others are formally coordinated into numerous subnetworks. The system is regulated by an interplay of governmental agencies and professional organizations and greatly dominated by the official representatives of the medical profession. Yet, the coordination of the numerous providers is unsystematic and ambiguous, resulting in redundant services in one place and in lack of services (of a needed kind) in another.

The principle of "fee for service" and entrepreneurial

competition for greater volume of patients permeates the whole system.[53] Every patient is supposed to select freely a practitioner or institution of his own choice or select none of them. On the other hand, every provider of health services is supposed to serve the needs of the entire community and offer institutional nurturance as well as therapy. Indeed, the patient who enters the network (or often is caught in it) expects to receive both during his diagnosis and treatment.

In actual functioning the system may fall short of the ideal. The free choice of a provider is greatly restricted by the patient's limited knowledge of the system and limited means to pursue his choices. Any provider, institution as well as individual practitioner, is just as greatly tempted to apportion its services unequally within the community and give better services to the privileged and the powerful. Finally, any large system develops its own work routine, which by its nature militates against individualized care and, at worst, may bring forth an assembly-line kind of health care.

The routinization of handling the patient begins with the diagnosis. The diagnostic procedures aim not simply for the exploration of possible organic disturbances but also for a convenient labeling of the patient, and such a labeling helps the communication among the members of the health care system. An English authority reminds us that "there is no disease of which a fuller or additional description does not remain to be written; there is no symptom as yet adequately explored."[54] In accordance with the available level of medical knowledge the diagnosis classifies the symptom into one of the professionally approved categories for which standard management procedures are available. The system of professional health care, in the effective discharge of its duties, has to follow a specific routine and categorize the personal complaint of the patient so it can be handled uniformly by any unit of the organization.

The diagnostic label imposes upon the patient an inhibitive system that controls his primary responses to anxiety and leads him toward a professionally approved, therapeutic management of the complaint. At the same time it enables the health care system to apply to the patient the standard treatment procedures, specified for the various illnesses and conditions. The standard procedures are likely to be efficient and competent, but they pose the danger of fragmented care for patients with several labels or with cases not fitting a label; moreover, they tend to neglect treating the highly subjective anxiety component. It hardly needs to be added that the shortcomings of the system are, again, not equally distributed within the community but weigh down upon the poor.

It is an often repeated statement that the system of professional health care is in a state of flux, although the same observation has been made in perhaps every epoch of medical history. At present the system provides for the patient's needs through three networks: private practice of physicians and other healers, public clinics maintained by institutions, and what can be best described as the first rudiments of a national health insurance scheme that the nation rather reluctantly is getting ready to adopt. The three networks are interlocked; they coexist in the same communities, often employ the same physicians, and just as often have the same patients using them alternately. Nor are they greatly different in getting paid for services; they are distinguished by differences of proportions rather than of substance. All three networks operate on a fee-for-service basis, although the private network is more likely to charge the patient directly, the public clinics are conspicuous for charging frequently to Medicare-Medicaid funds, while in the third network (which experiments with new forms of health care delivery) financing through direct governmental grants and prepayment plans looms large.

In their service pattern, however, the networks differ strikingly. Private practice is utilized mainly by patients in higher income brackets (the so-called middle class) who desire personal relationships with a specific health professional, continuity of services, as well as individualized care concerned with the totality of the morbid episode. Public clinics tend to be parts of welfare medicine and are used by patients in the lower income brackets who, as a rule, receive there competent but impersonal, discontinuous, and fragmented care. The third network came into existence to experiment with new forms of health care delivery and promises to find solutions to the inequities of the two other networks; at this point it may be too early to judge its achievements.

There is no reason to believe that public clinics deliver health care at a lesser cost than private practice; the former, as a rule, do not charge less, and often more. It is not the cost factor in itself but rather a long-standing social usage that sorts out the patients by social class and maintains a separate network of services for the lower or poverty class. During its social development the practice of medicine has generally come to be geared toward middle-class life and has developed public clinics and related institutions as dispensers of care to the lower class. Thus, the lower-class patient is apt to feel a social distance when facing a physician, experiencing it more acutely in the setting of private practice than in public clinics.[55]

POVERTY AND THE HEALTH CARE SYSTEM

It is a natural consequence of our health care system that the private practice of medicine is sensitive to the patient's personal anxiety and is willing to consider his wishes regarding therapy; it functions in a way as to complement and accommodate the patient's manipulative actions. The public clinic system, lacking the needed time, facilities, and privacy, cannot develop a similar personal relationship with the patient and cannot pay due regard to his manipulative actions. Frequently, it leaves a gap between the professional and the lay system of manipulating health disturbances; in particular, it is likely to leave unattended the problems of anxiety.

In spite of such differences, private practice and public clinics exert the same kind of control over the morbid episodes of the public. One line of control is implied in their service pattern, which, in face of the haphazard needs of the public, sets up a systematic routine-like cooperation of many agents in the management of diseases, the schedules and circumstances of physician-patient contacts, and the preventive measures applied to the general population. The routine eliminates wasteful individual variations, increases the efficiency of organized work, and insures a fairly uniform treatment of a large mass of patients. The popular joke about hospital patients being awakened to receive their sleeping pills caricatures the general shortcomings inherent in every routine; but, as more positive achievements, the same routine enables us to administer various screening tests to large populations or to obtain comparable tests and analyses from almost any agent of the health care system.

As another line of control, professional health care influences the public toward adjusting the lay system of manipulating health disturbances to the professional standards of therapy. This is mainly done through the formal and informal teaching that members of the health professions carry out in public as well as in private contacts with patients—for example, with the aim of making patients keep the regimen for the prescribed time even when the distressing symptoms disappear.[56] This teaching furnishes another inhibitory system to the emotional responses to health disturbances. The routine and the inhibitory system of professional health care carry the danger of ignoring the anxiety element of morbid episodes; any increase in routine and efficiency tends to exacerbate this danger and cannot fail to evoke criticism from patients.[57]

Cure is the ultimate aim of every manipulative action, but one should remember the saying of the wit, "When trying to cure illnesses, medicine sets its aim too high." Cure indeed is an ancient concept, coined in those times when life-threatening infectious diseases accounted for the far greater part of morbidity, when in the common cases of dysentery, scarlet fever, plague, only two outcomes—cure or death—were possible. But at present degenerative diseases, congenital and age-connected disabilities, constitute a great part of the morbidity. In their case cure (in the sense of a complete restoration of health) is an often unattainable goal. Accordingly, professional health care aims for a control, or arrest, of the health disturbance and accompanying anxiety, as well as for a similar control over the physical and social disabilities that serious illnesses are prone to leave behind.

The current standards of medicine try to adjust the professional practices to this complex aim. They recommend treating the patient rather than the symptom and utilizing the whole process of social interaction for the achievement of the medically ascertainable cure. In any case they use relatively objective criteria in judging whether a cure has been accomplished.

The layman, however, applies more subjective standards to his judgment of what constitutes a cure. For him the morbid episode for all practical purposes ends at a psychological threshold where he does not discern any anxiety-arousing health disturbance or where his felt anxiety is at a level comparable to the level that existed before the perception of the disturbance. In case of minor symptoms this state is often achieved "naturally," and the patient claims that the cold or other ailment "has gone." More serious illnesses require a more careful assessment of whether or not a cure has been achieved. Since gratificatory manipulations often alleviate the symptom and bring results which by lay standards come near to cure, the patient feels healed and may end the therapy without completing the cure. At other times, however, the patient is willing to make a more balanced judgment of whether or not he has been cured, and in this judgment he is led by his medical knowledge and feelings of anxiety. Thus his perception of being cured is a psychological counterpart of his initial perception of a health disturbance, an assessment of the comparative difference between the previous (sick) and the present (cured) functioning of his health. In any case the discrepancy between the professional and the lay definition of cure carries its own dangers. On the one hand it may lead to breaking off the professionally recommended treatment procedure and, on the other, it may lead just as frequently to hypochondria and search for miracle cures.

To summarize the reasoning above, Chart II-2 gives a schematic representation of the place of morbid episodes in the social interaction pattern. It indicates that the morbid episode, individualistic and unique in its physiological as well as psychological origin, in the course of its treatment and cure has to be fitted into the social interaction pattern of the patient with his primary group (as represented by the family) and his secondary group (as represented by the system of professional health care). Both groups have their routines for dealing effectively with morbid episodes, and, in order to obtain their help, the patient has to comply with the demands originating in the inhibitory system and other stable features of the social organizations.

In the present state of morbidity and health care the

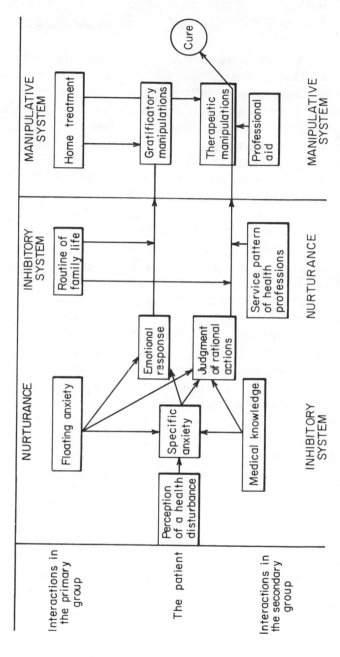

II-2. The place of morbid episodes in the social interaction pattern

desirable resolution—cure—of any morbid episode cannot be attributed to the control of purely pathological factors; rather it depends to a very great extent upon the apt or inapt use of the social interaction process. The structure of the total health care system suggests that poverty as a rule cannot maintain a fully efficient interaction pattern, and every step of the process restricts its felicitous use. Speaking of the primary group (see Chart II-2), the poverty family with its specific nurturance, inhibitory, and manipulative systems is more predisposed toward undesirable outcomes than the well-to-do family which in times of morbid episodes can, and does, mobilize a greater array of means, privileges, education, and other resources. Hence, the poverty patient in his perception of health and illness, in his management of anxiety, frequent emotional responses, and gratificatory manipulations is likely to fall short of the professionally recommended standards and find it more difficult to reach the medically desirable cure.

When it comes to interactions in the secondary group, the poverty patient is at a particular disadvantage. The service pattern of the health professions and general professional aid are not equally available to all. Their ready availability is greatly dependent upon all those privileges that in their totality make up social and political power, those with more privileges and power having a better access to health services. Most countries provide very good health care to the military and often a better one to the officers than to the privates. This ancient and ubiquitous inequality has not been fundamentally changed by the recent reform actions in the American health care system—the development of the experimental network of services.

The latter network operates mainly through institutions and organizations which interact with their patients in an impersonally regulated way, defined by their policy. As a rule, institutional policy aims for a large volume of standardized services that precludes any dyadic relationship between doctor and patient; it aims for institutional growth as the proof of its success and creates giant-size hospitals and health empires; it aims for efficiency and relegates the authority of making decisions to a small group of insiders, excluding the public. Institutional medicine always runs the danger—and the larger the institution, the greater the danger—of neglecting the personal humanistic aspects of health care; in fact, it has been repeatedly accused of dehumanization.[58]

Many reform movements of the last few years have assumed that good health care for the nation and especially the poor is simply a matter of finances and that every shortcoming can be righted by changing the "payment mechanism"—for example, by giving somewhat more money to welfare recipients or establishing special institutions for their health care. But an examination of the total system suggests that finances will solve, at best, half of the present shortcomings. The other, and perhaps greater part, centers around two objectives: that the consuming public should have its voice in the management of health institutions and that the institutions should deliver a personal health care comparable to what is given in the private practice of medicine. At this writing no nationwide solution of the two objectives has been attempted.

The systematic interaction of the patient, his family, and the health care system assures the best resolution of morbid episodes that our medically advanced age can offer. But our experiences with poverty give a warning that the interaction of the three parties works optimally for the patient with means and privileges, while the poverty of the patient tends to detract from the smoothness and efficiency of the interaction.

It would be easy to verify this assumption and compare how the poor and non-poor fare in illness and health if there were a uniform index of health that could measure in a simple way all the differences that can be observed in the course of morbid episodes. But no such index exists because the pathological, psychological, and social components of any episode are to a great extent individualistic and independent and cannot be reduced to a common denominator.

Therefore a more difficult path has to be taken. The following chapters will investigate the social implications of morbid episodes as they appear in the schema of interaction pattern: the observable differences among the poor and non-poor in physical and mental health (Chapters III and IV); in preventive behavior (Chapter V); the seeking of help by the poor (Chapter VI); the functicning of the manipulative system in treating and rehabilitating the sick (Chapters VII and VIII); the institutional operation of the health care system (Chapter IX); and finish with an analysis of the present efforts and future possibilities for providing better health care (Chapter X).

III. Social Differences in Physical Health

by Monroe Lerner

The object of this chapter is to provide a conceptual frame-work, or model, for comparing the level of physical health of the poverty population, as currently defined, with the health level of the rest of the population of this country. According to this framework, however, the "rest of the population" should not be considered as a single homogeneous entity. Rather, it is most meaningfully classified, for purposes of considering the level of physical health as the dependent variable in the relationship, into two large categories or strata defined by socioeconomic status (SES). It is suggested in this chapter that identifiable social factors affect these strata of the population very differently, resulting in correspondingly dissimilar levels of physical health.

The conceptual framework presented here is buttressed, in some degree at least, by the use of some small proportion of the empirical data comparing the physical health of the poor in the United States with that of the rest of the population. For this purpose existing data are used; no "original" data were collected especially for the analysis. The discussion focuses on the United States, and within this country its primary emphasis is on the national health

Monroe Lerner is Professor, Department of Health Care Organization, School of Hygiene and Public Health, the Johns Hopkins University, Baltimore, Maryland.

situation. However, local data are used to clarify relationships in those instances where appropriate national data are not available. Although the poor are treated as an overall category, this chapter does include some consideration of the Black population as a specific subcategory of the poor. It does not include, however, separate discussions of other subcategories, e.g., the Puerto Rican, Mexican-American, or other generally poor ethnic minorities, the aged, migratory laborers, or the rural poor in Appalachia or the Deep South.

Measuring the level of a population's physical health is a complex conceptual problem, not unlike that of measuring socioeconomic status.[1] In part, the difficulty stems from the apparent multidimensionality of health, but also from the absence of any widely accepted, standard definition of this characteristic. Health appears to be socially defined, with its definitions varying according to the specific social and/or professional setting. The definition of health used by the practicing physician, a major provider of health services, apparently differs widely from lay definitions, and there appears to be a wide range of cultural variation in the meaning of the concept. For example, some conditions defined as illness in some settings are accepted as "natural" in others.

But even if a standard definition existed, two larger philosophical questions remain. First, can we really separate, in any meaningful sense, the physical from the mental or emotional aspects of health? Second, should the health of individuals in a community be considered apart from the health of the community or society as a whole? Can a *healthy* population exist in a *sick* society, or vice versa, and, if so, for how long? The level of health of a community or society may differ, in an as yet unspecified way, from the aggregate total of the health of individuals comprising it.

Our inability to answer either of the above problems in an absolute sense may constitute a limitation to any conclusions that might be derived from the present discussion. Nevertheless, for pragmatic reasons and in the absence of any better procedures, simple answers are provided here for these complex questions. For example, levels of physical health will be the prime focus of the present discussion. These are considered as adequately measured by mortality rates and by that proportion of this nation's morbidity, impairments, and the resulting disability manifesting itself directly as, or due directly to, physical as opposed to mental or emotional illness. This decision eliminates from the present discussion the whole notion of mental and social well-being as formulated in the World Health Organization's definition of health. Similarly—again a simple answer—the health of individuals comprising a community and the health of the community as a whole will be considered as identical in the present discussion.

Mortality rarely, if ever, has other than a physical condition as its *immediate* cause, at least in the philosophical sense in which the concept of "cause" is customarily used in mortality statistics. As a result, mortality rates can quite legitimately be used as partial indicators of a population's level of physical health. However, the distinction between physical and mental or emotional causation or involvement is much less clear with regard to morbidity, impairments, and disability; it is extremely doubtful whether in real life the physical aspects of these conditions can be neatly disentangled from their emotional aspects. Thus, the decision to confine the present discussion to their physical aspects is purely arbitrary, justified only by the apparent usefulness of the distinction for analytical purposes. Finally, no attempt is made in the present discussion to combine mortality rates (essentially a measure of the duration or quantity of life) with any indicators of morbidity, impairments, or disability on the one hand, and "social well-being" on the other (essentially measures of the quality of life), into a general index or ratio. Each of the two characteristics customarily used as major dimensions of physical health, mortality and morbidity, will be considered separately.

A similarly complex conceptual and measurement problem concerns the classification of any community's population into socio-economic strata. On what basis should populations be classified into strata: i.e., what dimensions or characteristics should be included in an index of socio-economic status, and how many strata should be delineated? The approach taken here is that this is best done by classifying populations into the minimum number of major socioeconomic strata that will be relevant to and predictive of the achievement of health levels, however the latter may be defined. For the United States, following this line of reasoning, the minimum number of major strata into which the population should be divided appears to be three.

What are the characteristics of the populations comprising these strata? Although the boundaries between the three strata are by no means sharp or clear-cut, and at their margins shade into one another, it is nevertheless possible to delineate their outlines, which are defined, in the most general terms, by *distinctive life styles*. These life styles are, in turn, dependent on or associated with the amount and the source of resources (income, wealth, and so on) available to the members of each stratum; their type of occupation and the prestige associated with each type; the type and value of their dwelling and neighborhood and possibly even the region of the country in which they reside; their level of knowledge and educational attainment; and their race or ethnic origin. This listing by no means exhausts all of the factors on which the life styles of these strata depend or with which they are associated. There may be a considerable amount of movement from one stratum to another, particularly because the boundaries between them are not clear-cut and no rigid legal distinctions exist, but also because there is a considerable degree of overlap in the factors on which these strata are dependent or with which they are associated. Nevertheless, this delineation corresponds essentially to the general perceptions of the American population and, in the sense of a self-fulfilling prophecy, it is at least possible that these strata may be tending in the general direction of becoming collectivities rather than mere aggregates of population.

The highest of the three socioeconomic strata delineated here consists of persons designated in both conventional sociological terminology and popular parlance as the middle and upper classes. This stratum includes families whose heads are engaged in salaried, white-collar occupations, usually those falling within the following general categories: professionals, small-businessmen, middle-level and junior executives, and even some categories of upper white-collar workers (e.g., technicians, salesmen, and the like). It also includes families above this in the social hierarchy, e.g., families of top-level business executives, high government officials, and college presidents, and some families below it, e.g., supervisors, foremen, and possibly even some members of the highest echelon of skilled blue-collar workers. Although engaged in industrial occupations, these skilled blue-collar workers and their foremen and supervisors are nevertheless exposed to relatively few industrial hazards; and although technically blue-collar, in many respects they follow a white-collar life style.

The range of variation within this stratum in health,

income, housing, and educational attainment is great; nevertheless, the group as a whole falls at the upper end of each continuum. Despite the range of variation within it, in very general terms its members share the essential elements of a "middle-class" way of life. They generally reside in the "better" neighborhoods of large and medium-size cities or in the suburbs surrounding them. They participate in the general affluence characteristic of this country as it enters the last fourth of the twentieth century, and they set the standards in general life styles for the rest of its population and, indeed, for the population of a large part of the world. This stratum will be called the "middle class."

The intermediate stratum in the three-tiered hierarchy proposed here consists of the population that can best be described as the "blue-collar working class," i.e., most of the skilled and semiskilled and many unskilled blue-collar workers and their families; small farmers and possibly even farm laborers and their families; and lower-level, poorly paid white-collar workers (often young clerical workers and their families). These people in general "work with their hands." They are likely to be employed in the mass-production industries, e.g., steel mills, automobile and air-craft factories, mines, smelters and refineries, and in such blue-collar service industries as transportation and communications. A large number in this stratum consist of the "respectable" working classes, including large nonpoverty ethnic groups (and their descendants) especially on the East Coast and in the Midwest, and dwellers in small towns and medium-sized communities of this country. Again, the range of income, education, and residence within this stratum is very great; nevertheless, like the upper stratum, they too share a general style of life, one which is distinctively different from that of either of the other strats considered

here. They share in the general affluence characteristic of
our society, although not to the same extent as the middle
class.

The lowest of the three strata is the poverty population.
Concepts of poverty are obviously relative, varying with
time and place, and numerous standards have been used to
define poverty and to measure the poor. Poverty may perhaps best be thought of as *relative deprivation,* using some
standard for comparison, and subjective elements enter into
the definition of its own situation by a nation, group,
family, or individual. This complicates the problems of
definition and measurement enormously. Nevertheless, the
poverty population may be described as the stratum that
does *not* share in the affluence characteristic of current
American society. This population is generally outside the
mainstream of American life and has its own distinctive life
style. Its levels of unemployment are typically high, with
income and educational attainment low. Its family structure
tends to differ from the rest, being marked among some of
its segments by a relatively weak paternal role, often involving prolonged absences, while among other segments the
paternal role may be overly "strong." It is often thought to
include substantial proportions (by no means all) of the
following population segments: the Black, Puerto Rican,
and Mexican populations, and the other relatively poor
ethnic minorities in this country; the poor in large-city
ghettos and the rural poor (residents of Appalachia or the
Deep South); Indians on reservations; the aged; migratory
laborers; and the dependent poor.

The three strata differ from one another in four specific
aspects of their life styles which, it is hypothesized, result in
the achievement of substantially different levels of health
among them. The four aspects are: level of living; degree of

Table III-1. Specific aspects of life-styles most relevant to the
achievement of health among the three major socioeconomic strata

Specific aspects of life-styles	Poverty popula- tion	Blue-collar working class	White-collar middle class
Level of living (food, housing, transportation, etc.)	−	+	++ --(?) (perhaps even dysfunctional)
Access to medical care within the private medical care system	−	+	++
Occupation of family head: sedentary or involving physical activity	+(?)	+	−
Nature of social milieu: degree of economic or social security	−	−	+

access to medical care *within the private medical-care system;* nature of occupation of family head, i.e., whether sedentary or involving physical activity; and the nature of the social milieu, i.e., its degree of economic or social security or protection against economic hazards. These relationships are shown in the paradigm of Table III-1.

Perhaps the most important specific aspect of the life style distinguishing the poverty population from the other strata is its relatively low level of living, specifically with regard to food, housing, transportation, and similar items. With regard to food, for example: while for most Americans diseases related to nutritional deficiency may be a thing of the past, this is probably not true to the same extent for the poverty population. The diet of the blue-collar working class probably compares favorably with that of the middle class. The middle class, in fact may actually eat too well, and too much. This may transform the two pluses in this classification into a minus. Poor housing appears to be correlated with poor health, and at least for some specific illnesses, correlations have been demonstrated and the mechanisms operating in the relationship are well understood.[2]

The medical care received by the poverty population, when they receive it at all, is often received in a setting that is definitely inferior to that of the rest of the country's population. Strauss uses the probably accurate term "medical ghettos" to describe the medical care situation of the poor.[3] However, even when technically good medical care is available to the poor, they generally do not avail themselves of this important resource to the same extent as the white-collar middle class. This has now been documented in many studies, and it appears to apply in some degree to the blue-collar working class as well as to the poor, although probably not to the same extent. After reviewing the many studies along these lines, Irelan has concluded that the poor and the working class tend to ignore minor conditions and seek treatment only at a relatively late stage.[4]

Generally, the working class does have access to the private medical care system in this country, and they are likely to be served by it. They are probably served inadequately by middle-class standards, it is true, and they certainly do not use the system as much in conformity with professional standards as the middle class does, but served they are, nonetheless. Possibly the single most important factor, over the last generation, in bringing this population into the private medical care system has been the phenomenal proliferation of voluntary health insurance and, more recently, possibly even Title XVIII of the Medicare legislation, at least for the substantial aged population who were formerly active members of the working class.

The middle class is generally likely to have access to a relatively high level—in quantity and quality—of medical care within the private medical care system, and they are usually educated enough to use it as it is intended to be used according to professional standards. In contrast, the poverty population has little command of resources except through public assistance programs; this applies especially to their relationship to the medical care system. Even when they do have access to medical care services and use them, they receive these services as an indigent population, a fact which has implications for both the quantity and quality of care they receive.*

The physical activity characteristic of an occupation is one aspect of life style that pertains only to male family heads. While there is clearly a continuum, generally persons engaged in salaried white-collar occupations—the middle class—lead sedentary occupational lives in contrast to the generally "physical" occupations of the blue-collar working classes. Moreover, persons within this group who occupy executive positions may be subject to particularly severe strains and tensions. Shepard, quoting a study by William H. Whyte, Jr., notes that executives are working as hard as they ever did, although other workers long ago cut their working weeks down to forty hours or less.[5] Even with the new emphasis on human relations and committee management in industry, executives are apparently subject to more tensions than ever before. The consequences in morbidity and mortality are thought to be particularly evident during the period of midlife and beyond.

*The subject of access to medical care is discussed extensively in other chapters.

The poverty population is most likely to resemble the working class in this respect, but the situation of this stratum is by no means clearly a benefit. A large proportion of family heads among the poverty population will more often than not be unemployed, a large proportion are female, and a large proportion are more likely than not to be engaged in service-type occupations, often domestic service.

Finally, an important element of life styles concerns the nature of the social milieu experienced by the three strata in terms of their degree of protection against economic hazards, particularly those of a short-term nature. The implication of this difference is that persons with a maximum amount of protection can afford to seek medical treatment for relatively minor conditions and to assume the sick role when occasion warrants.

THE CONCEPTUAL FRAMEWORK:
HEALTH AND SOCIOECONOMIC STRATA

Mortality in the Poverty Population

It seems reasonable, *a priori,* to expect that complex human societies, that is, human societies which contain reasonably well-defined socioeconomic strata, would exhibit substantial differentials in health levels among the various strata. This must have been true under almost any set of historical circumstances yet encountered by human societies, and it appears to derive from the following set of considerations.

In any society, whatever the prevailing system of social stratification, the desired "goods" of life, by definition "scarce," are likely to be distributed unequally among the various strata, however these strata are defined. These goods of life are likely to include at a minimum the necessities required by man for life sustenance and the maintenance of health among the living—food, clothing and shelter. The upper strata of any society will in all likelihood and at all times have the power and means to obtain a larger share of the total of these scarce goods than their sheer numbers would warrant, while in contrast the lower strata are generally likely to be able to obtain less than an "equal" proportion. To the extent that these goods are in fact life-sustaining and do contribute to the maintenance of health among the living, health—defined here to include both duration of life and freedom from illness—is also likely to be unequally distributed. At a somewhat higher level of societal complexity, the ability to avoid a hazardous occupation (except perhaps the occupation of military command) is also likely to be desired and considered a scarce good, and therefore to be distributed unequally, thus also contributing to the disparity.

But another scarce good consists of the society's and/or community's health services. These can be public (goods and services provided by the community as a whole or at least provided under its auspices, and generally directed to the community as a whole or to specific segments of it, and where the entire community is believed to benefit by this diversion of resources from the whole to some of its segments) or personal (goods and services provided by health practitioners *directly* to families and/or individuals). These health services, whether public or personal, are specifically assumed to maintain or promote health and to prevent "premature" death. All societies provide services of these types to their members (although public health services—as opposed to collective effort in the provision of food supplies and military protection and security—may be provided only in the more advanced societies), and to the extent that these services do actually maintain or promote health and prevent premature death, this situation also is likely to result in better health for the upper strata.

Do health services actually maintain or promote health and prevent premature death? There really is not much question in this regard about public health services; the record of history provides eloquent testimony to their beneficial effects in prolonging life and maintaining a healthy environment. The aqueducts of Rome present merely one example of this. Even with regard to personal health services, it seems unreasonable to suppose that there would be no correspondence between these two, i.e., that there would be no beneficial effects. Clearly, some individuals must always benefit from some contacts with some providers of health services, or else new providers would be sought and would, indeed, emerge.

However, what has the balance been? Have the contacts with providers been on the average beneficial or detrimental? We have no way of knowing what the situation was in the past in Western society, or what it is even today where non-Western systems of medicine are practiced. According to as eminent an authority as L. J. Henderson, it was not until early in this century that an individual in this country taken at random stood a better-than-even chance to benefit from an encounter with a professional in the health establishment. But this situation does appear to be much improved today. Nevertheless, to say that the balance is beneficial is not to say that complete control of an individual's health by health practitioners is possible. There are far too many lacunae in medical knowledge to make this even a remote possibility. There are still too many unknowns in the etiology and/or therapy of the major illness conditions to assume that patients will always benefit from contact with a medical practitioner or with some other part of the health establishment. Too often the opposite may result;

iatrogenic conditions may be more significant than is commonly supposed. Also, and to understate the case somewhat, the present organization of the health services' system in this country may not always optimize conditions for the practitioner to render the highest quality of care.

In some instances, even if all etiological factors of all illness conditions were known and therapy were available for all of them, complete control might still perhaps be impossible, since massive changes in the customary behavior patterns of the population might have to take place. Smoking, and eating habits directly conducive to obesity, are perhaps only the better known instances of this seeming irresponsibility and/or urge toward self-destruction on the part of the general population. Although good health is surely a universal value, evidently our attachment to this value is not strong enough to orient our behavior, at the expense of alternative satisfactions, toward the attainment of perfect health.

Social position and health levels have been closely related, certainly in our immediate past. This has been especially true for the ill health attributable to the major communicable diseases, leading causes of death until very recently, and possibly through the first quarter of this century in the United States. Pond has reviewed some of this literature:

Historically, the healthiest nations have been those with the highest incomes and the lowest illiteracy rates. At the beginning of this century life expectancy at birth was greater in the United States, Great Britain, and the Scandinavian countries than it is today in many parts of the world. . . .

Throughout history communicable diseases have struck most severely among the poor. Even today, it is the serious communicable diseases that present the greatest threats to the health of people in underdeveloped lands. Many diseases that are virtually unknown or non-existent in the United States and other economically favored nations are the main causes of death and disability among large population groups elsewhere on the globe.[6]

Typhoid fever and tuberculosis are obvious cases, but the same is true also for the communicable diseases of childhood, gastrointestinal diseases, and—earlier—leprosy and plague, smallpox, typhus, and other louse-borne diseases, and syphilis.[7]

During the periods when the communicable diseases were the major causes of death, they must also have been the major causes of morbidity, impairment, and disability. If this is indeed the case, and there seems to be little reason to doubt it, then the poor, most affected by these diseases, must have been less healthy than the well-to-do along the entire measurable spectrum of ill health. The major health problems of the entire population of each community must have been public health problems of the traditional kind—poor sanitation and impure water supplies, and the like. The more well-to-do populations might have been able, at least in some degree, to counteract their poor sanitary environments by availing themselves of better nutrition, better access to medical care, less crowded housing, and better working conditions.

Does poverty cause ill health or does ill health cause poverty? While the form of social organization is surely an intervening variable, it does not seem unreasonable to suppose that there is a large degree of interdependence between these factors, with each reinforcing and even feeding upon the other. Each can usefully be considered, according to this formulation, as either the dependent or the independent variable in relation to the other, and something like a vicious circle must result. Undoubtedly, much the same situation must have obtained both today and in the past, whenever and wherever ill health and poverty are found.

These conditions clearly still obtain in large parts of the world, especially where public health facilities remain inadequate, where water supplies are contaminated, or food impure. But it is probably also still true for some populations even where public health facilities and services are relatively adequate as, for example, in the slums of large cities in this country today. Here the symbiotic relationship between poverty and ill health continues to exist. Mortality rates, especially during infancy, childhood, and even the younger adult ages, appear to be higher here than for the rest of the population, again especially from the communicable diseases. Morbidity, impairments, and disability must also be more prevalent here than in the surrounding areas. The same is likely to be true for other pockets of poverty in this country—the Deep South, Appalachia, Indian reservations, and elsewhere. By and large, whatever the public health situation of these populations may be, they surely do not have access to adequate personal health services equal to that of the rest of the population, nor do they have adequate nutrition and housing. But in addition to the economic factors that condition this lack of availability, cultural factors and knowledge of how to use personal health services and other welfare services are all relevant in this context. Their lower level of use of primary health services is perhaps most clearly evident with regard to dental care, possibly the most neglected aspect of the health of the poor.

Mortality in the White-Collar Middle Class

During the second quarter of this century the major communicable diseases declined as leading causes of death in this country, to be replaced by the degenerative diseases—heart disease, cancer, and stroke—and accidents. Medical advances, especially the development of the antibiotics, and the improving social conditions of the general population played major roles in this transformation. In contrast to the communicable diseases, which took their major toll of life during the younger years, heart disease, cancer, and stroke are largely associated with the aging process, and death rates from these diseases are highest at the older ages. What is most important for this discussion, however, is that by and large the overall burden of these conditions as expressed in excess mortality may be approaching the point where it does not fall much more heavily on the poor than on the rich. There are many exceptions to this emerging relationship, especially among various components of the broader disease categories, e.g., cervical cancer, cancer of the digestive system, vascular lesions of the central nervous system, infectious diseases of the heart, and others, but it appears to be generally true of the broad disease categories.

As perhaps a partial explanation of these statements, which seemingly fly in the face of common sense, some of the newer and more important forms of ill-health may to some degree be an actual concomitant of the affluent life styles of the middle class in the United States. Members of this stratum may be subject more than others to some forms of social stress. Perhaps in recalling past deprivations, whether real or imagined, or for other reasons, they may overcompensate in their drive to achieve, and once achieved maintain, high status; there may be some selection for personality types here. High status, in turn, so often involves sedentary (executive and white-collar) occupations, mechanized transportation (two or even three cars), and richer foods. The unintended consequences of affluence may well include obesity, excessive strains and tensions, excessive cigarette smoking, and, resulting from these, perhaps ultimately premature death from coronary artery and arteriosclerotic heart disease or from respiratory cancer.*

Males in the forty-five to sixty-four age category, especially white males, appear to be particularly vulnerable to coronary artery disease and respiratory cancer. Women in the middle and upper strata, on the other hand, appear to be less affected by these affluence-related forms of ill health than men, possibly because of an innate resistance to coronary artery disease and lung cancer, for example; possibly because of greater social pressures upon them to avoid obesity and perhaps to take better care of their health generally; possibly because they smoke less or, at least, do not inhale cigarette smoke as men do; possibly because they may lead generally less stressful lives; or perhaps because of some combination of these factors.

During infancy and the younger years, however, while differentials in mortality among the various socioeconomic strata of the nonpoverty population have probably narrowed, those between the poverty and nonpoverty populations have probably continued to be substantial, despite the decline in absolute mortality rates for both groups. For example, Robert M. Woodbury, studying infant mortality during 1911-1916 in seven cities in this country, found that infants born to families with an annual income of $1,250 or over had an almost three times better chance to survive their

---

*This may not be the first time in history that upper-class life styles (or cultural patterns or status symbols) may be detrimental to health and/or life-shortening (e.g., foot-binding among women of the Mandarin class in imperial China; obesity in some parts of the ancient Middle East).

first birthday than infants in families whose annual income was less than $450; the infant mortality rates were 59 and 167 per 1,000, respectively. When infants in families with no income at all were compared to the highest income group, the comparative ratio was 3.5 to 1; the infant mortality rate in the no-income group was 211 per 1,000.[8] While these rates are nowhere near as high today for either high- or low-income groups, the comparative ratio between them continues to be substantial. The sharpest contrasts today in infant mortality and in mortality during childhood and the younger years are probably between the nonwhite population, in both the Deep South and the large-city poverty areas, and the white nonpoverty population, especially its more affluent strata.

If these hypotheses are correct, the poverty population is likely to experience a relatively high level of mortality, i.e., higher than the level for the total population. Its mortality rates, especially from the communicable diseases, and during infancy and at the younger ages, are likely to be high. At the older ages, its mortality record may be relatively good, possibly because poor risks have already been selected out at the younger ages. The upper stratum (middle class) is also likely to experience a relatively high level of mortality, i.e., higher than that for the total population, but from very different causes of death. Death rates from degenerative diseases and at the older ages are likely to be high among this group, while during infancy and the younger ages its mortality record is likely to be excellent.

Mortality in the Blue-Collar Working Class

The working class is likely to have the best overall mortality record of the three strata. Its mortality rates from the communicable diseases and from various causes during infancy and the younger ages are likely to be as low, or at least nearly as low, as the rates of the middle class, and much lower than those for the poverty population. On the other hand, its mortality rates during the older ages and from the diseases associated with the aging process are likely to be as low, or nearly as low, as the rates of the poverty population, and much lower than the rates for the middle-class population. The hazards specific to blue-collar industrial occupations have declined sharply in this country since the early years of the century, undoubtedly due in large part to the industrial hygiene movement. Industrial hazards probably no longer constitute a significant factor in the overall picture of mortality in this country, certainly not sufficient to raise the mortality level of blue-collar workers above that of the other strata.

Morbidity, Impairment, and Disability

Differentials in the prevalence of morbidity, impairments, and disability between poverty and nonpoverty populations, apparently quite clear and well-defined during the era of communicable disease, are considerably less clear today *unless* relatively severe and relatively minor conditions are considered separately. Thus the prevalence of morbidity, impairments, and disability, particularly chronic conditions causing activity restriction for long periods of time, is probably highest among the poverty population. This follows from the higher prevalence of severe communicable diseases as causes of death in the poverty population. However, unlike the mortality rate, higher in the poverty population during the younger years, the prevalence of morbidity, impairments, and disability is likely to be higher for the poverty population especially during the later years of mid-life and old age.

The poverty population experiences more severe illness to begin with, or is more vulnerable to it when it does appear.

But even if this were not the case, if they experienced only the same amount of illness and had the same degree of vulnerability as everyone else, because they generally remain outside the private medical-care system their illnesses are much more likely to remain untreated and consequently ultimately to increase in severity, often resulting in higher mortality among them than for other segments of the population. With severe illness, it is likely that the traditional poverty-nonpoverty differentials still exist today, although it is possible that the comparative excess of severe illness among the poverty population may not be as high as in former years.

For minor illness, however, especially for those conditions which by their very nature are self-limiting and do not result in mortality, the situation may be considerably different. For example, considering the United States population as a whole and with no distinction between rich and poor, there appears to be relatively more minor illness today than in former years, at least as reported in household interviews. This was one of the principal findings emerging from an earlier study by Lerner and Anderson of acute disabling illness in the United States.[9] For serious acute illnesses, on the other hand, that study found that there had been a substantial decline in prevalence, especially for the communicable illnesses serious enough to be reported to the U.S. Public Health Service. However, as part of the general decline in the major communicable diseases, the proportions of many of these illnesses terminating in death (their case-fatality rates) had declined sharply.

The Lerner and Anderson study also compared 1958-59 data on the prevalence of acute disabling conditions derived from the household interviews of the U.S. National Health Survey with combined data from five separate periodic-visit household enumerations of illness in this country between

1928 and 1943, compiled by Selwyn D. Collins. According to this comparison, the prevalence of acute disabling conditions in this country had risen substantially—more than a 200 percent increase—from the earlier to later surveys (about a generation), but as a counteracting tendency the average duration of each illness had declined sharply, by almost 50 percent. Thus many more disabling conditions of relatively short duration were being reported in the later survey. Was this a "real" increase, or merely an artifact of better data-gathering techniques or improved survey procedures? The suspicion that it may have been real was strengthened by the findings of a series of data on illness among industrial employees in this country, which showed that their annual rate of illness cases involving disablement for one day or longer was substantially higher in 1952 (when the series was terminated) than during the 1930s.[10]

The notion that there may have been a real increase in the volume of minor illness in this country over the last generation is very difficult to accept, at least at first glance, because it implies that the efforts of the whole health establishment over the last generation to reduce the prevalence of illness may have had no appreciable effect or, even worse, that these efforts may have boomeranged and may actually have produced a larger volume of illness in the general population. How can this iconoclastic notion be explained?

The following statement is offered as at least a tentative hypothesis in explanation of a *real* increase: The increase in the prevalence of minor illness may have resulted from a whole complex of changing social conditions and structural features of society. More liberal policies regarding sick leave, the growth of insurance against medical costs and loss of income due to illness, relatively full employment since World War II—all of these may have reduced the economic and social penalties for short absences from employment or other restrictions on usual activities. The average person is better educated, more sophisticated about medical care, and probably far more aware today than in former years of the need to acknowledge and seek treatment for even minor cases of illness. Finally, the increased use of physicians' services and the increase in hospital admissions, along with shorter stays, may both indicate a larger volume of illness episodes, at least as defined in terms of people's awareness of illness and perceptions of their need for services. All of these factors, plus others not specified here, may add up to a real increase in the volume of illness, but especially in those relatively minor conditions which are by their very nature self-limiting.

To some degree the suspicion that the increase is real was strengthened also by the data regarding the "condition group" (diagnostic condition) of illness. Thus the largest increases in prevalence from the earlier Collins surveys to the later National Health Survey were for upper respiratory conditions (common cold, acute sinusitis, pharyngitis, tonsillitis, laryngitis, tracheitis). The prevalence of these conditions increased by over 500 per cent; they accounted for almost 40 percent of the episodes of all illness conditions in the National Health Survey data. Large increases were also registered in the prevalence of lower respiratory conditions (influenza and grippe, bronchitis, pneumonia, and pleurisy), and of accidental injuries. Within accident group in the National Health Survey data, about 60 percent of the illness episodes consisted of fractures, dislocations, sprains, strains, contusions, and superficial injuries. The prevalence of the infectious-parasitic condition group also increased, but again the increases were confined to the relatively minor conditions within it. The prevalence of the more serious of the conditions in this group—smallpox, pertussis, typhoid fever, diphtheria, scarlet fever, malaria, undulant fever, and some others—actually declined sharply. In contrast to prevalence, the average duration of illness declined for each of the major condition groups enumerated in these surveys.

The hypothesis of this discussion is that these increases in relatively minor illnesses are real, for the reasons enumerated above. Most important, the major changes that have been specified here have taken place primarily in the middle-class population. This group is generally likely to have the fewest social and economic penalties levied against it for relatively short excursions into the sick role. In general, the middle class tends to work in more protected jobs than either the working class or the poverty population, and it is likely to be better educated, more sophisticated about the uses of medical care, and on the whole more aware of the need to acknowledge and seek treatment for even minor cases of illness than the rest of the population. The result of all of this is that this group is likely to perceive and experience more relatively minor illness than the others, although the others, and particularly the poverty population, are likely to experience more relatively severe illness.[11] The higher level of minor illness in the middle class should be particularly evident at the younger ages. In contrast, the higher level of relatively severe illness among the poverty population is likely to be evident at the later years of midlife and during old age.

The working class is not likely to respond in the same fashion as the middle class to minor illness, especially because sickness has a different set of consequences for workers in blue-collar occupations. Sickness resulting in absence from employment is likely to entail economic penalties that will have far more severe consequences for this group than comparable penalties might have for the middle class. On the other hand, the working class, because it is included in the private medical care system, is likely to have its severe illnesses attended to, while minor illnesses are also likely to be treated before they build up into severe illnesses. Moreover, the success of the industrial hygiene movement during this century has substantially reduced the prevalence of severe illness due to occupational hazards (industrial injuries, silicosis, pneumonia and other respiratory conditions, industrial poisonings, dermatitis, cancer, tuberculosis, and many other disease conditions). As a result of these factors, the working class is likely to have less minor illness at the younger ages than the middle class, and less relatively severe illness at midlife and during the older ages than the poverty population.

DIFFERENTIALS IN MORTALITY

Mortality in this country, has declined substantially during the twentieth century. This is true regardless of whether crude or age-adjusted mortality rates are used to measure the decline, and it appears to be true also for both the total population of the country and for each of its major segments, however these are defined. Nevertheless, a leveling off began to take place prior to 1954 in the downward trend of the crude rate for the total population, and since that time this rate has more or less rested on a plateau. Thus the crude mortality rate for the total population of this country dropped from 17.2 per 1,000 population in 1900 down to 9.2 in 1954, but it has fluctuated between 9.7 and 9.3 since that time.* In 1971 the provisional rate was 9.3. [12] While the severe influenza epidemic of 1918-19 caused the

---

*The rate for 1900 was based on data from the "death-registration states" only (ten states and the District of Columbia in that year). However, for comparison purposes this rate is customarily taken to represent that of the entire country.

mortality rate to rise sharply, the rise was only temporary. The mortality rate fell at a particularly rapid rate after 1939, largely in response to the introduction of new medications (sulfas, antibiotics), but also because of other life-extending medical advances.

The "crude" mortality rate of a population is clearly inadequate in most instances as a basis for comparing mortality experiences (whether of the total population of a country or merely a segment of it), and even of the same populations at different points in time. This is primarily so because mortality is definitely a function of age and age-compositions often vary substantially among populations. As a result, it is customary to compare populations in terms of age-adjusted mortality rates, and this is usually done by using the 1940 population of the United States as the standard population to which adjustment is made. The change in age-composition of the United States population between 1900 and the present was generally in the direction of an increase in the proportion of the total population constituted by the high-risk groups at the expense of the low; thus the age-adjusted death rates prior to 1940 were much higher than the crude rates, while since that time age-adjusted rates have been much lower. The decline in age-adjusted death rates from 1900 to the present has therefore been much sharper than the comparable decline in crude rates; even so, there has been little or no decline in age-adjusted rates since 1960.[13]

Unfortunately for the present purpose, no mortality statistics have ever been collected specifically for the poverty population of the entire United States; furthermore, it is unlikely that such statistics will be collected, at least in the near future. To obtain data for this population separately would require that death certificates contain the information necessary to classify the deceased in terms of at least some objective indices of socioeconomic status, i.e., income, educational attainment, occupation during the major portion of their working lives, and size of family. An innovation of such major dimensions in the vital-statistics record-keeping system on a nationwide basis is unlikely to occur. As a result, it is unknown whether the poverty population in this country has shared equally with the rest of the population in the overall mortality decline since earlier in this century. Also, comparisons of the mortality experience of the poverty population with the mortality experience of the rest of the country even at this point must necessarily rely on the results of studies of limited populations. In the present instance, much of the discussion is based on a study of the mortality experience of poverty and nonpoverty populations in Chicago (the Chicago poverty study).[14] This, however, is supplemented by a study of mortality contrasts in high- and low-income states and by another study of mortality in three geographic divisions of this country.

The Chicago Poverty Study

For the purposes of the Chicago poverty study, an earlier division of the city into poverty and nonpoverty areas by the Chicago Committee on Urban Opportunity (CCUO) was used as the basis for analysis. Poverty was defined by CCUO as the concentration within specific areas of the city of populations with low income, low education, poor housing, large proportions on public assistance, and high unemployment and juvenile delinquency rates. On the basis of this definition, Chicago's seventy-five community areas were divided into twenty-four poverty and fifty-one nonpoverty areas. The residents of the poverty areas were, on the average, considerably younger than the nonpoverty population, and about one half were nonwhite.

Since the population of Chicago's poverty areas was, on the average, younger, it would be expected, if poverty made no difference and if the age-specific or real mortality experience of these two groups was identical, that the crude mortality rate in the poverty areas should be much lower than the comparable rate in the nonpoverty areas. This proved not to be the case. Against an overall crude mortality rate of 11.9 for the city (see column 1 of Table III-2) the overall crude mortality rate in the poverty areas (12.1 per 1,000 population) was actually slightly higher (by less than 3 percent) than the comparable rate of 11.8 in the nonpoverty areas (see columns 2 and 3 of Table III-2). It seems that if age-adjusted mortality rates had been computed for this study, a substantial differential would have been found, with mortality rates much higher among the poverty population.* The conclusion on the basis of these data is that poverty *does* make a difference in the risk of mortality.

This contrast in overall mortality rates between the poverty and nonpoverty areas is confirmed and made much more clearly evident in the age-adjusted mortality data for 1960 available from the *Chicago Local Community Fact Book,* and adapted for present purposes.[15] These data are expressed in terms of the standardized mortality ratio, a measure of the extent to which the age-adjusted mortality rate for community areas exceeds, or is less than, the comparable rate for the city as a whole. The age-adjusted mortality rate in the poverty areas exceeded the comparable rate for the entire city of Chicago by about 23 percent, while the age-adjusted mortality rate in the nonpoverty

---

*Age-adjusted mortality rates could not be computed for Chicago in 1964 because mortality rates specific for age were not available.

Table III–2. Selected measures of overall mortality (all ages combined) and infant mortality by place of residence of (poverty and nonpoverty areas) and race, Chicago, 1964

Selected measures of over-all and infant mortality	All races			White population			Nonwhite population		
	1	2	3	4	5	6	7	8	9
	All places of residence	Poverty areas	Non-poverty areas	All places of residence	Poverty areas	Non-poverty areas	All places of residence	Poverty areas	Non-poverty areas
Over-all mortality (all ages combined) rates per 1,000 population									
All causes of death	11.9	12.1	11.8	12.6	14.0	12.2	10.0	10.7	7.4
By cause									
Heart disease	4.6	4.4	4.7	5.1	5.7	4.9	3.1	3.3	2.4
Cancer, all sites	1.7	1.5	1.8	1.8	1.7	1.9	1.2	1.3	1.0
Cancer, by site (rate per 100,000 population)									
Colon	19.2	15.9	21.2	21.2	20.4	22.4	12.1	12.0	12.6
Breast	16.0	11.1	18.7	17.8	11.2	20.3	9.7	10.5	3.8
Cervix	4.4	6.6	3.2	3.6	5.3	3.0	6.9	7.2	6.0
Infant mortality rates per 1,000 live births									
All causes of death									
Entire year of infancy	30.0	38.5	22.2	22.2	25.1	21.3	43.0	45.5	29.6
Neonatal period	21.1	25.6	17.0	16.6	17.3	16.4	28.7	29.9	22.0
Post-neonatal period	8.9	12.9	5.2	5.6	7.8	4.9	14.3	15.6	7.6
Entire year, by cause									
Influenza and pneumonia	5.0	7.9	2.2	2.6	4.4	1.9	8.9	9.8	4.4
Congenital malformations	1.1	1.3	1.0	0.9	0.6	1.1	1.5	1.6	1.1
Gastroenteritis, colitis	_a	1.3	_a	_a	0.6	_a	_a	1.6	_a

Source: Chicago Board of Health, Planning Staff of the Health Planning Project, A Report on Health and Medical Care in

areas was less than the comparable rate for the entire city by about 12 percent. To put this in other terms, the *age-adjusted* mortality rate in the poverty areas exceeded that in the nonpoverty areas by about 40 percent.

To return to the Chicago poverty study, the effect of differences in age-composition are evident also in the comparison between the entire white and the entire nonwhite population of the city (columns 4 and 7). The crude mortality rate for the white population (12.6) exceeds that for the nonwhite (10.0) by about one fourth. Again the implication is clear that age-adjusted mortality rates would have shown an entirely different picture. Finally, when race is held constant (and this holds some proportion of the age differences constant also), the effect on mortality of residence in the poverty areas is seen. The crude mortality rate for the white population only was 14.0 in the poverty areas as against 12.2 in the nonpoverty areas, an excess of 15 percent in the poverty areas, while for the nonwhite population the comparable rates were 10.7 and 7.4, respectively, an excess of almost 50 percent in the poverty areas. Again, these differences would clearly have been of much greater magnitude if age-adjusted rates had been used.

The figures in Table III-2 also show some data for mortality rates from two major causes of death—heart disease and cancer. The rates are shown only for these two because, among the major causes, they alone had mortality rates of at least 0.05 per 1,000 population in this experience. Both of these causes of death are strongly associated with the aging process. Because of this, as well as because of the older average age of the nonpoverty population compared to the residents of the poverty areas and of the white population compared to the nonwhite, the mortality rates from heart disease and from cancer (all sites) were found to be higher for the nonpoverty population and for the white population than for their opposite numbers. Thus the mortality rate from diseases of the heart in the nonpoverty areas, 4.7 per 1,000, exceeded the comparable rate in the poverty areas, 4.4, although only by a relatively slight margin (about 6 percent). The comparable figures for the mortality rates from cancer of all sites were 1.8 and 1.5 per 1,000, respectively. The very narrowness of these differentials, despite the wide differences in age-composition of the two populations, suggests that the influence of poverty on the population residing in the poverty areas raises the mortality rates of this group and from these causes of death far above where they would otherwise be in the absence of poverty. Considering the nonwhite population only, those residing in the poverty areas had substantially higher mortality rates than those residing in the nonpoverty areas. These same relationships held for the white population, at least for heart disease; for mortality from cancer of all sites, however, the white population residing in the nonpoverty areas had somewhat higher rates.

The statistics for mortality from cancer of three specific sites—the colon, breast, and cervix—are particularly interesting. It is generally agreed that a very large proportion of all deaths from cancer of these sites is preventable, given the proper application of modern medical knowledge. Only for cancer of the cervix was the mortality rate for the poverty population (6.6 per 100,000) clearly and substantially higher than the comparable rate for the nonpoverty population (3.2 per 100,000), and the rate for the nonwhite population (6.9) clearly and substantially higher than that for the white population (3.6). For cancer of the colon and the breast, the higher average age of the white population than of the nonwhite, and of the nonpoverty population than of the poverty, could have resulted in higher mortality rates among the white and nonpoverty populations, and therefore evaluation is difficult. An excess mortality risk comparable to that for cancer of the cervix, however, was clearly not demonstrated for cancer of these other two sites.

The limiting of the mortality rates shown in Table III-2 to data for only two of the major causes of death, heart disease and cancer, obscures the importance of the communicable diseases as major health problems in the poverty areas of Chicago. Andelman has pointed to the magnitude of tuberculosis as a problem in that city:

> ... We look at the new case rate of 75 in the city under consideration and learn that in some parts of the city there are no new cases or only one or two a year, while in some community areas there is a new TB case rate anywhere from 150 to 200 per 100,000 per year. This analysis points up the real tuberculosis situation in the city. It shows that there are well-defined pockets of tuberculosis. ... This condition prevails in nearly every big city in the nation, with the rare exception of cities in the most predominantly agricultural states with nontransient populations.[16]

High- and Low-Income and Geographic Divisions

It may be useful to supplement the data from the Chicago poverty study with data from a study of mortality in high- and low-income states in this country. This study, reported in full elsewhere, compared the mortality patterns of the ten states (including the District of Columbia and excluding Hawaii and Alaska) ranking highest in average per capita personal incomes with the ten lowest during 1930, 1940, 1950, and 1957.[17] The composition of these groups of states varied somewhat over the years, but in general the high-income group consisted largely of the most industrialized and urbanized states, especially those in the Northeast but also including some in the Middle and Far West. In contrast, the low-income states were generally but not exclusively in the South, much more rural in character, and with large nonwhite populations. The range between these groups of states in average per capita income narrowed between 1930 and 1957, as did also the differentials in at least some of the health facilities available to their respective populations.

The generally superior health facilities available to the population residing in the high-income states were reflected in lower mortality rates only to a relatively small extent even in 1930, but since then this differential has actually declined. Thus, in 1930 the age-adjusted mortality rates of the low-income states exceeded the comparable rates in the high-income states by 13 percent, but by 1940 this margin had dropped to 7 percent, to 5 percent in 1950, and to less than 1 percent in 1957. However, the trends and differentials in mortality rates between these two groups of states varied sharply in accordance with the ages of their populations. In 1930, for example, mortality rates had been substantially higher in the low-income states for ages under forty-five, and especially for childhood and infancy; by 1957, although these differentials were much reduced, they were nevertheless still substantial. At ages forty-five to sixty-four, mortality rates had been somewhat higher in the low-income states in 1930; by 1957 there was almost no difference. Finally, at ages sixty-five and over, relatively little difference in mortality rates between the two groups of states had existed in 1930; however, by 1957 the low-income states were favored with a substantially lower mortality rate.

The changing relationship of mortality in the low- and high-income states has resulted largely from the general decline of the major communicable diseases (influenza and pneumonia, tuberculosis, gastritis and other major infectious diseases of the gastrointestinal system, the major communicable diseases of childhood, and certain diseases of early infancy) as leading causes of death. These diseases were primarily responsible during the early years of this century for the higher mortality rates prevailing in the low-income states; in later years they were replaced as leading causes of death by heart disease, cancer, and stroke, among others. The latter conditions, strongly associated with the aging process, were generally far more prevalent in the high-income states. Because of these trends, the rates for the leading causes of death converged in the two groups of states.

This convergence in the overall mortality rate was accompanied by a parallel convergence in mortality from some of the leading causes of death. Thus the mortality rate from diseases of the heart in 1930 was only 71 percent as high in the low-income states as among the more well-to-do states; by 1957, however, this ratio had risen to 86 percent. The comparable rise (in ratio of rates in low-income to high-income states) for mortality from cancer was from 59 to 77 percent; for mortality from diabetes mellitus it was from 57 to 80 percent; and for suicide it was from 59 to 91 percent.

A similar study of three geographic divisions compared mortality rates of the heavily urbanized Middle Atlantic states (New York, New Jersey, and Pennsylvania), the relatively prosperous and rural West North Central states (Minnisota, Iowa, Missouri, North and South Dakota, Nebraska, and Kansas), and the relatively poor and rural East South Central states (Kentucky, Tennessee, Alabama, and Mississippi).[18] Between 1940 and 1959 age-adjusted overall mortality rates were converging among these three groups of states; nevertheless, in 1959 the relatively well-to-do rural states of the Midwest still had the lowest mortality rates, while the heavily industrialized and urbanized northeastern states had the highest mortality rates. Mortality rates in the East South Central states were close to those of the Middle Atlantic.

In general, the relatively well-to-do rural midwestern states had not only the lowest overall mortality rates, but their experience was uniformly favorable at all ages and from the leading causes of death. Thus in 1950 (the latest year for which these data were available, they had the lowest mortality rates not only from the major communicable diseases (influenza and pneumonia, tuberculosis, major communicable diseases of childhood, certain diseases of early infancy) generally most prevalent at the younger ages, but also from the degenerative diseases associated with the aging process (heart disease, cancer, stroke). These states consisted largely of relatively well-to-do populations, even though rural, with relatively small proportions of "poverty" populations.

The relatively poor, rural southern states, on the other hand, had the highest mortality rates at ages under forty-five, and especially during infancy and childhood. Their mortality rates were highest at all ages from the major communicable diseases and from accidents; however, their mortality rates among the population aged sixty-five and over and their overall age-adjusted mortality rates from heart disease, cancer, and stroke were not as high as the comparable rates in the Middle Atlantic states. Their mortality patterns—for the entire geographic division—were characteristic of rural poverty populations. Although these patterns tend to be similar in most respects to those of urban poverty populations, the latter constitute only part of the total population in the Middle Atlantic states, so that the overall mortality patterns within the two divisions accordingly differed somewhat.

Finally, the heavily urbanized and industrialized Middle Atlantic states had the highest mortality rates at the middle and upper ages, especially from heart disease, cancer, and stroke. Their mortality from accidents was lowest among the three groups of states. And because large poverty populations resided in these states, even as far back as 1950, their mortality from influenza and pneumonia and from tuberculosis was substantially higher than in the West North Central states, i.e., the relatively well-to-do midwestern states.

DIFFERENTIALS IN INFANT MORTALITY

Perhaps the most sensitive single index of health conditions within a community is its infant mortality rate (deaths of children under one year of age per 1,000 live births). This rate has traditionally been very widely used to classify communities or populations in terms of their overall levels of health, particularly where morbidity data have not been available. Further, it has generally been used also as an indicator of the level of social and economic well-being within a country.

The Chicago Poverty Study

In Chicago in 1964, according to the data of the Chicago poverty study shown in the lower tier of Table III-2, the differential in infant mortality between the populations residing in the poverty and nonpoverty areas was substantial. For example, the infant mortality rate for the population residing within the poverty areas, 38.5 per 1,000, was about 75 percent higher than the comparable rate of 22.2 within the nonpoverty areas. Moreover, the differential by racial group was also substantial. Thus considering the population of the city as a whole, the infant mortality rate of the nonwhite population was almost double that of the white,

43.0 and 22.2, respectively. The same relationship—higher infant mortality rates among the nonwhite than among the white population—was evident in both poverty and non-poverty areas. The nonwhite infant mortality rate of 29.6 in all nonpoverty areas combined exceeded the comparable rate of 21.3 for white persons residing in these areas by about 40 percent. For residents of the poverty areas, the comparable rates were 45.5 and 25.1, an excess in nonwhite infant mortality over white of about 80 percent. Thus, to judge by these figures, the impact of race alone, at least with regard to infant mortality, was greater on the residents of the poverty areas. That is, the disabilities usually associated in our society with membership in a minority group—discrimination and inability to obtain access to adequate medical care, and so on—fell relatively most heavily on the nonwhites residing in poverty areas.

However, racial group membership alone did not account for the differentials in the infant mortality rate within Chicago because, even with each racial group considered separately, there was still a substantial differential in infant mortality between those persons residing in the poverty areas and those in the nonpoverty areas. Thus the infant mortality rate of the nonwhite population residing in all poverty areas combined was over 50 percent higher than the comparable rate of the nonwhite population residing in the nonpoverty areas; for the white population, however, the comparable excess was only about 18 percent. These figures indicate that the impact of residence in the poverty areas on the white population of the city, although by no means negligible, was far greater on the nonwhite population. In short, it is clear that the nonwhite population residing in poverty areas experienced the combined impact of both major social disadvantages—minority group membership and residence in poverty areas—and as a result this group had by far the highest infant mortality rate of the four population groups considered here.

Even though the infant mortality rate is generally considered to be very sensitive as an indicator of health levels, the post-neonatal mortality rate (deaths of infants who have survived their first month of life per 1,000 live births) is perhaps even more sensitive. The greater sensitivity of this measure occurs essentially because it eliminates from consideration the large number of deaths of newborn babies, either at birth or shortly afterward, some proportion of which results from biological factors whose control is either extremely difficult or impossible in the present state of medical science. These deaths occur apparently in almost equal degree among babies born to mothers of all social classes. That is, they appear to be largely independent of social and economic status.

The post-neonatal mortality rate for Chicago in 1964, considering its entire population, was 8.9 per 1,000 live births. Post-neonatal deaths thus accounted for about 30 percent of all infant deaths. As expected, the rate for residents of the poverty areas, 12.9 per 1,000, was more than double the comparable rate of 5.2 for residents of the nonpoverty areas. Similarly, considering the experience of residents of poverty and nonpoverty areas combined, the rate for the nonwhite population, 14.3 per 1,000 live births, was 2.5 times the comparable rate for the white population, 5.6. The highest rate among the four population groups was, again, that for the nonwhite population residing in poverty areas, 15.6; this rate was double that of the white population residing in poverty areas and just over double that of the nonwhite population residing in nonpoverty areas.

Much the same pattern, although in lesser degree, was evident when only the neonatal mortality rate (deaths of infants during their first month of life per 1,000 live births) was considered. Thus the neonatal mortality rate was again highest for the nonwhite population residing in poverty areas and lowest for the white population residing in non-poverty areas. However, the differential between the poverty and nonpoverty areas was not substantial when the white population alone was considered. Thus the neonatal mortality rate of the white population residing in poverty areas, 17.3 per 1,000, was only about 5 percent higher than the comparable rate for the white population residing in the nonpoverty areas, 16.4 per 1,000.

Among the major causes of infant death, the combined disease category of influenza and pneumonia played a leading role for all population segments. This category accounted for 5.0 infant deaths per 1,000 live births in the city as a whole. However, and as a clear indication of the extent to which mortality from influenza and pneumonia reflected social and economic conditions, the comparable mortality rates from this cause in the poverty and non-poverty areas were 7.9 and 2.2, respectively, while for the nonwhite and white populations in the city as a whole they were 8.9 and 2.6, respectively. These are substantial differentials. The nonwhite population in the poverty areas, least well off socially and economically of the four population segments, had the highest rates, while the white population in the nonpoverty areas, living under the best conditions of the four population groups, had the lowest rate. The rate of the former population was more than five times the rate of the latter. Influenza and pneumonia accounted for over 20 percent of all infant deaths among the nonwhite population in the poverty areas, against less than 10 percent of all infant deaths among the white population in the nonpoverty areas.

Congenital malformations as a cause of infant death also reflected differences in social and economic conditions in the city, but not nearly to the same extent. Nevertheless, the rate in the poverty areas was 1.3 infant deaths from this cause per 1,000 live births, compared to 1.0 in the non-poverty areas. Similarly, the infant mortality rate from this condition was 1.5 for the nonwhite population, compared to 0.9 for the white population. Somewhat surprisingly, the infant mortality rate from this condition among only the white population was higher in the nonpoverty than in the poverty areas. Finally, gastroenteritis and colitis as a cause of infant deaths is shown in the table only under the poverty areas because the rate in the nonpoverty areas and in the city as a whole was less than 0.05 per 1,000. In the poverty areas the nonwhite rate, as expected, was considerably higher than the comparable rate for the white population.

The Ten Largest Cities

The relationships between poverty and infant mortality found in the Chicago poverty study above correspond generally to those between racial group membership and infant mortality found in a study of the experience of the ten largest cities in this country during 1962.[19] While the nonwhite and poverty populations in this country by no means coincide, there is of course a good deal of overlap; the analysis in the following pages is offered as suggestive rather than definitive, and perhaps useful only because of the leads it may offer for further research. The data from this study by cause of infant death are shown in Table III-3.

Thus in 1962, according to these data, the nonwhite population of the ten largest cities in this country experienced an infant mortality rate of 39 per 1,000 live births compared to 23 per 1,000 for the white population in these cities, an excess of 67 percent. (As reported earlier, the comparable figures in Chicago during 1964 were 38.5 per

Table III–3. Infant mortality by cause, 1962, in ten largest cities (according to 1960 U.S. Census)[a]

Cause category[b]	Category number[b]	Deaths under 1 year per 10,000 live births		
		White	Non-white	Percent excess of nonwhite
All causes	–	230.8	386.0	67.2
Prenatal and natal	–	154.6	230.4	49.0
Immaturity and certain other prenatal and natal causes	769,774,776	44.0	87.8	99.5
Postnatal asphyxia and atelectasis	762	48.9	81.4	66.5
Congenital malformations	750–759	36.0	31.8	–11.7
Birth injuries	760–761	18.8	25.7	36.7
Hemolytic disease of newborn (erythroblastosis)	770–771	6.9	3.7	–46.4
Postnatal	–	76.2	155.6	104.2
Ill-defined, peculiar to early infancy	772–773	18.0	30.6	70.0
Influenza and pneumonia (except newborn)	480–493	18.5	41.3	123.2
Certain infections	053,340, 470–475 500–527, 763–768	17.0	41.8	145.9
Disease of digestive system	530–587	7.8	11.7	50.0
Accidents	E800–E962	3.8	10.1	165.8
Other postnatal causes, including residual	–	8.2	10.8	31.7
Symptoms and ill-defined conditions	780–795	3.0	9.5	216.7

Source: Eleanor P. Hunt and Earl E. Huyck, "Mortality of White and Nonwhite Infants in Major U.S. Cities," Health, Education, and Welfare Indicators (January 1966), p. 15.

[a]Baltimore, Chicago, Cleveland, Detroit, Houston, Los Angeles, New York, Philadelphia, St. Louis, and Washington, D.C.

[b]According to the Seventh Revision of the International Statistical Classification of Diseases, Injuries, and Causes of Death, World Health Organization, 1955. Categories are listed in rank order according to United States rates, 1962, for corresponding categories.

1,000 for the poverty population and 22.2 for the non-poverty, an excess of 73 percent, and 43.0 for the nonwhite population compared to 22.2 for the white, an excess of 94 percent.) The comparable ratio (of nonwhite to white infant mortality rates) was larger among the deaths due to factors presumed to be of postnatal origin (an excess of 104 percent) than among those due to prenatal or natal origin (a comparable excess of 49 percent). Again, the general direction of this relationship was similar to that found in the Chicago poverty study.

Among the mortality factors of postnatal origin, the ratios were particularly high for accidents (166 percent), certain infections (146 percent), and influenza and pneumonia, except of the newborn (123 percent). Among the factors of prenatal and natal origin, the ratio was particularly high for immaturity and certain other prenatal and natal causes (almost 100 percent), and postnatal asphyxia and atelectasis (67 percent). The high ratios for the categories lacking in diagnostic content—symptoms and ill-defined conditions, and immaturity and certain other prenatal and natal causes—indicate a lower degree of completeness of reporting of causes of death for nonwhite infants. This incomplete reporting may also have been a partial factor in the lower rates for nonwhite than white infants of the somewhat more specific diagnostic categories "hemolytic disease of the newborn" and "congenital malformations."

DIFFERENTIALS IN MORBIDITY, IMPAIRMENTS, AND DISABILITY

In contrast to death, by its very nature a clearly defined event, morbidity and impairments, as well as the disability associated with these conditions, are often relatively nebulous categories, and therefore difficult to measure. They may be thought of as states of being that lie beyond a point on a continuum. Often the continuum is multidimensional, including subjective and socially defined components along with the physiological, and there may be a considerable degree of overlap among them. The states are frequently of long duration, and many separately identifiable states may coexist within the same individual and at the same time; in some instances it may be very difficult, if not impossible, to classify these separately identifiable states in a hierarchy of importance. Partly for these reasons, and because of the resulting difficulties of measurement, but also because death has important legal consequences so that records of it have to be kept in any well-ordered society, the development of statistics on morbidity, disability, and impairments has lagged far behind the development of mortality statistics in this country and, indeed, in the Western world generally. However, this situation has improved greatly within recent years, at least in the United States and due largely to the efforts of the National Center for Health Statistics (NCHS). For the first time some systematic data on these conditions are available.

For the purpose of comparing the health levels of poverty and nonpoverty populations, the adequacy of morbidity data still leaves much to be desired. For example, in contrast to the relative availability of mortality statistics, there are no series of data on morbidity, disability, or impairments by state or by any geographic area smaller than national. Data along these lines are fragmentary, scattered among a number of different sources, and in many instances collected on different bases. As a result, we cannot as yet directly analyze differentials in these conditions by state or within a state, and certainly not between poverty areas within a city.

However, some data on morbidity and disability by family income are available from the National Health Survey of NCHS. These data are based on household surveys of the civilian noninstitutional population, and the ability to generalize from them is limited. These data may also gloss over differences that are germane to the present comparison, since they do not pinpoint the poverty population accurately. To do this, for example, family income ought ideally to be related to such characteristics as size of family, place of residence (rural, urban, suburban, by geographic area), race, availability of health facilities, and costs of services. These adjustments were not made in the present data; nevertheless, they are by far the best available at present.

One of the best-known tabulations of data demonstrating a reasonably clear inverse relationship between disability (restricted activity and bed disability) and family income among the civilian noninstitutional population of the United States during 1968 is shown in Table III-4. According to the table, days of restricted activity per person per

Table III–4. Days of disability per person per year by type od disability and family income, United States, 1968

Type of disability	Family Income					
	Less than $3,000	$3,000– 4,999	$5,000– 6,999	$7,000– 9,999	$10,000– 14,999	$15,000 or more
	Days of disability per person per year					
Restricted activity	25.4	17.5	14.3	13.9	12.8	11.0
Bed disability	10.2	7.1	6.1	6.2	5.3	5.1

Source: U.S. National Center for Health Statistics, "Disability Days, United States, 1968," *Vital and Health Statistics: Data from the National Health Survey,* ser. 10, no. 67 (Washington, D.C.: U.S. Government Printing Office, January 1972), p. 7. Based on household interviews of the civilian noninstitutional population and adjusted to the age and sex distribution of the total civilian noninstitutional population of the United States, 1968.

year dropped from 25.4 among persons in families with incomes less than $3,000 to 11.0 at incomes of $15,000 or more. However, the break was fairly abrupt between those with family incomes under $3,000 and those with $3,000–$4,999, and between those in the latter category and the rest of the population. (This latter abrupt break is, very roughly, at the poverty cut-off line.) At the higher incomes,

Table III–5. Days of disability per person per year by type of disability, age group, and family income, United States, 1968

Type of disability and age-group	Family Income					
	Less than $3,000	$3,000–4,999	$5,000–6,999	$7,000–9,999	$10,000–14,999	$15,000 or more
	Days of disability per person per year					
Restricted activity						
Under 5	13.0	10.5	11.2	9.5	11.0	9.3
5–14	11.1	9.0	9.3	10.4	9.2	9.1
15–24	13.3	10.2	11.1	9.8	10.1	9.2
25–44	26.2	18.1	12.3	11.9	10.3	10.4
45–64	44.3	27.3	18.3	17.4	15.5	12.1
65–74	41.4	27.1	24.5	24.0	21.5	15.4
75 and over	46.5	38.5	40.8	42.4	35.0	28.0
Bed disability						
Under 5	8.0	4.4	5.1	4.3	4.1	3.8
5–14	5.5	3.9	3.8	4.6	4.1	4.2
15–24	5.1	4.1	4.8	4.5	4.8	5.3
25–44	11.2	7.4	5.3	4.7	4.2	4.4
45–64	15.8	10.8	6.6	6.6	5.3	5.1
65–74	14.5	9.8	11.1	10.8	8.0	8.6
75 and over	17.6	19.4	22.8	27.3	18.6	13.5

Source: U.S. National Center for Health Statistics, "Disability Days, United States, 1968," *Vital and Health Statistics: Data from the National Health Survey,* ser. 10, no. 67 (Washington, D.C.: U.S. Government Printing Office, January 1972), p. 7. Based on household interviews of the civilian noninstitutional population.

in contrast, the decline with rising incomes was much more gradual (14.3 days at $5,000–$6,999 dropping only to 11.0 at $15,000 or more). For days of bed-disability, the data show a relatively abrupt break at annual income of less than $3,000, and only a gradual decrease with rising income for the higher income groups. When the data are examined by age, the inverse relationship—decrease of disability days with rise in family income—seems to be most consistent during the adult years, beginning with the twenty-five to forty-four age group and ending at sixty-five to seventy-four (see Table III-5).

Another well-known set of tabulations demonstrating relationships along the lines of those discussed above is shown as Table III-6. This table shows the percent distribution of persons by chronic condition and mobility limitation status according to family income in the United States from July 1965 to June 1967. Among persons having one or more chronic conditions (a category considered here to include both relatively severe and relatively mild conditions) and among those with one or more chronic conditions but with no limitation of mobility at all (relatively mild conditions), no clear pattern of relationship to family income was evident. But it was evident among persons with the more severe handicaps. Thus 2.8 percent of those with family incomes of less than $3,000 had trouble getting around alone, but at $15,000 or more the comparable proportion dropped to 1.0 percent. For the category "needs help in getting around," these proportions were 1.5 and 0.8 percent, respectively, and for "confined to the house" they were 1.4 and 0.4 percent. In each case the proportion was substantially higher in the low-income group.

Data from the same source show that the proportion of persons with one or more chronic conditions causing activity limitation was clearly related inversely to family income

Table III-6. Percent distribution of persons by chronic condition and mobility limitation status, according to family income United States, July 1965–June 1967

Mobility limitation status	Family Income					
	Less than $3,000	$3,000–4,999	$5,000–6,999	$7,000–9,999	$10,000–14,999	$15,000 or more
	Percent distribution					
All persons	100.0	100.0	100.0	100.0	100.0	100.0
With no chronic conditions	48.2	51.8	51.9	50.1	49.2	50.0
With 1 or more chronic conditions, total	51.8	48.2	48.1	49.9	50.8	50.0
With no limitation of mobility	46.2	44.7	45.3	47.3	48.1	47.9
Has trouble getting around alone	2.8	1.8	1.4	1.3	1.4	1.0
Needs help in getting around	1.5	0.9	0.7	0.8	0.6	0.8
Confined to the house	1.4	0.7	0.7	0.5	0.6	0.4

Source: U.S. National Center for Health Statistics, "Chronic Conditions and Limitation of Activity and Mobility, United States, July 1965–June 1967," *Vital and Health Statistics: Data from the National Health Survey,* ser. 10, no. 61 (Washington, D.C.: U.S. Government Printing Office, January 1971). Based on household interviews of the civilian noninstitutional population, and adjusted to the age distribution of the civilian noninstitutional population of the United States.

for at least these major chronic illness conditions: heart conditions, arthritis and rheumatism, mental and nervous conditions, high blood pressure, visual impairments, and orthopedic impairments (except paralysis and absence of limbs). Each of these conditions was far more prevalent among the older than among the younger population but the inverse relationship to family income was evident among all age groups except children under fifteen where the prevalence of these conditions was too small for any relationship to family income to be evident.

For acute conditions receiving medical care or resulting in activity limitation, unlike the situation for chronic illness and disability, a consistent inverse relationship to family income was clearly *not* evident in the data collected by the National Center for Health Statistics. In fact, inference can be made more readily from these data to a *direct* than to an *inverse* relationship. For example, the age-adjusted incidence of medically attended or activity-restricting acute conditions per 100 persons per year in the United States during July 1962 to June 1963 dropped from 215.9 at incomes under $2,000 to 204.5 at $2,000–$3,999, but thereafter the rate rose to 216.2 at $4,000–$6,999 and to 232.5 at $7,000 and over.[20] This overall inverse relationship, however, did not hold for all condition groups and among all age groups of the population. By specific condition group, there was clearly a rising rather than a falling gradient with family income for infective and parasitic diseases and for upper respiratory conditions, but no gradient at all for influenza and for other respiratory conditions. Only for acute conditions of the digestive system was there a clear inverse relationship to family income.

By age group, and again considering all medically attended or activity-restricting acute condition groups combined, an inverse relationship to family income was much more pronounced at the older ages (sixty-five and over) than during midlife (ages forty-five to sixty-four). During early adulthood (ages fifteen to forty-four), family income was apparently unrelated to the incidence of acute conditions, but during childhood the incidence of these conditions rose sharply with income. Thus children in more well-to-do families experienced many more acute conditions than the children of lower-income families.

Dental Morbidity and the Unmet Need for Dental Care

The level of a population's dental health is today widely recognized as an important aspect of its general level of health and well-being. Nevertheless, in many nations of the world today, but especially where modern health facilities are poor or virtually nonexistent and where inadequate nourishment and highly debilitating communicable diseases are endemic, infections of the teeth and oral tissues represent a considerable burden on the population and depress the general level of its health substantially, representing a not inconsiderable factor even in the general toll of death. In the United States, because dentistry has attained a high level of development, critically serious sequelae of dental disease are seen infrequently and the major dental diseases, dental caries and periodontal disease, are rarely direct causes of death.

Despite this, however, the sheer accumulation of untreated dental conditions in the population is staggering, and they are among the most common of all diseases afflicting the American people. One authority has estimated that in 1960 the average American had four unfilled cavities in his mouth, while current evidence suggests that this figure has continued to increase, rather than decrease, with the passage of time.* Dental morbidity is not self-limiting, i.e.,

*If only those with one or more primary or permanent teeth in their mouths are taken as the base for this computation, the figure is 4.5. The figure of 4 was

neither dental caries nor periodontal disease are likely to cure themselves in the absence of care, except that uncared-for teeth may either have to be extracted or else may fall out by themselves—for example, as the result of severe periodontal disease. In either case, missing teeth should be considered as a morbid condition.

Because dental morbidity is not self-limiting, it seems reasonable to expect that persons who do receive care are likely to be in better dental health than those who do not. Considering the entire population as a whole, poverty and nonpoverty alike, there is clearly a considerable disparity between the need for dental care and what is being done about it. In part this comes about because Americans apparently set a low priority on dental care, although this may be less true of the more well-to-do than of the rest of the population. Other factors here may be the shortage and maldistribution in the number of practicing dentists, and the inability of many people to pay for the comprehensive dental care that they should be receiving. The burden of these factors would, of course, fall most heavily on the poverty population.

The state of dental morbidity is somewhat confused when the dental health level of the poor is compared to that of the non-poor, because the addition of fluoride to a community's supply of drinking water materially lessens the total amount of dental decay among children in both primary and permanent teeth. This simple preventive measure—convenient, inexpensive, and safe—benefits the poor and the affluent alike. It is performed by the community, requiring no effort on the part of the individual. As a result, it is entirely conceivable that the segment of the poverty

derived by using the entire population as the base for the computation. See Wesley O. Young, "Dental Health," in Commission on the survey of Dentistry in the United States, *Survey of Dentistry, Final Report,* Byron S. Hollinshead, (Washington, D. C.: American Council on Education, 1961).

population which drinks fluoridated water may have a lower level of dental caries than those of the non-poor who live in areas not served by a fluoridated community water supply; this would be true at the younger ages, and before the lack of care received by the poor could make its influence felt. With the effects of fluoridation held constant, however, the impact of socioeconomic status should be considerable.

A study of nearly 4,000 five-year-old children of Contra Costa County, California, showed that the prevalence of dental caries was inversely related to socioeconomic status.[21] Children in the lowest of five socioeconomic groups had 60 percent more carious teeth (decayed, teeth indicated for extraction, and filled teeth) than those in the highest group, while a much lower proportion were free of caries altogether. Similar results were found in a survey of school children in Buffalo, New York.[22] The same author studied the caries experience of white and nonwhite children, at ages six through eleven and of differing socioeconomic backgrounds, in both a fluoridated and nonfluoridated community in North Carolina.[23] In the nonfluoridated community, the white children of upper socioeconomic status had a much lower dental caries rate than children of either race in the low socioeconomic group. In the fluoridated area, there were only negligible differences in the permanent teeth of all groups; among the primary teeth, however, the caries rate for the upper socioeconomic groups was better than that for the others.

The amount and type of dental care that a person receives varies significantly by family income. For example, according to data from the National Health Survey for the twelve-month period ending June 1969, the rate of dental visits per person per year for persons in families with annual incomes of $15,000 or more (2.5 visits) was over three times the rate for persons with less than $3,000 family income (0.8 visits). For children five to fourteen years old the comparable ratio was about four times as high for the $15,000-and-over income group as for the under-$3,000 group; for persons aged twenty-five to forty-four, about two and a half times as high; and for persons sixty-five and over, again about four times as high. Similarly, while in the highest income families 33 percent of those interviewed had not visited a dentist during the year, the comparable proportion was 73 percent in the lowest income group.[24]

What kinds of services do people receive when they see a dentist? According to National Health Survey data for July 1963-June 1964, preventive care services such as fillings, cleanings, examinations, and straightenings accounted for a much larger proportion of the visits by persons in upper-income families than those with lower incomes, while for therapeutic work—extractions and other surgery, and denture work—the reverse was true. Generally, although there are some irregularities in the progressions, the percentage for each of the items classified as preventive care increased as family income rose. For example, for persons of all ages the proportion of visits for fillings rose from 31.4 percent at under $4,000 to 36.1 percent at $10,000 and over; for cleaning and examinations, the comparable percentages were 27.2 and 41.4; and for straightenings they were 3.3 and 8.8 percent. For extractions and other surgery, in contrast, the comparable proportions dropped from 26.0 to 8.5 percent; and for denture work from 18.0 to 13.0 percent. There was some variation by age, but on the whole the patterns were remarkably consistent.[25]

PATTERNS AND TRENDS

The framework and the hypotheses developed here are only tentative. The major concepts that have been used to develop the framework include such social factors as style of life, inclusion or exclusion from the private medical care system, engaging in physically active versus sedentary occupations, whether or not social protection exists which permits the luxury of reacting in the sick role to minor illness, and inclusion or exclusion from the general affluence characterizing current society. Each factor represents a way in which the social system impinges on segments of the population. The use of these concepts, and relating them to one another, appears to require the use of no more than three major socioeconomic strata to derive gross differences in the levels of physical health, as expressed in mortality and morbidity, which are large enough to be significant or even measurable by present imperfect measurement methods.

What emerges, for mortality and morbidity alike, appears to be an essentially U-shaped curve; however, the reasons for the shape of the curve are different for mortality than they are for morbidity. The age patterns of mortality in the three strata are also likely to be different, and this would be reflected in different patterns of cause-of-death. For morbidity, severity of condition is likely to be the most important differentiating factor among the three strata, and this too is likely to be reflected in different age patterns. At least two implications of this are worthy of note: for one thing, the poverty population in this country is still clearly and by a considerable margin the least healthy of the three socioeconomic strata discussed. What happens to the level of health of this population as the programs to alleviate poverty, or at least to raise the level of living of the poverty population, succeed (if in fact they ever do)? Obviously, the patterns of mortality and morbidity of the poverty population will shift in the direction of those now prevalent in the working class. This means essentially lower mortality for the poverty population, especially from the communicable diseases and during the younger ages, and much less severe illness, especially during midlife and the later years. However, a condition which is essential before this change in mortality and morbidity patterns can occur is that the poverty population be brought into the mainstream of the medical care system.

What will happen to the mortality and morbidity patterns of the members of the working class if their level of living is raised and if they concomitantly adopt middle-class life styles? Will their patterns begin to resemble those of the middle class? If so, it means that their overall mortality rate may actually increase, although this would be the result of increases only during midlife and the older ages, and only from the degenerative diseases. It is very likely that their mortality rates during the younger ages and from the communicable diseases will continue to improve, as they have been doing throughout this century. But as larger proportions of this stratum presumably with less innate resistance, survive to midlife, their mortality rates may be expected to increase at these years. A similar change with regard to morbidity seems likely. While the prevalence of relatively severe illness among them may be expected to decrease, the prevalence of relatively minor illness may increase.

Will the working class then become a healthier population than it is now? At this point the second implication of the U-shaped curve emerges. The very concept of health needs reexamination. On a population or statistical basis, improvements in level of living may actually result in a higher mortality rate, although only during midlife and the older ages and from the degenerative diseases, and in a greater prevalence of morbidity, although again due to only relatively minor, self-limiting conditions and primarily at the younger ages. But if these statements are even partially true, it is obvious that no general index of health could ever be anything like a simple summing of mortality and morbidity (or disability) rates, no matter how complex the weights to be used for each component of the index. One must ask: Mortality at what ages and from what causes? And morbidity (or disability) with what degree of severity and at what ages? Health is socially defined, varying among the diverse social strata of the community, and among various cultures. While death may be considered, independently of social or cultural definition, as a negative element in the assessment of health levels, the circumstances under which death occurs are not similarly independent. Perhaps different indexes should be used for different cultures and possibly even for different population groups within the same culture. It seems clear that intensive scrutiny of the concept of health is required in order to construct a satisfactory index of health.

IV. Social Differencs in Mental Health

by Marc Fried

The evidence is unambiguous and powerful that the lowest social classes have the highest rates of severe psychiatric disorder in our society. Regardless of the measures employed for estimating severe psychiatric disorder and social class, regardless of the region or the date of study, and regardless of the method of study, the great majority of results all point to this fact clearly and strongly. It is striking that, despite the strength and consistency of this finding and the infrequency of such results in the social sciences, it remains in the limbo of facts that continue to be understated, challenged, and rarely examined for clarification.[1]

Although the evidence is clear, it is not nearly so well known as one might hope. Thus, we shall first review the literature showing the consistencies and inconsistencies in gross results and shall then examine the limits within which the finding can be generalized and understood. Once the facts have been reviewed and qualified, we can examine the more difficult problem of underlying sources of the relationships, the intricacies of causal interpretation, and the implications for our understanding of mental health.

Marc Fried is Professor, Institute of Human Sciences, Boston College, Chestnut Hill, Massachusetts.

Whenever we consider the problem of mental health, we are forced into either of two contrasting and equally unsatisfactory positions. We can elect to formulate an ideal type either as a composite image of health or as a set of variables signifying attributes we regard as healthy. This is a procedure that has been used in numerous psychological studies. Some of these are based on clinical experience and represent an effort to formulate those characteristics that seem to be associated with effective performance or with some highly respected accomplishment like creativity. Others are based on an analysis of data from a less highly selected population.[2] Even the proponents of this "ideal" approach often recognize the cultural, subcultural, situational, and temporal limitations of an ideal for mental health. They pursue it, however, in trying to establish a basis for evaluating the positive, healthy, competent, or creative end of a hypothetical spectrum of psychological or social accomplishments.

Another approach involves backing into the problem by delineating the more easily defined and more readily studied problem of mental illness, treating the problem of mental health as a by-product. Generally, studies in the epidemiology of mental illness do not give much attention to mental health but focus on the more limited and more readily defined problem of illness. Indeed, this is part of the reason that a fairly substantial empirical foundation exists for reviewing this interrelationship. These findings determine the initial approach of the present discussion. Although we will consider primarily problems of mental illness, we shall subsequently turn to the implications of the data about social class and mental illness for the small but important contribution they make to our understanding of social class, social process, and mental health.

EMERGENCE OF CONTEMPORARY CONCEPTIONS OF MENTAL HEALTH

In recent years, the fields of mental health have developed a more substantial appreciation of the social processes that confound distinctions among a variety of forms of deviant behavior. Thus, emotional difficulties, intellectual dysfunctions and deficits, antisocial behavior, social incompetence, and other types of malfunction have frequently been clustered for study or treatment. The community mental health movement is one of the most striking examples of this trend. Coupled with this has been a continuous growth of a literature dealing with the social forces that influence potentials for malfunction, that define acceptable and unacceptable behavior in the community, that produce resources differentially for different communities and subpopulations, and that affect the paths to treatment and the outcome of diagnosed malfunction. Nonetheless, we are still far from an integrated understanding of malfunction, of its social origins and correlates, or of its relationships to social class differences.

In the past the social forces that affected social class differences in malfunction were all too evident. Despite differences in manifest behavior, great masses of the lowest strata experienced similar maltreatment through incarceration in punitive, custodial, and work institutions of a society on the verge of massive industrialization. Although this problem is most familiar through Dorothea Dix's attack on the imprisonment of lunatics and through the widespread impact of the Elizabethan Poor Laws, the use of the same institutions for a variety of forms of deviance associated with poverty was widespread. It appears to have been characteristic for most Western European countries and the United States.[3] The vast mass of people incarcerated in asylums, workhouses, and prisons were drawn from the poverty-stricken lower classes. Alienated both from their preindustrial communities, which were in the process of disintegration, and from the rudimentary industrial society, which could not yet provide adequate roles or opportunities for them, the poor were both numerous and a potential threat to the precarious stability of rapidly changing societies. In the face of promiscuous disregard for the misery of a large proportion of the population in Western Europe, the professionalization of psychiatry offered a new and more sensitive conception of psychopathology. By the end of the nineteenth century, the sharp distinction between mental illness and other social problems was effectively drawn, paving the way for the advances of Charcot, Janet, Kraepelin, and Freud.

During the last half of the nineteenth century, the growing field of psychiatry made several important contributions toward a reconceptualization of mental illness.

1. In providing a new system of classification, Kraepelin (and later Freud) helped to give some sense of scientific order to superficially irrational and apparently nonpatterned behaviors.

2. Charcot and Janet helped to develop a wider appreciation of the milder disorders, to reveal the compelling and involuntary character of psychological malfunctioning, and to provide a more sympathetic framework for understanding the suffering associated with psychopathology.

3. In developing a systematic etiological formulation, Freud provided both a generic and a differentiated understanding of intrapsychic and developmental forces associated with psychological disorder, and introduced an awareness of the widespread nature of psychic conflict,

conceived as a continuum extending from health through mild mental disorder to the most severe and bizarre forms of psychosis.

Freud satisfactorily established the fundamental developmental importance of "internalization" processes relatively early in his work, and then turned to intrapsychic processes as the focus for subsequent theoretical clarification. While his rejection of the importance of social determinants in adult behavior (indeed, his rejection of his own prior concern with overt traumata) may seem cavalier, it allowed Freud to develop formulations of human functioning to which we must constantly return on the basis of wider knowledge about environmental influences on behavior. Perhaps his single most general contribution consisted of a theoretical framework tracing neurotic and psychotic disorders of adults and children to a long, premorbid history. While psychoanalysis has never altogether succeeded in demonstrating the distinctive developmental sequences that make for symptom formation, it provides a theoretical basis for understanding important liaisons between early experience and later psychic structure. Despite the relatively meager attention Freud gave to the importance of the social environment, it is largely on the basis of his theoretical framework that we can meaningfully speak of mental illnesses as disorders of living.[4] As we pursue the association between social class position and mental illness, the appreciation of malfunctioning as disorders of living provides both a basis for more dynamic analysis of social variables and a link between social and psychological processes.

DEFINITIONS AND EMPIRICAL DATA

The most unambiguous data on mental illness and social class concern those severe psychiatric disorders referred to as psychosis. The total situation, however, in which an individual comes to psychiatric notice and is diagnosed contains many ambiguities. An extreme view maintains that these uncertainties do not affect the psychoses: that individuals who are psychotic may remain in the community for different periods of time but sooner or later will come to psychiatric attention, will be properly diagnosed, and will most often be hospitalized.[5] This view contains several underlying and unsubstantiated premises: that psychosis is a persistent disorder, that community tolerance varies only within a narrow range, and that there is widespread agreement on the criteria for diagnosis and hospitalization regardless of the severity of the psychosis.

Much of the growing evidence concerning psychiatric disorders points to a rejection of this view. First, social factors, particularly differences in the social class position of the patient, affect diagnostic decisions; second, with new conceptions of a patient, many individuals with severe psychiatric difficulties, including those diagnosed as psychotic, can remain outside the hospital and may require little assistance; and third, a great many transitory psychotic states appear among individuals with relatively stable functioning and a great many diagnosed psychotics recover during relatively brief periods of time.[6] More generally, it is clear that incipient tendencies to disorganization can be exacerbated by social stress or lack of resources leading to psychotic states and that, conversely, social processes may compensate for and stabilize precarious psychological states and result in effective functioning. In the course of a few decades, a number of dramatic changes have taken place in psychiatric ideology that must inevitably affect criteria for diagnosis and treatment, changing conceptions of hospital care, increased awareness of the role of the family in individual functioning, greater sensitivity to the influence of the natural environment of home and work on psychological adaptation. While we may be far from an adequate understanding of either the social or psychological processes involved and their interrelationships in producing effective or ineffective adaptive patterns, this broader perspective modifies the conception and definition of psychosis.

These and many theoretical and empirical considerations suggest that (1) communities vary considerably in their levels of tolerance and in whether or not they view a particular behavior as severely disordered; (2) that the initial response to disordered functioning, either within the community or during early contacts with professionals, can entail either further disorganization leading to psychotic manifestations or provide support and stabilization leading to the maintenance of ego boundaries; (3) that the very path to treatment, due to availability of resources, initial professional contacts, or community and familial preferences will further serve either to disorganize or to stabilize disordered functioning and will influence the diagnosis; and (4) that whether an individual is hospitalized or not, with or without the diagnosis of psychosis, will determine his subsequent level of organization and functioning and will vary for different patients, different professionals, and different institutional settings.[7] That there may be a small proportion of extreme cases of very high vulnerability, minimally affected by current environmental transactions, negates neither these propositions nor their explanatory value for the great majority of cases.

From this point of view, the justification for considering psychosis or psychiatric hospitalization an adequate subject for empirical study is itself open to challenge. Indeed, in the absence of adequate data for extricating these variables, considerable interpretative caution is essential in dealing with data about severe psychiatric disorders. Nonetheless, there is ample justification for treating severe psychiatric disorders as a meaningful category, provided we utilize the data for continuing clarification of meaning. At the very least, within short periods of time and within similar professional environments, we can expect the differences in criteria for seeking professional assistance, in diagnosis, and in treatment to be smaller than for any other category referring to less severely disturbed behavior.

Above all else, the analysis of relationships between psychiatric disorders and social class are legitimate to the extent that we treat the diagnosis or treatment as a *social* fact. We do not need to concur in the diagnostic or treatment decision in order to recognize that similarities in social conditions may or may not lead to similarities in social outcome. The purpose of such study is to determine whether these similarities in social condition, in this case social class, operate to produce similar effects because of or in spite of vast differences in other variables that may also affect the outcome. This is precisely the argument Durkheim employed in his analysis of suicide.[8] He did not purport to bypass psychological processes or psychological selection in determining individual instances of suicide; he wished to focus on social conditions and social outcomes. A rate of psychiatric hospitalization or of diagnosed psychosis is precisely such an outcome. Granting the complexity of factors influencing this outcome, we want to know if there are any overriding consistencies associated with social class. If the outcome is treated as a social fact, we must still determine the ways in which other forces, psychological processes, familial relationships, community values, or professional orientations contribute to this social fact and, thereby, to the existence of the relationship itself.

PSYCHOSIS AND SOCIAL CLASS POSITION

Although only a small number of studies have been responsible for the public and professional awareness of the relationship between social variables and mental illness, the relationship between social class and mental illness has been studied and documented extensively.[9] The earliest studies were theoretical and were often beset with unsolved problems of epidemiological analysis. Yet the fact that the available studies go back as far as 1917 and include patient populations from several decades before, provides us with a relatively long period for analysis.[10]

From the early study by Nolan (1917) until the recent study by Dunham (1966), the largest body of data on psychiatric disorders and social class have important similarities. They generally use records of psychiatric hospitalization and rates based on the number of patients in a given demographic category, employing census calculations of the population at risk in these categories as denominators. And they more often deal with occupational distributions than with any other social class indicator. On the other hand, there are also a number of important differences among them. They vary in the use of controls (or rate adjustments) for such variables as age and sex; they vary in the completeness of coverage of patients within a given geographical region; they vary from the inclusion of schizophrenia alone to consideration of other psychoses, or of all hospitalized patients; and they vary greatly in the statistical methods employed for the analysis of results and evaluation of data. Finally, there are a large enough number of studies using variant methods to allow further comparisons. There are a number of ecological studies, using hospitalization rates and social class indices for geographical regions (generally census tracts); there are several "community" studies based either on household interviews or on selective service evaluations; there are several studies that combine psychiatric hospital information with massive efforts to obtain data about non-hospital psychiatric contacts for the population at risk; and there are a number of studies that use education, income, residential housing characteristics, and color, which provide additional comparative materials.

Nolan's 1917 study, based on 7,026 first admissions for dementia praecox (schizophrenia) to New York Civil State hospitals between 1909 and 1916, was not directly concerned with occupation as an indicator of social class. [11] Nolan was led to examine the relationships between different aspects of occupational functioning and dementia praecox since "among the many methods of reeducation the most effectual seems to be systematic instruction in simple, interesting work" (p. 128). Although his analysis shows markedly higher rates for unskilled laborers than for any other occupational group among males (210 per 100,000 compared to 166 per 100,000 for clerical service, 149 per 100,000 for domestic and personal service, to 47 per 100,000 for trades at the low extreme), his conclusions at the end of his detailed article never mention the implicit class or status distribution of the findings.

Starting with Nolan's pioneer study, there have been at least thirty-four studies that have presented relevant data on severe psychiatric disorders and social class indices, excluding those that deal only with Negro-white differences. Limiting the first review of these data to studies based on evidence of psychosis and/or psychiatric hospitalization for mental disorder by occupational status, education, income, rental costs, or dependency as social class indicators, we shall ask three major questions: (1) What proportion of these studies provide evidence that the lowest status group or groups, by any social class indicator, have the highest rate of psychosis and/or psychiatric hospitalization? (2) What proportion of these studies provide evidence of an inverse linear relationship of psychosis and/or psychiatric hospitalization with social class indicators? (3) Are there differences in findings associated with the different indicators used for social class or for severe psychiatric disorders? Once these issues are clarified, it will be possible to turn more systematically to several other important questions concerning differences in the findings associated with different dynamic features of social class, comparative data for Negroes and whites, variables that modify or are modified by these relationships, and causal implications. For the time being, we assume that social class differences form the independent variable and psychosis or psychiatric hospitalization the dependent variable, although the interpretation of causal priority is itself a major issue in this field.

The gross question, do the lowest social class groups show the highest rates of severe psychiatric disorder, must be answered clearly in the affirmative. Indeed, among thirty-four studies that provide answers to this question, the results shown in Table IV-1 appear:

Table IV—1

	Number of studies	Proportion of studies (%)
Lowest-status group has highest rate of psychosis and/or hospitalization	29	85
Data ambiguous or contradictory findings with different indicators	4	12
Lowest-status group does not have highest rates of psychosis-hospitalization	1	3
N =	34	100

Considering only social class indicators and omitting Negro-white differences and unemployment, 85 percent of the studies clearly support the proposition that rates of severe psychiatric disorder are highest among the lowest social class groups. Two of the four studies listed as ambiguous present positive support for this proposition with one social class indicator and negate the proposition with another social class indicator.[12] The two other studies, although classified as ambiguous, provide more supportive than contradictory evidence.[13]

The significance of a finding that the lowest social class group by education, occupation, income, rental, or any other characteristic has the highest rate of severe psychiatric disorder will be considerably affected by a number of other considerations. Few of the studies present statistical tests of the differences between social class groups, although inspection reveals that rates for the lowest groups are quite considerably higher than the rates for groups of higher position. Several of the studies that do employ tests of significance reveal that the difference between the lowest-status category and all others are statistically significant. The differences are not only quite pervasive; they are frequently quite powerful.

The other question of importance is the extent to which these differences are linear. The data for this question are more difficult to evaluate because a new judgment is required for which there is no empirical basis. We must now estimate how much linearity is linear and how many deviations justify an overall categorization of the pattern as nonlinear. The question is complicated by other factors: the lack of clarity, in several instances, of placing different occupations along a simple scale (e.g., are agricultural laborers or unskilled workers the lowest category or how do we compare the category "trade" with the category "skilled workers"?); the different numbers and types of categories used in different studies; and the comparison of studies that use rates for different social class frequencies with those that use some measure of association. Naturally, the results depend on how we deal with each of these issues.

For these thirty-four studies the results, shown in Table IV-2, are only a little less striking than for the comparison of rates between the very lowest-status groups and all others:

Table IV—2

	Number of studies	Proportion of studies (%)
Linear trend with inverse relationship between social class and severe disorder	24	71
Data ambiguous or contradictory findings with different indicators	8	23
Nonlinear relationship between social class and severe disorder	2	6
N =	34	100

The evidence is clear that most studies show a fairly continuous linear pattern of inverse relationships between severe psychiatric disorders and social class indicators. The greatest difference from the previous result arises in the loss of clarity and the increase in the number of reports that are ambiguous. In fact, none of the reported studies shows a perfect linear relationship either supporting or contradicting the inverse association between social class and mental illness. Nonetheless, while the evidence for a linear, inverse relationship between social class and rates of severe disorder is not entirely consistent or uncontrovertible, the data point quite clearly toward support of the proposition.

The relationships presented above hold either for a total

count of all psychotic disorders or for schizophrenia alone. The fact that schizophrenia accounts for the largest proportion of psychotic disorders means that we may get different social class patterns for other psychotic disorders without affecting the overall trend. The most notable deviation from this pattern is to be found for the manic-depressive or affective disorders. The eight studies that give separate rates for these disturbances are approximately evenly distributed between those that show weak positive associations with social class indicators and those that show weak inverse associations with social class indicators.[14]

Most of the thirty-four studies are based on psychiatric hospital records. However, a number of studies use other methods either to implement these data or in lieu of psychiatric records, trying to replicate the same diagnostic criteria. There are studies that utilize contact with psychiatric facilities other than hospitals to screen a population, studies based on selective service psychiatric evaluations, and a few studies using a field screening instrument for evaluating levels of psychiatric impairment. The results based on these different approaches are shown in Table IV-3.

Apart from studies based on psychiatric hospitalization, the number of studies using other criteria is too small to provide an adequate basis for interpretation. However, it is evident that studies based on a case count from a wider array of facilities and those that have used a screening instrument in the community do not as clearly substantiate the proposition that there is an inverse, linear relationship between social class and severe psychiatric disorder.[15] But while these studies must qualify the nature of the relationship between social class and psychiatric disorder, they do not entirely negate the other evidence. The three ambiguous studies using data that are not limited to the records of psychiatric hospitals support the proposition of a strong

Table IV—3

Criterion employed	Linear trend	Am- biguous	Non linear
Psychiatric hospitalization for psychosis	17	5	1
Hospitalization and diagnosis of psychosis in other facility	1	1	1
Selective service psychiatric evaluation	2	0	0
Level of psychiatric impairment from field screening instrument	4	2	0
N =	24	8	2

relationship between social class and psychiatric disorder to a considerable extent. One of these studies rejects the hypothesis of an inverse linear relationship but finds the highest rates among the lowest status groups. Another shows a clear trend toward an inverse class relationship although the lowest-status group does not have the highest rate of impairment. And one of the community studies indicates that there were higher rates of nonhospitalized psychosis in communities of higher status but these did not compensate for the higher psychiatric hospitalization rates in the lower-status community.

The different results obtained with different methods suggest that some of the relationship between social class and severe psychiatric impairment may be artifactually produced by selective forces in psychiatric hospitalization, but when this is taken into account an important residual relationship between social class and psychiatric disorder becomes apparent. Moreover, two studies based on selective service evaluations that represent a community sample of males both found increasing rates of psychosis with decreasing social class position. These discrepancies are not readily explained. Some of the studies are based on state psychiatric hospitalization, and these may reveal linear relationships between social class and psychiatric disorder because of bias in the case load.[16] Moreover, lower-class patients are undoubtedly seen less often in private practice, are more likely to receive severe diagnoses, and are more readily hospitalized in psychiatric institutions.[17] But if discriminatory diagnosis is built into psychiatric practice, it should affect psychiatric assessment whether this is done in a hospital, in private practice, or in the community. And the distorting effects of uncounted cases seen in private practice or the greater tendency to hospitalize patients of lower status should be eliminated as sources of bias in any study using a wider community sample. Yet discrepancies remain even among these studies. A large number of studies based on hospitalization, however, report figures of prevalence rather than incidence. If lower-class people are retained in the hospital for longer periods of time, as seems to be the case, this alone should produce an unknown inflation in the rates of psychiatric disorder at lower-status levels. But, as some of the data indicate, this factor alone is not sufficient to account for the rate differentials by social class. While precise estimates of class differentials in psychiatric disorder are not possible under these circumstances, the weight of evidence is unambiguous in its support of the general proposition that there is an (imperfect) inverse relationship between total rates of psychiatric disorder and social class position.

The majority of reports support the inverse relationship between social class and severe psychiatric disorder. However, the findings are most ambiguous for occupation (5 out of 14 reports do not support the proposition) and income-dependency (3 out of 7 reports do not support the proposition). Although these results do not lead to any noteworthy conclusions, they do offer an interesting suggestion for subsequent consideration. Occupational achievement among adults is clearly more responsive to situational changes than educational achievement; and income or dependency status is more immediately responsive to temporary changes in economic situation than is rental cost. Does this point to a more dynamic feature of social class position as the source of these relationships than would be indicated by a stable conception of social class status as the critical dimension? We shall address this question as we accumulate more data.

NONPSYCHOTIC DISORDERS AND SOCIAL CLASS POSITION

Many difficulties attend the study of the most severe psychiatric disorders but empirical study of the wide variety of other mental and emotional disorders is even more problematic. Data are rarely available to permit the study of milder disorders in the entire population of a geographical region. A wider variety of resources are available for the care and treatment of milder disorders, many of which may not involve any psychiatric personnel and may not eventuate in a psychiatric diagnosis. Movement between geographical regions for treatment may lead to the disappearance of a great many cases, which means that not only is the case count inaccurate, but there is no adequate basis for determining the appropriate population at risk. Finally, the gross behavioral criteria on which a diagnosis of psychosis or a decision for psychiatric hospitalization can be based are much clearer than the more subjective and variable criteria for seeking evaluation or treatment in the milder disorders. For mental retardation and suicide we may approximate adequate rate analyses but for childhood or adult neuroses, psychosomatic symptoms, or behavior disorders we cannot hope to find a sufficient base for conclusions.

In spite of the many inadequacies in available sources, the data on social class and suicide are of particular interest. There is a widespread impression that suicides are most frequent among the highest-status groups and least frequent among those of lowest status. Durkheim contributed to this view: "So far is the increase in poverty from causing the increase in suicide that even fortunate crises, the effect of which is abruptly to enhance a country's prosperity, affect suicide like economic disasters."[18] Dublin, moreover, suggested that a sudden loss of status and position among high-status people, that is, severe relative deprivation, was one of the most frequent causes of suicide in situations of economic depression.[19] However, the facts do not consistently support the view that "more suicides occur among persons who have every financial facility to enjoy life than among those with barely enough to keep body and soul together."[20]

Following Durkheim's concept of anomie and his analysis of anomic suicide, the early sociological literature gave particular attention to social disorganization. Ecological analyses revealed a high correlation between residence in underprivileged areas and suicide but this was generally interpreted as a result of social disorganization rather than of poverty or lower-class status. A more recent study tried to reformulate the problem of anomie and suicide by developing a conception of status integration.[21] This study does not present separate analyses or controls for social class status but social class position as a determinant of suicide is implicated since it contributes to the measures of status integration.

The most substantial analyses of empirical data are those

by Dublin and Sainsbury.[22] Dublin presents data from several sources. Concerning England and Wales in the years 1949–1953, he shows that the lowest social class category has the highest rates of suicide although it is closely seconded and, from ages 35 to 64 is surpassed, by the highest social class. Thus, were we to formulate the proposition as we did for social class and severe psychiatric disorders, we would find support for high rates in the lower class but no evidence of a consistent inverse relationship. Recent United States data support the British results of high rates in the lowest class but reveal no differences among all the other class groups. Finally, a study covering the period 1910–1960 compares the per capita gross national product and the age-adjusted suicide rate and, despite a number of discrepancies, finds a significant negative correlation between prosperity and suicide rate. The finding provides an important clue to much of the literature on suicide and social class position. Although the literature on severe psychiatric disorders emphasizes class position per se, the literature on suicide stresses the importance of rapid and generally downward changes in position. Sainsbury's study of suicides in London points up factors of change and reveals the difficulty in assessing this from ecological correlations. His ecological analysis revealed that suicide was inversely correlated with poverty but showed little relationship with other indices of status or unemployment. A closer analysis, however, indicated that many of the higher-status suicides were living in poverty, suggesting loss of status as an important factor, and showed significant correlations between suicide and unemployment. Other studies have also stressed the high correlation between unemployment and suicide. [23] The importance of the occupational role, in its social class implications and psychological ramifications, particularly when associated with downward mobility or major social transitions, has been repeatedly pointed up.[24] Clearly, however, and in contrast to the data on psychiatric hospitalization, the weight of evidence points toward the importance of loss of status or inadequacy in coping with status demands rather than poverty or stable social class positions as the critical determinants of suicide rates.

Mental retardation is another disorder in which social class differences have long been suggested. Despite the realization that only a relatively small proportion of retardates, generally the most severe ones, have clear evidence of organic impairment, there has been considerable reluctance to undertake large-scale epidemiological studies of mental retardation. In recent years, however, increasing attention is being devoted to social factors, and among them class differences, in the development of retardation. After reviewing the meager literature relevant to this problem, Perry concludes that the vast majority of retardates present problems related to the sociocultural background of lower-class populations.[25] Similarly, Wortis points out that "by almost every available measure: correlation with family income, with social class, with parent's vocation, by comparison of white with Negro, white with Puerto Rican, white with Mexican-American, white with native Indian, we find this same marked tendency to higher concentration of the retarded in the more disadvantaged sections of our population."[26] Unfortunately, beyond so gross a statement, the data are inadequate for assessing any other features of the distribution of mental retardates.

If the data for evaluating the relationship of social class to suicide and mental retardation are inadequate, we can well anticipate that the materials will be inadequate for examining social class differences in any other form of mental disorder. One observation stands out: the greater frequency of mild mental disorders (neuroses, personality impairments) among higher-status groups found in studies based on psychiatric treatment is contradicted by the higher rates of mild impairments (along with higher rates of severe impairments) among lower social class groups found in studies based on field interviews or mental health screening instruments.[27]

The existing studies, however, present no adequate empirical or rational grounds for the analysis of social class and psychiatric impairment. Under conditions of professionalization in the mental health fields of an affluent society, the difficulties that lead to psychiatric treatment for mild disturbances or to the evaluation of mild psychiatric impairments are based on complex but highly subjective and often transitory experiences. This, of course, does not rule them out as subjects for study but they present great difficulties for analysis. The significance of social class differences in mental disorder must, then, rest upon the substantial results based on severe psychiatric disorders. We have found these results to be striking both in their consistency and strength. On this basis, we can turn to a more analytic effort at extricating the components of social class position that appear to be most important in producing these relationships.

DYNAMIC RELATIONSHIPS BETWEEN POVERTY AND MENTAL ILLNESS

Race

It is an open question whether Negro-white differences are most meaningfully treated within the social class framework or as an aspect of race relations and discrimination. On empirical grounds, it is clear that the lower social class categories are disproportionately represented by Negroes. The justification for viewing the situation of the Negro within a traditional social class framework does not lie, however, in the data on the disproportionate number of Negroes in lower social class positions but rather on whether a shift in these positions has the same consequences for Negroes as for whites. In view of the severity of discrimination and uniquely severe forms of segregation, do the factors that follow from social class positions affect the Negro in roughly comparable degrees? Even if we regard the situation of the Negro as that of an underclass or caste group, with unique experiences of degradation and relatively impermeable barriers to acceptance and absorption, the data on Negro-white differences in mental disorders are useful for clarifying the relationship between social class and severe psychiatric disorders. On the other hand, if we regard the situation of the Negro as primarily that of a newcomer to an urban lower class, we must confront similarities and differences in patterns of mental disorder as issues that help to elucidate the dynamics of social class that affect rates of psychiatric illness.

Some of the same unfamiliarity that characterizes public and professional knowledge about social class and mental illness obtains for the data concerning Negro and white differences in psychiatric disorders. A total of twenty-one studies report on Negro-white differences in rates of mental disorder.[28] The conclusions begin to become clear as soon as we look at the distribution of findings. In order to simplify some of the issues, the twenty-one studies are divided into those based only on psychiatric hospital data, those that include nonhospital cases but limit themselves to severe psychiatric disorders, and those that include nonhospital cases with a wider range of personality disorders (See Table IV-4).

The results are only slightly less consistent than those for social class differences in severe psychiatric disorder; they

Table IV—4

	Negro rates higher	Differences ambiguous	White rates higher
Psychiatric hospital data only	8	0	0
Additional screening for severe cases	5	1	2
Additional screening for all disorders	2	1	2
All methods N =	15	2	4

show some striking similarities to the previous social class findings. Seventy-one percent of the studies point to higher rates among Negroes than among whites, and two ambiguous studies also point toward higher rates for Negroes. The four studies that show higher rates for whites involved locating patients in addition to or in lieu of psychiatric hospitalization for psychosis. Thus, the consistency of the results based on psychiatric hospitalization may, in part, be due to disproportionately high rates of hospitalization for Negroes in relation to actual levels of severe psychiatric disorder among Negroes in the community. This supposition is supported by Dunham's finding of a much smaller gap between initial onset of symptoms and the decision to seek treatment or extrusion from the community for Negroes than for whites. That is, the shorter community residence of disturbed persons implies lower community tolerance for psychiatric symptoms among Negroes than among whites.

The issues, however, are more complex than is suggested by the contrast between studies based on psychiatric hospitalization and those which use other means for locating patients. As Dohrenwend points out in a comparison of eight studies, three of the four studies showing higher rates for whites were conducted in the South and the fourth included the South; on the other hand, three of the four studies showing higher rates for Negroes were based in the North.[29] The significance of this observation can be interpreted in numerous ways but its importance is supported by several other findings that have pointed to the disproportionate increase in first admissions to psychiatric hospitals among Negroes.[30] By 1922 Negro and white rates reached parity for the United States as a whole, a result produced by disproportionately high rates for Negroes in the North along with low rates for Negroes in the South. From these data, Malzberg concluded that "the low rates of mental disease among Negroes in the South is to be found in the lack of adequate provision for their treatment in institutions."[31]

Since 1922 Negro rates of psychiatric hospitalization have continued to increase more rapidly than white rates. A similar trend is found in the data for first admissions to psychiatric hospitals of Negroes and whites in Virginia.[32] The hypothesis of differential treatment facilities is illuminated by a comparison of patients admitted to psychiatric services in Maryland and Louisiana.[33] This study points out that in Louisiana first admission rates to all psychiatric facilities were higher for whites than for nonwhites with a major exception for schizophrenic reactions. In Maryland, however, nonwhite rates were higher than white rates for a number of conditions, including schizophrenic reactions. More generally, rates for nonwhites were consistently higher in Maryland than in Louisiana, particularly among the urban population. There are a number of possible explanations, all equally plausible and all equally consonant with these few fragments of data. Thus, it is possible that greater opportunity along with persistent impediments to actual achievement for Negroes in the North (or in Maryland compared with Louisiana) leads to higher rates of malfunctioning.

In spite of qualifications based on the results of nonhospital psychiatric data, the findings remain quite striking that there are overwhelmingly higher rates of psychiatric hospitalization for severe disorders among Negroes. The weight of evidence continues to support the proposition that these high rates represent greater prevalence of severe psychiatric disorders among Negroes. It should also be noted that a number of the studies comparing psychiatric hospitalization of Negroes and whites have used extensive controls and the finding is maintained when such factors as migration, education, and occupation are taken into account. Indeed, among all the factors considered in several studies, the Negro-white difference is the largest and most consistent.[34]

If we consider only the disproportionately high rates of psychiatric hospitalization for Negroes, we are faced with the same analytic uncertainty presented by the data on social class. Extrinsic factors can probably account for some portion of the difference: higher rates of extrusion from the community, difficulty in access to outpatient facilities, more severe diagnoses for comparable symptoms, readier hospitalization, less adequate treatment, and longer retention in the hospital. But there is reason to believe that intrinsic differences in the situation of lower-class groups and of Negroes compared to higher-status groups and whites could explain the largest part of the difference in rates of severe psychiatric disorder. Most of the forms of situational stress—for example, marital disruption, migration, and forced residential relocation, physical illness, and unemployment—occur with disproportionate frequency among lower-class populations and among Negroes. If these bear any relationship to the occurrence of mental disorder, we can expect higher rates of psychiatric disorder regardless of the extrinsic influences that make them more visible or translate malfunctioning into psychiatric disorder and hospitalization. We must now turn to these factors in an effort to extricate some of the dynamic forces that are associated with social class and color in our society and are responsible for the more striking experiences of deprivation and crisis.

Migration and Social Disruption

The earlier ecological studies of mental disorder, showing higher rates of psychiatric disorder (and particularly schizophrenia) in deteriorated central city areas, led to considerable controversy about the importance of geographical drift among schizophrenics.[35] This controversy gradually gave way to studies that implicated social isolation as a factor in the areal distribution of schizophrenics and in rates of psychiatric hospitalization among minority groups.[36] Both social isolation and minority status are, in large part, the product of geographical and social transition and can best be viewed in the context of the widespread experiences of change that characterize complex modern societies.

The most characteristic experiences of change that directly affect the lives of individuals are migration and residential displacement. The effect of migration on mental disorder has been extensively studied and its causal implications vigorously debated.[37] The argument need not be recapitulated since no bases internal to the data provide adequate grounds for discriminating between the selection hypothesis or the transition-stress hypothesis. However, the data continue to accrue revealing the persistence of a relationship between migration and severe psychiatric disorder in spite of changes in pattern from one period of study to another.

The data are remarkably consonant in showing higher

rates of psychiatric disorder for migrants than for non-migrants. As with several other variables (social class differences, Negro-white differences), Jaco's Texas data diverge from the majority of studies and, in this instance, represent the only clear negation of an association between migration and mental disorder.[38] In the recent studies based on psychiatric hospitalization in the United States, one of the most interesting shifts is the diminution in the differential rates of severe psychiatric disorder for the foreign born compared to natives. By contrast, the rates of severe psychiatric disorder for interstate migrants are disproportionately high compared to nonmigrants, although a recent study of Negroes in Philadelphia presents contradictory evidence.[39] The increased use of controls or adjustments for intercorrelated variables further reveals that the high rates of psychiatric disorder for interstate migrants revealed by most studies hold up for Negroes and whites and within education, occupation, and age subcategories.

With social class variables controlled, the fact that the disproportionate rates of severe psychiatric disorder are maintained indicates that migration does not, in any simple way, explain the relationship between social class and mental illness. Although shorter range, intracommunity movements have not been adequately studied, these are unlikely to account for social class differentials. Such movement is disproportionately frequent among higher-status groups, and the little evidence available suggests that short-distance moves are less clearly associated with mental disorders than large moves.[40] Lower-status migrants have greater difficulty and assimilate more slowly into the new environment, and this might provide a basis for linking social class, migration, and mental disorder.[41] Moreover, none of the data allows for an analysis of the level of urbanization or industrialization from which migrants derive, or of the degree of transition necessary for adaptation to the new society.

Minority Status

Another factor worthy of consideration and related to the readier assimilation of higher-status migrants is the effect of minority status on mental disorders. Faris and Dunham had originally mentioned the possible significance of minority status in pointing out the high rates of disorder for whites living in Negro areas and for Negroes living in white areas.[42] Strikingly, the issue received little further attention. One study implicated the factor of disparities in parental background or between parents and neighborhood mode as a determinant of schizophrenia.[43] Other studies focused attention on the influence of disparities between family and community on rates of psychiatric hospitalization. A comparison of rates of schizophrenia and manic-depressive psychosis among Italians in metropolitan Boston points quite unambiguously to the fact that the higher the proportion of Italians in a community, the lower the rates of these psychoses among Italians.[44] The use of simple demographic indices (the conceptual significance of which, as "minority status" variables, is often tenuous) indicates that people with a particular personal characteristic living in communities where that characteristic is less common have disproportionately high rates of psychiatric hospitalization.[45]

These studies do not go very far in explaining the relationship between social class or poverty and mental illness. They do suggest that the minority status of newcomers to a community (as newcomers, as foreigners, as less urbane, as preindustrial, as minorities) may be a central factor in the relationship between migration and mental illness. This hypothesis receives support from a comparison of migration to different countries suggesting that the receptiveness of the host society is a major determinant of high or low rates of psychiatric disorder among migrants.[46] It may also account for the high rates of psychiatric disorder among

Negroes who move to the North, not merely as members of a minority population but as strangers and aliens by virtue of unfamiliarity, less urbanized backgrounds, poverty, and low status.

Marital Status

Family disruption is another form of transition experience that is correlated, on the one hand, with social class position and, on the other, with hospitalization for psychiatric disorder. It warrants attention as a potential basis for explaining a greater proportion of the variance than we can now achieve. The findings are, with a few minor variations, probably the most consistent in the epidemiology of mental illness.[47] The most stable finding is that married people living with spouse show by far the lowest rates of psychiatric hospitalization, while those who are divorced or separated show by far the highest rates.[48] The major variations in the data occur in the rank order of single persons and of widowed persons. Both single and widowed people have considerably higher rates than the married and considerably lower rates than the divorced or separated, but show relatively similar rates to one another and change rank positions from one set of data to another. Despite high rates of divorce and separation among Negroes, the same pattern of marital status and psychiatric disorder obtains with smaller differences between the extremes.

Although these findings on migration, minority status, and marital disruption offer only suggestive clues to the relationship between social class position and mental disorder, they point up some interrelated factors that affect the distribution of psychiatric disorders. Thus there are marked differences in the patterns, conditions, and auspices of migration for lower- and for higher-status groups, and these differences may affect the distribution of disorders.[49]

Lower-status groups more often leave a region because of inadequacies in the community of origin while higher-status groups more frequently seek opportunities otherwise unavailable to them. Moreover, lower-status people are far less likely to have a clear idea about the work they will do, the place in which they will live, or the people with whom they will associate. At the same time, the psychological requirements of lower-status people for environmental support and dependability are great. Marital disruption, more frequent among lower-status people, can only intensify the need for external resources. The combination of a pervasive sense of inner uncertainty and inadequate social resources for stabilizing immediate life situations is likely to be a major factor producing the phenomena of psychiatric disorder. On this basis, migration, marital disruption, or any other form of major social transition may produce differential rates of psychiatric disorder at different social class levels and, in particular, are likely to increase the vulnerability of low-status persons.

Work and Unemployment

While complex theoretical considerations prove fundamental in the design of studies to extricate the causal sequences linking social class and mental disorder, several simpler relationships may prove more immediately useful and empirically verifiable in accounting for these associations. In most instances the studies are inadequate for providing conclusive evidence, but several investigations of the effects of employment status and of social mobility on psychiatric disorder provide a more meaningful basis for translating social class and Negro-white differences in mental illness into the dynamics of social processes. In view of the critical importance of occupational performance in modern societies, the large differences in the work situation of people at different social class levels, and the associations between occupational status and severe psychiatric disorder, the potential significance of work and unemployment for mental health and illness is apparent. Nonetheless, very few studies have examined this relationship.

Only two of the thirty-four studies dealing with social class and mental illness report rates of psychiatric disorder for the unemployed. Granting the technical difficulties of assessing unemployment for a person who is hospitalized after some period of serious malfunctioning, and the analytic difficulties of interpreting the association causally, the data are striking. The technical problem of assessing unemployment is minimal for the first of the two studies since it is based on selective service registrants. This study found by far the highest rates of rejection for mental and personality disorders (excluding psychoneurosis) among the category of unemployed and emergency (presumably temporary or transient) workers.[50] This category showed a rate of 84.8 per 1,000 compared to an overall rate for all occupations of 50.1 per 1,000 and a rate of 24.7 per 1,000 for professional and managerial occupations. Similarly, Jaco found extremely high rates of psychosis among the unemployed in his occupational analysis of three subcultural groups in Texas.[51]

It may well be that unemployment is a major precipitating factor in psychiatric disorder and that status differentials in rates of unemployment account for some of the relationship between social class and psychiatric hospitalization.[52] Rates of unemployment for the population of the United States as a whole increase quite markedly with decreasing occupational status. Thus, in any distribution by occupation, it is likely that the lower occupational statuses will contain higher proportions of unemployed persons. The few studies that do isolate rates of severe psychiatric disorder for the unemployed certainly indicate their enormous preponderance over rates for the employed at any occupational level. It is quite reasonable, then, to extrapolate from these relationships in the data the likelihood that unemployment among lower occupational status groups accounts for some proportion of the high rates of severe psychiatric disorder at lower-status levels.

In cross-sectional studies, however, it is impossible to extricate the causal priority of psychiatric disorder and unemployment. On logical grounds alone it is reasonable to assume either that psychiatric disorder leads to unemployment or that unemployment engenders psychiatric disorder. Time series data, on the other hand, do allow us to make estimates of the major direction of causality. The trend data on employment levels reveal that increases in unemployment (or decreases in employment) precede increased rates of psychiatric hospitalization with a period of lag ranging from several months to several years. These relationships are evident in Dayton's data for the Great Depression and are presented for long series of economic upturns and downturns in Brenner's sophisticated statistical analyses of psychiatric hospitalization in the state of New York.[53] These powerful findings lend considerable support to the importance of economic conditions and, particularly, of employment status as major determinants of psychiatric hospitalization.

Other data also provide support for the significance of unemployment as a cause or, at least, as a mediating factor in psychological malfunctioning. Data on suicide present evidence of high rates of unemployment among people who subsequently commit suicide.[54] While there is ambiguity about whether prior psychological difficulties were implicated in both the loss of employment and in the act of suicide, these data provide circumstantial support for the view that unemployment either precipitated the self-destructive act or exacerbated prior social or psychological problems. However, even if we conclude that unemployment is a major determinant of psychiatric hospitalization, this does not preclude the priority of psychiatric difficulties as determinants of unemployment for some proportion of cases. One study in particular provides some useful data on this point. In an examination of the work histories of a sample of male schizophrenic patients, Cole and co-workers found a high level of stable occupational careers in the past experience of people who were subsequently hospitalized.[55] Immediately prior to hospitalization, however, many of those who had previously maintained long-term job stability began to have lengthy periods of unemployment. On the other hand, after psychiatric hospitalization, there was a gradual attrition in levels of employment among this sample, indicating great inroads on work functioning as a consequence of psychiatric difficulties or of the labeling implications of hospitalization or, most likely, of both. It is noteworthy that even in this study of prehospitalization and posthospitalization work experiences, those former patients who were of lower status experienced more frequent subsequent hospitalizations as a result of unemployment.

We can tentatively conclude that unemployment almost certainly accounts for some substantial proportion of severe psychiatric disorder; that it may well be one of the significant components linking lower social class status with high rates of psychiatric disorder; and that the very high rates of unemployment among Negroes may readily account for a significant portion of their high rates of psychiatric disorder. At the other end of the scale, a number of studies show increasing rates of work satisfaction with increasing occupational status.[56] At least one study shows an association between work satisfaction and mental health ratings.[57]

With these results, one can begin to clarify the dynamic factors in occupational position and employment status that account for a persistent but otherwise unexplained relationship.

Social Mobility

Although the potential importance of downward social mobility as a factor in explaining the relationship between social class and mental illness is self-evident, the literature in this area is moderately weak. Not only are there very few studies but the samples are small, and insufficient consideration is given to the population base against which mobility rates can be evaluated. Which are the most appropriate indicators? Should intergenerational or intragenerational mobility be considered? What life-cycle status of parents or patients should be used? How should the social mobility status of women be evaluated? How is individual change estimated in light of the large-scale structural changes over time that have upgraded the entire occupational distribution? An analysis of social mobility necessitates an adequate estimate of the frequency of upward and downward mobility and of status stability in the population at·risk. Even those studies that compare the occupational distributions of sons and fathers do not take full account of occupational opportunities relative to achievements for the populations during the two periods a generation apart. Nonetheless, the issue is of such central importance that we cannot neglect it.

There are only ten studies of the relationship between social mobility and psychiatric disorder.[58] Among these, seven suggest that there are higher proportions of downward social mobility (and/or lower proportions of upward social mobility) among the psychiatrically disturbed than are to be expected. Three suggest that upward social mobility is not disproportionately low nor is downward social mobility disproportionately high among people with severe psychiatric disorders.[59] Two of the studies are totally inadequate for drawing conclusions about social mobility and mental illness. One study that contradicts the hypothesis warrants rejection not only because of the great loss of cases but because of the many unjustified assumptions implicit in the use of an index based on residential changes classified according to median monthly rental.[60] The other study, supporting the hypothesis, must be excluded because of its lack of controls and its reliance on addresses and ratings of housing quality.[61] Dunham's recent analysis and support for the hypothesis cannot be included because of the absence of controls or of any other basis for comparing rates among psychiatric patients with rates for the population at risk. Clausen and Kohn's rejection of the hypothesis must be reinterpreted in light of the fact that, given the categories they employ (consistent downward mobility, consistent upward mobility) their findings provide more support than contradiction for a relationship between social mobility and psychiatric disorder.[62] Thus, the percentage of consistent upward mobility among the control group is twice as great as among the schizophrenic group (16 percent against 8 percent), and a much smaller proportion of the controls fall into the category "fluctuation in level" than of the schizophrenics (2 percent against 8 percent). On the other hand, the fact that more than 50 percent of both the schizophrenics and controls fall into the category of "all jobs— same occupational level" indicates that, at best, the relationship between psychiatric disorder and social mobility does not account for the majority of cases.

Despite reservations, we can tentatively sustain the hypothesis that individuals with severe psychiatric disorders show either disproportionately low rates of upward mobility or disproportionately high rates of downward mobility.

With the rejection of three reports and the reinterpretation of the findings in one report, there remain six instances of support for the hypothesis contrasted with one instance of rejection. There are a number of additional studies, using selected samples, which tend to give further support to the hypothesis as well as more recent evidence that has not been included in the actual count.

Although sufficient evidence exists to demonstrate the relationship between social mobility and psychiatric disorder that may partially account for the differential rates of psychiatric hospitalization among different social classes, the mechanisms involved are less evident. Moreover, it is quite likely that no single mechanism explains this relationship but rather several quite different processes culminate in the same cross-sectional result. From Turner's findings one can conclude that low rates of upward intergenerational mobility and high rates of downward intergenerational mobility among people with psychological difficulties swell the rates of psychiatric problems at lower status levels. At the same time, it is evident that some proportion of these cases move into low-status positions relatively early in their careers. Whether this is itself a product of prior personal difficulties or reflects situational factors that disproportionately affect people from low-status origins and results in psychological problems remains an open question. There can be little doubt that some people who subsequently become hospitalized have had personal difficulties quite early in life that affect their occupational careers and that alone or in conjunction with occupational stresses result in later psychiatric problems. One study based on earlier school records reveals a high frequency of such difficulties during school years among those who subsequently were diagnosed as schizophrenic.[63] Another study reports greater discrepancies between education and occupation for schizophrenic sons than for their fathers, a pattern that was significantly different among controls. Still another study reveals that early school careers of schizophrenic patients compare favorably with the national average but begin to deteriorate at the secondary school level.[64]

While all of these studies imply the early onset of problems that might eventuate in psychiatric disorders and, at the same time, may account for occupational failures, the conclusions one can draw are quite limited. In the first place, they do not account for a sufficient amount of the variance to be considered as exclusive explanations. In the second place, even when we push back the problem of causality to these earlier years, similar problems arise in separating these intertwined causal phenomena. We cannot say much more than that psychological deficits lower the threshold for situational problems *and* situational deficits lower the threshold for psychological problems.

It is unfortunate that we try to seek in cross-sectional statistical analysis singular explanations for extremely complex phenomena. More often than not, social and psychological processes occur in spiral and mutually reinforcing or counteracting events. Only rarely are results so overwhelming that a single variable or process accounts for even the largest part of the variability in the dependent variable. There is no reason for assuming that because some proportion of the cases, even enough to affect a statistically significant difference, reveal patterns of early disorganization, this explanation precludes the existence of an alternative or opposite pattern. One clinical study of schizophrenic patients, for example, distinguishes four different patterns of work experience in a sample of schizophrenic patients. The distinctions indicate that less than 25 percent of the patients fall into the pattern of early onset and chronic difficulty, although for the group as a whole downward social mobility and high rates of prehospitalization unemployment were extremely frequent.[65]

The difficulties of data interpretation are thus clearly manifest. If we accept the proposition that severe psychiatric disorder is associated with downward social mobility, to what extent does downward mobility play the critical causal role leading to psychiatric disorder? If this were the case, downward mobility as the determinant of psychiatric disorder would be an important factor in explaining the relationship between social class and mental illness. Conversely, to what extent does psychiatric disorder play a critical causal role in downward social mobility? If this were the case, it would also contribute to an explanation of the relationship between social class and mental illness. If both of these sequences operate, how much of the total variance is accounted for by each dynamic? The data do not come very close to answering these fundamental questions.

From the vantage point of the larger question, however, it becomes clear that disproportionately low rates of upward social mobility and disproportionately high rates of downward social mobility among persons with severe psychiatric disorders do help to account for the highly consistent and frequently powerful association between social class and mental illness. Along with such other factors as unemployment and marital disruption, which may also serve as either cause or effect of psychiatric disorder, the significant implication of social mobility begins to transform a static conception of the relationship of social class position to mental illness into a framework for understanding the social dynamics of this relationship.

POVERTY AND POWERLESSNESS

It is hardly accidental that a discussion of the relationship between poverty and mental health should deal neither with poverty nor with mental health. The reasons for focusing primarily on mental illness, and, within this broad category on severe psychiatric disorders, have already been mentioned. The reasons for discussing social class rather than poverty are similar. Poverty is an empirical category, not a conceptual entity, and it represents congeries of unrelated problems: unemployment and underemployment, the condition of the aged, the situation of the Negro, the consequences of physical illness, inadequacies in welfare policy and migration, inadequate preparation for the urban environment, changes in agriculture, and the deterioration of rural areas. The problems posed by poverty are not readily accessible for study or resolution in the name of poverty. Like psychiatric disorder, poverty is a social fact that requires explanation. It can serve as an entry into a set of issues that can be examined and changed. The use of poverty or income levels in studies of social behavior is infrequent largely because such studies have revealed fewer uniformities than other indicators of social class.[66] Even those forms of social behavior that presumably are more directly responsive to available financial resources, like consumer behavior or choice of housing, educational achievement, occupational status, or cultural orientation, are more likely to be closely implicated than is income as such.

Some of the issues involved in the relationship of poverty as an empirical phenomenon to social class as a conceptual entity can only be clarified by extensive theoretical discussion. Even if we translate the conception of social class into empirically definable phenomena like educational attainment and occupational status, there is little enough data on which to base detailed analysis. These variables show moderately high intercorrelations but we cannot go much beyond this. To a considerable extent, therefore, just as we have implied a relationship between poverty and mental illness in discussing social class and mental illness, we will base our discussion of poverty largely on what is known about low educational and occupational status.

All of the variables considered so far have been objective social events. In this sense we have been dealing with objective social phenomena to explain objective social events and a straightfoward association between two sets of social facts. Although it is not theoretically necessary that intervening psychological processes mediate these events, with phenomena so complex it seems essential to assume internal responses to these events, responses affecting the likelihood that particular consequent events will occur. It would be difficult to explain psychiatric disorder on the basis of prior unemployment without assuming that unemployment is experienced as a threat, loss, disruption, or provocation. Similarly, in explaining that unemployment sometimes leads to psychiatric disorder, other times to halfhearted job-seeking or increased determination to find a job, we imply that unemployment is experienced differently by different people and/or that the necessity, possibility, and desirability of employment are differently perceived. The framework may be one of motivation, cognitive orientation, and attitudinal disposition, or it may be formulated as feedback processes in an information network. But the central importance of a psychological organism experiencing and responding to social events is common to these formulations.

From this psychological point of view, what are the components of social class generally and of poverty specifically that are likely to explain the disproportionate frequency of psychiatric disorder at lower levels of the status scale? Haggstrom states the issues most cogently:

The situation of poverty ... is the situation of enforced dependency, giving the poor very little scope for action, in the sense of behavior under their own control which is central to their needs and values. This scope for action is supposed to be furnished by society to any person in either of two ways. First, confidence, hope, motivation, and skills for action may be provided through childhood socialization and continue as a relatively permanent aspect of the personality. Second, social positions are provided which make it easy for their occupants to be implemented in their futures. Middle class socialization and middle class social positions customarily both provide bases for effective action; lower class socialization and lower class social positions usually both fail to make it possible for the poor to act.[67]

Haggstrom stresses powerlessness as the critical factor in the psychology of poverty, mirroring the enforced dependency of the poor on the agencies of society. Powerlessness can be quite general or highly specific. Poverty as the absence of power to control goods and services represents only one form of powerlessness. For a college student, or for a religious man who has taken vows of poverty, this form of powerlessness may be quite specific and limited. For those people who represent the largest proportion of the poor, powerlessness in the market is coupled with most other forms of powerlessness in society and becomes a highly general phenomenon.

Powerlessness and a corresponding *sense* of powerlessness may attend an individual's economic situation, his social status, or his political control. Lower-class persons most frequently and quite vividly sense their powerlessness in economic choices, in social and occupational decisions, and in political access. Negroes, for whom the avenues to modest power are often closed, have given increased emphasis to "Black Power" and community-wide efforts to alter their powerlessness in all these spheres. Strikingly, however, the emergence of lower-status groups as "countervailing powers" does not readily alter the widespread sense of powerlessness among the rank and file who now must deal with a new, if more responsive and more closely identified, bureaucracy or leadership. Perhaps the reason for this lies in the immediacy and urgency of economic powerlessness which, even if welfare agencies are available to stave off starvation, allows virtually no options and no sense of self-esteem and participation in one's own fate. It is an ultimate form of enforced situational dependency.

The sense of powerlessness provides an important hypothetical link to the development of psychiatric disorder. Most of the social factors that help to explain the association of social class and psychiatric disorder can readily be understood as stimuli to an increased sense of powerlessness. Whether this is the single most general and useful conceptual formulation is not altogether clear. However, the sense of powerlessness can potentially include these diverse social events, and there are few alternative psychological variables that meet this qualification. In the absence of relevant data the adequacy of this variable can be examined by simulating imaginary examples. Let us consider, as one example, a situation in which unemployment leads to psychiatric disorder. For the person who is unemployed, a number of options exist. In order to accept the precarious and threatening option of psychological and behavioral disorganization leading to psychiatric disorder, he would have to find other options completely intolerable and feel powerless either to expand the range of options or to alter the definition of the situation that makes other options intolerable. Alternatively, we might say that he feels hopeless rather than powerless. He might, of course, be hostile or diffident but these appear to lead to determined or sporadic efforts to find another job. Hopelessness implies the expectation that no external change will occur; powerlessness implies the expectation that one has no control over his own destiny.

Another hypothetical situation may help to discriminate between these conceptions. Imagine a case in which, with no prior evidence of malfunctioning, the incompatibility of two marital partners leads to divorce, which eventuates in psychiatric disorder for one of the partners. As the statistical findings indicate, this is considerably more likely to occur to husbands than to wives. Hostility or diffidence is likely to be a frequent response but would not account for increasing disorganization. Hopelessness is certainly a possibility, assuming the man's thoughts tend toward remarriage coupled with feelings of inadequacy. With these feelings of inadequacy, of course, we approach a sense of powerlessness. But why is psychiatric disorder associated with marital disruption more frequently for women than for men? Are men more likely to feel hopeless in response to marital disruption than women? This seems unreasonable, particularly since the realistic situation of the divorced or separated women, who must often maintain the children, is more complex, more difficult, and more realistically hopeless. It is not obvious that men are more likely to feel powerless than are women in this situation except for the fact that, in our society, divorce or separation implies that the man has not maintained adequate control over the marriage, even if the immediate cause is the wife's dissatisfaction, her sexual inadequacy or infidelity, or her desire to attain greater independence and freedom. And this conception of the man's responsibility for the inviolability of the marriage is more frequent at lower social class levels.

It would be pointless to go beyond these few imaginary examples. Clearly, we cannot expect to obtain conclusive evidence nor even a clear delineation of the alternative psychological processes that might intervene between social disruption and psychiatric disorder. In the absence of virtually any effort to link a relationship between social class factors and psychiatric disorder through intervening psychological processes, and in view of the lack of any attempt, in the data on psychological processes in psychiatric malfunctioning, to tie these processes to antecedent social events, some initial formulation seems essential. The sense of powerlessness appears to be a potentially important psychological variable that is meaningfully tied to social class position and to social disruptions and transitions that are frequent among lower social class poeple. At the same time, it provides a useful bridge to the development of psychiatric disorder. The primary purpose of this imaginary simulation, however, is as much methodological as substantive. It serves to indicate the ways in which psychological processes can implement and further clarify the analysis of relationships between an antecedent and a consequent social event.

Even assuming the substantive importance of a sense of powerlessness as a consequence of lower social class position and as a determinant of psychiatric disorder, there is no reason to believe that the form of powerlessness associated with poverty is of any greater significance in this sequence than the forms of powerlessness associated with deprivations of social position and opportunity. On the one hand, as this review of the data has indicated, the relationship between income variables and psychiatric disorder is, if anything, more tenuous than the relationship of psychiatric disorder to other social class factors. On the other hand, there is a wider variety of resources available for emergency and longer-term assistance with poverty than for other forms of deprivation. One of the merits of the conception of a sense of powerlessness is that it provides a common psychological base for the impact of different forms of deprivation. In the light of current data, one can only conclude that if poverty per se is closely linked to psychiatric disorder, it must be through some intervening psychological mechanism which also bears the burden of other forms of deprivation.

PSYCHIATRIC DISORDER AND HOSPITALIZATION

Considerably more attention has been given to the variables we have regarded as independent or antecedent than to those we have viewed as dependent or consequent. Apart from an initial formulation posing a social view of psychiatric disorder, we have not dealt with class differences in the manifestations, the processing, or the consequences of psychiatric malfunctioning. While this is a large and complex subject for review in its own right, it is essential that we consider at least some of the more promising directions of current investigation.

Relatively little attention has been devoted to social class differences in the phenomenology of psychiatric disorder. Two major contributions to the literature devote most of their analysis to early experience and precipitating events that distinguish people with effective functioning from those with psychiatric impairments.[68] One of the few findings beginning to emerge with some degree of consistency is the emphasis on physical symptoms, physical interpretations of psychological symptoms, and an organic conception of psychiatric disorder and treatment among lower class patients. This difference appears to be quite general and holds for different degrees of psychiatric impairment.[69] The explanation for this finding is not clear. To what extent is there a difference in organic symptomatology, in preimpairment experiences of organic illness, in understanding and conceptualization of psychological processes, in the forms of defense and the denial of mental illness, in the bases for legitimizing sick roles? Some data from Puerto Rico point to striking differences between schizophrenic and control families in physical illness, hospitalization for physical illness, and experiences of illness and death in the family.[70] It is reasonable to interpret these findings to suggest that recent histories of severe or protracted illness, more frequent among the lowest-status groups, color the experience of mental illness and may more often initiate psychological disorganization among lower-class people. Unfortunately, there is nothing in the available data to preclude the opposite interpretation: that early signs of psychological disorganization are viewed as physical illness and that psychosomatic pathways for the expression of malfunctioning are more readily available to lower-class people.

Class differences in psychiatric disorder may be affected by social and professional responses to malfunctioning. The data concerning social class differences in response to disordered behavior suggest that, whatever the intrinsic differentials in rates of disordered behavior, individuals from the lower social classes are more likely to be extruded and hospitalized, and more likely to receive more serious diagnoses and inadequate treatment. Several studies suggest that lower-class families and communities have lower levels of tolerance for disordered behavior and more readily seek hospitalization for malfunctioning family or community members.[71] In view of results indicating minimal class differentials in tolerance and different paths to treatment in different social classes, we may wonder whether the fairly evident difference in extrusion is due to different tolerances in family and community or, rather, to the different role of public representatives and professionals in encouraging higher rates of psychiatric hospitalization.[72]

Differences in diagnosis due to implicit or explicit social

class characteristics have only recently become evident. Hollingshead and Redlich hypothesized and several studies demonstrated this effect. Thus, Haase has shown remarkable discrepancies in the interpretation of paired examiner-constructed Rorschach protocols when these were associated with different social histories stressing the different social class background for each pair of protocols.[73] A careful analysis of casework records similarly reveals that social workers' evaluations of the treatability of clients is inversely related to the social class position of clients and similar orientations of psychotherapists lead to fewer recommendations of psychotherapy for patients of lower status.[74] Perhaps the most striking finding was that the lower the social class of patients coming to the emergency ward of a general hospital, the more likely he was to be diagnosed as alcoholic even when identical signs and symptoms of alcoholism were reported by the intake physician for people in other social class positions.[75] Differences in treatment-experience by social class were also first reported systematically by Hollingshead and Redlich. Although this issue has been accorded little replication, several studies agree with their data in showing the diminished expectations of treatability for lower-class patients, a lower rate of acceptance for treatment; and a higher dropout rate from treatment.[76] It seems most likely that the same unconscious discriminatory factors that exacerbate psychiatric hospitalization rates, severe psychiatric diagnoses, and inadequate treatment among lower-class patients also have similar consequences for Negroes and other minorities, producing a disproportionate appearance of psychiatric disorder. On the other hand, it is unlikely that these factors can entirely account for the size and persistence of differences between people in different social classes or between Negroes and whites in indices of psychiatric malfunctioning.

For a fuller explanation of differences in observed rates

of psychiatric disorder, we must investigate the vast differences in social and economic conditions and opportunities that so drastically differentiate social classes and people of minority status in our society. However, the data are clearly inadequate for any discrimination between the social events surrounding psychiatric malfunctioning that may lead to psychiatric hospitalization and the social factors antecedent to malfunctioning in accounting for the observed relationship between social class and mental disorder. They are, however, sufficiently striking to warrant greater attention and encourage more carefully designed studies in which several explanatory variables can be examined simultaneously.

INTERRELATIONSHIPS BETWEEN FORMS OF DISORDERED FUNCTIONING

As we move from relatively simple efforts to study the relationship between two variables such as social class and mental illness to more complex relationships that not only deal with a large number of variables but attempt to delineate sequences of determinism and directions of interaction, the theoretical formulation begins to approximate a reasonably lifesized conceptualization. The methodological and analytic problems, however, become enormous. Indeed, only in passing have we suggested some of the complexities that go far beyond any we have discussed in detail. Some of these warrant discussion if only to point up the great need for analytic models that more closely approximate, not merely our theoretical wisdom, but some self-evident aspects of the processes of development of illness and disorder. Two of the most critical of these issues are (1) the interrelationship between different types of pathology and disordered functioning and the different patterns of health and welfare services associated with them; and (2) the cumulative and spiraling effects of deprivations, problems, stresses, and crises which culminate in the situation of families with multiple, chronic problems.

Little research has been done on the interrelationships between different types of disordered functioning or on the interrelationships between different patterns of health and welfare agency usage. The literature is barren and leaves the issue open to wholly unsupported conjectures. Indeed, not only are these interrelationships important in their own right but the absence of information raises serious questions about any study in which the dependent variable is either some form of malfunctioning or some form of contact with professional health and welfare resources. If we make several conventional and unsubstantiated assumptions about malfunctioning and the use of professional services, of course, this problem does not arise. These assumptions are (1) that different forms of malfunctioning like mental disorder, physical illness, drug addiction, alcoholism, delinquency, and social problems are discrete, conceptually unrelated to one another, and technically distinguishable one from the other; and (2) that specialized professional health and welfare services are designed to deal with specific forms of malfunctioning and, through distinguishable paths to treatment and proper diagnosis, an accurate sort is made between the form of malfunction and the service speciality. These assumptions are probably more widespread among professionals working in the health and welfare fields than most social scientists are wont to imagine and enter into the scientific study of these problems.

If one makes these assumptions, some contrary evidence invariably intrudes. Over the past few decades it has gradually come to be accepted that a very large proportion, probably more than half, of the persons coming for medical assistance have no physical illness or disability but show signs of emotional impairment or behavioral malfunction. For the most part, juvenile courts have accepted the necessity of having a court psychiatrist who could distinguish the psychiatric from the delinquent case. Most social agencies maintain an extensive roster of medical and psychiatric consultants, not merely for general consultation but quite specifically for help with cases in which the predominant form of malfunction is physical or psychological. Similarly, social workers in psychiatric services have long served multiple functions, including greater attention to the social background of mental illness. One could expand this list but there is, to our knowledge, not a single piece of research that carefully documents this problem with respect to multiple forms of malfunctioning and multiple forms of services used or to the relationship between paths to treatment and characteristics other than intrinsic features of the disordered functioning.

If it is the case, however, that many individuals show multiple forms of disordered functioning, and there is a great likelihood that any one form of disordered functioning will show up in individuals who already show other forms of disordered functioning, then our empirical and analytic categories for disordered functioning must be revised. If a large proportion of the population falls either into the "no professional services" category or into the "multiple professional services" category, and relatively few in the "one professional service" category, then our conceptions of health and welfare services have to be reviewed.

If most professional services deal with a multitude of different problems, many of which might be more appropriate to another service, then studying a particular form of disorder through any case count based on a discrete conception of disorders or on discrete services is bound to fall victim to serious miscalculations due both to false positives (cases counted which do not properly belong) and to false negatives (cases uncounted). If any of these contentions is correct, it suggests that, in addition to independent estimates of disorder and of health or welfare agency contact, we must take account of the potential "false negatives"— those individuals who might have been counted but are using a different kind of service. This means that most of our estimates of the relationship between social or psychological variables and disordered functioning should be made against a background of all forms of disordered functioning or all forms of health and welfare service contact.

For purposes of understanding the relationship between social class and mental illness, these considerations provide us only with suggestive clues. Most forms of disordered functioning show some relationship to social class differences. The lowest social class groups have the highest proportions of disorder for suicide and mental retardation, while delinquency, crime, alcoholism, drug addiction, and other social problems show some association with social class. Kadushin argues that this inverse relationship no longer holds for physical illness in modern societies but the data he presents are ambiguous, and important technical questions raise doubts about his argument.[77] He questions the accuracy of disability days lost as indicators of physical illness but accepts the data for chronic illness as an accurate count of illness. Is the diagnosis of chronic illness completely independent of reactions to illness, and are disability days lost solely a consequence of such reactions? It may be that low-status people more readily stay away from work on minimal physical grounds, as Kadushin implies and, at the very same time, fail to recognize, and seek, professional attention for, chronic illnesses. If this is so, the data on chronic illness are subject to as many questions as are the data on time lost due to illness. Indeed, statistics from the National Health Survey indicate that the social class (income) difference for disability days is far greater for the categories "restricted activity" and "bed disability" than for "work loss," and the category "hospital" shows almost no class difference and includes an extremely small proportion of the cases in any income group.[78]

On this basis, it seems reasonable to include physical illness among the list of disorders which show the highest rates among the lowest social class groups. The essential point is that the congruence of these findings necessarily implies either or both of two conclusions: that the overall relationship between social class and all forms of disordered functioning is far greater than the relationship between social class and any single form of disordered functioning, and/or that the likelihood of multiple contacts with professional services is disproportionately high among lower social class groups.

CUMULATIVE IMPACT IN THE DETERMINANTS OF PSYCHIATRIC DISORDER

These considerations lead quite naturally to the problem of the multiple or cumulative effects of diverse forms of deprivation, disruption, and disordered functioning. If the literature on disordered functioning were scanned for all the factors that have been implicated for a particular form of disordered functioning, we might well collect a volume of substantial size. Undoubtedly a large proportion of these factors would disappear with a few careful studies devoted to the exclusion rather than the inclusion of variables. Nonetheless, even those studies that control for a modest number of variables rarely emerge with single variables that would account for most of the variance. But it seems that a large number of theoretically independent but empirically intercorrelated forms of deprivation and disruption during all phases of the life cycle contribute to psychiatric disorder and that, in turn, psychiatric disorder contributes to, or exacerbates; many different situations of deprivation and disruption.

The Midtown study is one empirical examination that presents controlled analyses of a wide variety of deprivations and disruptions during childhood and adulthood. [79] While it could dismiss many variables as spurious, there remained a huge number of variables that separately bore modest relationships to impairment ratings, and a fairly large number showed strong, independent relationships to psychiatric impairment. In addition to age, socioeconomic status, and marital status, there were eight composite childhood factors and six composite adult factors. The sheer number of negative sociocultural background factors (mainly deprivations and disruptions) reported by individuals showed the strongest relationship to mental health risk. No single experience was implicated either as a primary cause or as a uniquely important precipitating event. It may be, therefore, that the usual expectation that a single major factor will account for a large part of the variance is inappropriate for the investigation of psychiatric disorder, that many diverse factors have minor and independent determining effects, and that only their cumulative effect serves as a potent and highly general determinant of mental illness.

Although experiences of deprivation and disruption were more frequent among the lower socioeconomic status groups, these differences were not sufficient to account for the great differences in mental health risk. With the number of stressful experiences held constant, the lower socioeconomic status groups showed much higher mental health risks. At the low stress extreme, where there were virtually no reported experiences of deprivation or disruption, the different social class groups showed almost identical (and low) mental health risks, but at the other extreme of high stress, the mental health risk among the lower social class groups was disproportionately higher than among the higher social class groups. Langner points to three alternative hypotheses that might account for these findings: (1) social class differences in inner personality resources with greater resilience and resistance to impairment among higher-status groups; (2) social class differences in external resources which are less frequently available to lower-status groups for help in stress; and (3) differences in meaning of the same reported experience for different class groups, with higher thresholds among lower-status people who might report only more pathogenic experiences.

It is not possible to discriminate among these hypotheses from the available data nor to support or reject several other relevant hypotheses. Three other hypotheses in particular warrant consideration in trying to interpose dynamic sequences in the relationship between social class and mental illness: the role of selective (pathological) factors in producing lower social class status as opposed to social class as a source of frequent pathogenic influences; the culmative impact of disruptions and deprivations; and the more complex formulation of converging psychological and social forces in producing psychopathology. We have already shown that many of the reported findings can be interpreted as consequences of pathological influences in producing lower social class status or as the particularly severe and pathogenic effects of deprivation and disruption on lower-class people. The evidence is quite unambiguous that selective factors cannot possibly account for all of the findings but, beyond this, the issue remains open. The most reasonable hypothesis is that both types of relationships operate. However, even if the alternatives can be stated in the form of a critical test, there remain serious problems in the differential definition and conception of symptoms and disorder in different social class and subcultural groups that lead to difficulties in the very categorization of the dependent variable, psychiatric disorder.[80]

The hypothesis that gives importance to cumulative effects of disruption and deprivation involves two components: that deprivation and disruption are more frequent among people in lower social class positions; and that these deprivations and disruptions are not merely additive but each additional stress has increasingly greater impact among lower-status people. Indeed, this is one way of interpreting the Langner and Michaels data, which show a steeper curve of increasing mental health risk with increasing numbers of stress factors among lower than among higher-status people. Clinical and participant observation reveal that, in addition to the generic importance of a sense of powerlessness associated with social class position itself, experiences of deprivation and disruption tend to intensify feelings that the total situation has gone beyond the point of control. Is there a point, differing by social class positions, at which this sense of powerlessness frequently becomes overwhelming and results in disorganized behavior? This seems to be a reasonable conjecture that bears closer examination in empirical study.

Closely related to the cumulative stress hypothesis but theoretically more complex is the formulation derived from a principle of psychosocial complementarity.[81] In an application to the development of psychiatric disorder, this formulation would hold the following:

1. Among adults, reliance on personality resources and

on social resources tend to be mutually exclusive, a pattern that results from structural features both of personality and of social roles.

2. Such predominance and acceptance of either role-determination or of personality-determination are complementary patterns and allow for modest, progressive change within a relatively stable context.

3. The simultaneous absence of opportunities for clear role-determination and for clear personality-determination or the simultaneous presence of powerful inner and outer resources are noncomplementary patterns which are inherently unstable and facilitate either uncertainty and withdrawal or anxiety-laden and nonrational actions.

4. Deprivation and disruption exacerbate rapid changes in role-demands and role-expectations and place increased burdens on either the supportive functions of external resources or the coping functions of internal resources.

5. People of lower social class backgrounds and statuses less frequently have developed the inner resources for rapid adaptation to changes in role-demands and, under conditions of severe stress, go beyond the resources of informal or formal social networks, organizations, and agencies in their needs for support and assistance.

6. Under these circumstances, given identical phenomena of deprivation and disruption, people in lower social class positions readily develop noncomplementary patterns while people in higher social class positions can maintain themselves at a more modest level of disorganization in relatively complementary (and, thus, stable) patterns.

This formulation implies that the situation of lower social class groups is more vulnerable by virtue of their intrinsic dependence on external support under conditions in which, at best, such support can be provided for short periods of time and quite conditionally. At the same time, the pace of modern social change frequently places large lower-class populations in situations which exacerbate the need for coping with changing role-expectations without preparation for the internal demands involved and without appropriate external facilities for assistance in adaptation. Most of the social factors that have been implicated as components or intervening factors in the relationship between social class and psychiatric disorder can be seen as precisely such forms of deprivation or disruption, changes that can be conceived as opportunities or threats depending on the inner prepared-ness and the external resources to facilitate their definition as meaningful options rather than as disorganizing threats.

We are far from an adequate theoretical or empirical appreciation of the complex processes that might meaning-fully account for the persistent finding that lower social class groups show the highest rates of psychiatric disorder. At the same time, the meaning of mental health cannot adequately be understood as a set of traits, competences, or achievements independent of the social matrix in which they function. The effort to develop a reasonable nosology and a fund of information concerning the attributes and consequences of those phenomena labeled physical or men-tal illness was a great achievement for the nineteenth and the early twentieth century. By the middle of the twentieth century it became increasingly evident that social factors were of such great importance in the definition, conception, symptomatology, visibility, diagnosis, and response to treat-ment that a fuller examination of the host of problems was essential.

The relationship between social class and mental illness is only one special aspect of this more general issue, of partic-ular practical and theoretical importance because of the needs of the population involved and because of the relative clarity of the relationship. But further development of our understanding demands a far more open conception and far greater challenge to existing conceptual investments. We have yet to learn about the dynamics of social class positions and their psychological implications and about the dynamics of psychological disorganization and its interrelationships with social processes in order to account more fully for massive findings that are all too often massively denied.

V. Prevention of Illness and Maintenance of Health

by Irwin M. Rosenstock

This chapter will explore the relationship between income and the seeking of preventive or diagnostic medical services, and the reasons such a relationship exists. In the present context poverty will be considered, as far as possible, in its literal sense: paucity of money. Thus, the effects of low income upon behavior will be separated from the effects of educational status upon behavior. But it is perfectly apparent that in reality income is not disassociated from other characteristics. Socioeconomic and racial characteristics are usually found in combination and only on the analytic level can they be separated.

There are striking correlations between poverty and health behavior. It is important, however, to go beyond a mere description of the associations and to consider whether income itself accounts for differential responses or whether personal and social factors related to income are also involved in the causal sequence. To the extent that the former is true, social policy in the health area could be based on the effort to make services available at ever decreasing financial costs in the confident expectation that this approach alone would be effective in stimulating the poor to obtain the needed health services. On the other

Dr. Irwin M Rosenstock is Professor of Public Health Administration, School of Public Health, University of Michigan, Ann Arbor.

hand, if it should be found that health behavior cannot be explained entirely by income, the social policy issues would be much more complex. Those factors associated with income that help to account for public response to health services would have to be identified, and intervention strategies developed either to alter these factors or obviate their role.

INCOME AND PREVENTIVE BEHAVIOR

Kasl and Cobb have distinguished among health behavior, illness behavior, and sick-role behavior.[1] The latter two refer respectively to behavior undertaken by persons who feel ill, for the purpose of defining the state of their health, or activities undertaken by persons who consider themselves ill, for the purpose of getting well. Health behavior, however, is defined as the activity undertaken by persons who believe themselves to be healthy, for the purpose of preventing or detecting disease in an asymptomatic stage. Although the distinctions among the three forms of behavior are not perfect, the intent in the present chapter is to focus principally upon health behavior.

Unfortunately, most of the relevant studies have focused on illness behavior or sick-role behavior.[2] They are either frankly restricted to the behavior of persons who believe themselves to be ill, or they include composite data on all three classes of health-related behavior. Thus, generalizations drawm from such studies cannot be readily applied to the description and understanding of the key questions in this chapter: do relatively poor people take asymptomatic health action less often than those who are less poor, and, if so, why?

A small number of studies have focused specifically and exclusively on such preventive or diagnostic health behavior.[3] But even these studies of preventive behavior are of limited value since they were performed on relatively small samples or in highly restricted geographic regions. Moreover, most of them obtained measures at only one point in time, precluding the analysis of behavioral consistency over time, and they dealt with responses to a single health condition, eliminating the possibility of assessing the consistency of behavior for several health conditions.

One study has attempted to overcome such limitations.[4] A nationwide study of health beliefs and health behavior was undertaken with a probability sample of the adult United States population living in private households. The interviews focused on beliefs and actions concerning dental disease, tuberculosis, and cancer—diseases selected to provide a range of clinical severity. The respondents were questioned about visits to physicians during the preceding five years for medical checkups or tests; visits to dentists during the preceding three years for prophylactic purposes in the absence of symptoms; frequency of toothbrushing practices; and frequency of examinations or tests for detection of tuberculosis or cancer during the preceding ten years.

Fifteen months later, a resurvey of half of the sample was taken, inquiring about the same aspects of behavior during the fifteen-month interval. The findings provide information on the extent of preventive actions, the consistency of preventive behavior, and the personal factors associated with taking such actions.

It was found that about one third of the eligible public had not visited physicians for checkups during the previous five years, about half had not made a prophylactic visit to the dentist within the last three years, and nearly half had failed to brush their teeth after a single meal on the day preceding the interview. Nearly half who could have taken voluntary tuberculosis tests in the absence of symptoms failed to take a single test in the past ten years, and only about one in twenty who could have taken a voluntary test for cancer while asymptomatic had received any such test in the same period. From these data it is clear that though each of the preventive health actions, except screening tests for cancer, was taken by a substantial proportion of the public, a sizable number who could have taken each of the preventive actions did not do so.

The issue of the consistency of health behavior was subdivided into two questions: did members of the sample display consistency of behavior across the different health actions, and did they behave consistently with respect to given actions over time? To answer these questions, persons who had taken and those who had failed to take a given action on a voluntary, asymptomatic basis were compared to determine the extent to which they had taken a combination of the other three actions. For example, those who had visited their physicians for a check-up and those who had not were compared for the total number of other actions they had taken. In each instance, those who took a particular action had significantly higher scores on a combination of other behaviors than those who failed to take the action, though the differences were modest in size. The fact that behavior in the various preventive actions was consistent beyond chance expectations can be regarded as supporting the idea that people displayed a generalized pattern of response concerning preventive health action. Such consistency, however, was present only to a moderate degree.

To determine whether people behaved consistently over time, voluntary actions reported in the original survey were compared with those reported in the resurvey. For one analysis, the four separate actions were combined into an overall index of preventive behavior with each action given equal weight. When the index scores of individual respondents on the two occasions were compared, a marked consistency of behavior was observed. In other analyses, a non-chance consistency of behavior over time for each of the four separate actions studied was found; that is, persons who reported in the original survey that they took an action also tended in the resurvey to report having taken that action again. Similarly, those who reportedly failed to take an action when originally questioned subsequently tended to report a similar failure. These data and those cited earlier support the tenability of a general behavioral orientation, although the strength of that orientation is limited.

The data also indicate that for differences associated with income and socioeconomic status a strong association exists between income level, other personal characteristics, and the proportion of persons visiting the physician for checkups, visiting the dentist for prophylaxis, and obtaining chest X-rays. However, the association between income and reported frequency of brushing one's teeth "yesterday after one or more meals," though statistically significant, was much smaller than the former associations. It seems reasonable to conclude from these data that where substantial cost is involved, those with more income are far more likely to use the service than those in poorer financial circumstances. But where the action in question, i.e., tooth-brushing, involves only minimal or no cost, such differences are greatly reduced though still present. This finding is consistent with Kadushin's observation that while there are consistent income-related differences in the obtaining of medical care in the United States, such differences occur less often in the United Kingdom, where care is available through the National Health Service.[5]

A number of studies of more limited scope, investigating the association between income and the acceptance of preventive and/or screening services, support the above findings consistently and to a remarkable extent. Level of income is positively associated with the proportion of persons seeking each of the several tests. It should be noted that educational level is also correlated with the frequency of taking preventive and diagnostic actions. Although it is difficult to separate the effects of education from those of income, nevertheless there is good basis for believing that the effects of education and of income upon preventive health behavior are at least partly independent. Two bases for this connection can be provided. One is found in the Kegeles study which shows that income accounts for a larger proportion of the variation in taking a Papanicolaou test than does education.[6] If the correlation between income and behavior were wholly or largely attributable to education, one would not expect the income association to be greater than the educational association. A second basis is the finding mentioned earlier, that income appears to make more difference for behaviors that usually entail expense. Again, if the income–behavior correlation were spurious and attributable to education, then the failure to show a high correlation between income and engaging in cost-free actions is more difficult to explain.

In summary, virtually all relevant studies lead to the conclusion that income and preventive behavior are positively related. The higher the income level of a group, the more will they follow recommended preventive or diagnostic recommendations. However, it has been noted that the correlation is drastically reduced for tooth-brushing, an item entailing minimal expense, although it remains statistically significant. The majority of the studies also show that even when direct cost is minimized or removed, as in the case of inexpensive or free chest X-rays or inoculations, income is still associated with health behavior. But it would be too simple to assume that cost has been removed in such cases, for there may be greater costs associated with taking inexpensive or even "free" actions than middle-class persons can readily appreciate. A one-dollar charge for a polio inoculation may seem small but, when multiplied by six children for a series of four inoculations each, it may represent one half to one percent of a family's annual income. The seemingly small cost of public transportation may impose considerable financial burden on the poor, and where paid babysitting is required the financial burden increases. Systematic studies have not been made of all of the costs of obtaining a so-called free service, but they exist in most circumstances where individuals desiring a service are required to obtain it at a facility some distance from their homes. Thus it is by no means certain that economic factors do not play a significant role even where direct cost has been removed.

It would seem fair to conclude that removal of all financial barriers to health service might immediately lead to an increase in the proportion of poor people who use such service, but the result would fall far short of what is usually desired because large numbers of people would still refrain from taking the recommended action. Even at the highest levels of income, large numbers of people—in one study as many as 37 percent—still fail to take the recommended action.[7] According to another study, as many as 40 percent of the highest income population failed to brush their teeth after one or more meals.[8] Thus, while income does provide a barrier to obtaining health services, the elimination of that barrier would by no means insure the desired response. It is necessary to look at the correlates of the decision to seek or not to seek a particular health service in the absence of symptoms.

HEALTH BELIEFS AND BEHAVIOR

Research demonstrates that those with lower income are less likely to accept or seek preventive or diagnostic health services than those with higher income, but it does not provide a simple explanation of why this is so. The cost of the service does not wholly account for the response of those at lower income levels since they are also more prone to avoid presumably free services and refrain to a great extent from personal health practices that can be undertaken at nominal cost. We are therefore left with a problem: poorer people are less likely than richer people to use inexpensive or free health services.

Several efforts have been made to explain the phenomenon. One of the most comprehensive proposes a model for explaining health behavior in individuals who believe themselves to be free of symptoms or illnesses. The major variables in the model are drawn and adapted from general social-psychological theory, notably from the work of Lewin.[9] The explanatory model links current subjective states of the individual with current health behavior.

It has become a truism in social psychology that motivation is required for perception and action. Thus, people who are unconcerned with a particular aspect of their health are not likely to perceive any material that bears on that aspect of their health; even if through accidental circumstances they do perceive such material, they will fail to learn, accept, or use the information. Not only is such concern or motivation a necessary condition for action; motives also determine the particular ways in which the environment will be perceived. That a motivated person perceives selectively in accordance with his motives has been verified in many laboratory studies as well as in field settings.[10]

The proposed model used to explain health behavior grows out of such evidence. Specifically, it includes two classes of variables: (1) the psychological state of readiness to take specific action; and (2) the extent to which a particular course of action is believed, on the whole, to be beneficial in reducing the threat. Two principal dimensions are presumed to define whether a state of readiness to act exists. They include the degree to which an individual feels vulnerable or susceptible to a particular health condition and the extent to which he feels that contracting that condition would have serious consequences in his case. Readiness to act is defined in terms of the individual's points of view about susceptibility and seriousness rather than the professional's view of reality. The model does not require that individuals be continuously or consciously aware of their relevant beliefs. Evidence suggests that the beliefs that define readiness have both cognitive (i.e., intellectual) and emotional elements.

Perceived susceptibility. There is wide individual variation in the acceptance of personal susceptibility to a medical condition. At one extreme stands the individual who may deny that there is any possibility of his contracting a given condition. In a more moderate position is the person who may admit to the possibility of the occurrence but who does not really believe it will happen to him. Finally, a person may express a feeling that he is in real danger of contracting the condition. In short, susceptibility refers to the subjective risks of contracting a condition.

Perceived seriousness. Convictions concerning the seriousness of a given health problem may also vary. There is reason to believe that the degree of seriousness may be judged both by the degree of emotional arousal created by the thought of a disease as well as by the kinds of difficulties the individual believes a given health condition will create for him.[11]

A person may, of course, see a health problem in terms of its medical or clinical consequences. He would thus be concerned with such questions as whether a disease could lead to death, or reduce his physical or mental functioning, or disable him permanently. However, the perceived serious-ness of a condition may, for a given individual, include such broader and more complex implications as the effects of the disease on his job, family life, and social relations. A person may not believe that tuberculosis is medically serious, but may nevertheless believe that its occurrence would be seri-ous by creating important psychological and economic ten-sions within his family.

Perceived benefits of taking action. The acceptance of one's susceptibility to a disease that is believed to be serious provides a force leading to action, but it does not define any particular course of action. The direction of the action is influenced by beliefs regarding the relative effectiveness of known available alternatives in reducing the disease threat. A person's behavior will depend on how beneficial he thinks the various alternatives would be. An alternative is likely to be seen as beneficial if it relates subjectively to the reduc-tion of one's susceptibility to, or seriousness of, an illness. Again, the person's belief about the availability and effec-tiveness of various courses of action determines the course taken.

Perceived barriers to taking action. An individual may believe that a given action will be effective in reducing the threat of disease but at the same time he may see that action as expensive, inconvenient, unpleasant, painful, or upsetting. Such negative aspects of health action arouse conflicting motives of avoidance. Several resolutions of the conflict are possible. If the readiness to act is high and the negative aspects are seen as relatively weak, an appropriate action is likely. If, on the other hand, readiness is low while the potential negative aspects are seen as strong, they function as barriers to action.

Where readiness and perceived barriers to action are great, the conflict is more difficult to resolve. The individual is highly oriented toward acting to reduce the likelihood of the perceived health danger. He is equally highly motivated to avoid action since he sees it as highly unpleasant. Sometimes, alternative actions of nearly equal efficacy may be available. For example, the person who feels threatened by tuberculosis but fears the potential hazards of X-rays, may choose to obtain a tuberculin test for initial screening.

But what can he do if the situation does not provide such alternative means to resolve his conflicts? Experimental evidence obtained outside the health area suggests that one of two reactions occur. First, the person may attempt to remove himself psychologically from the conflict situation by engaging in activities which do not really reduce the threat. Vacillating between choices may be an example. Consider the individual who feels threatened by lung cancer and believes that to stop smoking cigarettes would reduce the risk. But if smoking serves important needs he may constantly commit himself to give up smoking soon and thereby relieve, if only momentarily, the pressure imposed by the discrepancy between the barriers and the perceived benefits. A second possible reaction is a marked increase in fear or anxiety. If the anxiety or fear becomes strong enough, the individual may be rendered incapable of thinking objectively and behaving rationally about the problem. Even if he is subsequently offered a more effective means of handling the situation, he may not accept it simply because he can no longer think constructively about the matter.

Cues to action. The variables that constitute readiness to act (perceived susceptibility and severity), as well as the variables that define perceived benefits and barriers to taking action, have all been subjected to research that will be reviewed subsequently. One additional variable is believed to be necessary to complete the model but it has not been subjected to careful study.

It appears essential to include a factor that serves as a cue or a trigger to set off appropriate action. The level of readiness provides the energy to act, and the perception of benefits (fewer barriers) provides a preferred path of action. However, the combination of these could reach quite considerable levels of intensity without resulting in overt action unless some instigating event sets the process in motion. In the health area, such events or cues may be internal (e.g., perception of bodily states) or external (e.g., interpersonal interactions, the impact of media of communication, knowledge).

The required intensity of a cue that is sufficient to trigger behavior presumably varies with differences in the level of readiness. With relatively low psychological readiness (i.e., little acceptance of susceptibility to, or severity of, a disease) fairly intense stimuli will be needed to trigger a response. On the other hand, with relatively high levels of readiness even slight stimuli may be adequate. For example, other things being equal, the person who barely accepts his susceptibility to tuberculosis will be unlikely to check upon his health until he experiences rather intense symptoms (e.g., spitting blood). At the same time, the person who readily accepts his constant susceptibility to the disease may be spurred into action by the mere sight of a mobile X-ray unit or a relevant poster.

Unfortunately, the settings for most of the research on the model have precluded obtaining an adequate measure of the role of cues. Since the kinds of cues that have been hypothesized may be fleeting and of little intrinsic significance (e.g., a casual view of a poster urging chest X-ray), they may easily be forgotten with the passage of time. An interview taken months or years later could not adequately identify the cues. Freidson has described the difficulties in attempting to assess interpersonal influences as cues.[12] Furthermore, it seems reasonable to expect that respondents who have taken a recommended action in the past will be more likely to remember preceding events as relevant than will respondents who were exposed to the same events but never took the action. These problems make it most difficult to test the role of cues in any retrospective setting. It would seem that a prospective design, perhaps a panel study, will be required to assess properly how various stimuli serve as cues to trigger action in an individual who is psychologically ready to act.

EMPIRICAL EVIDENCE AND THE MODEL

Evidence for the importance of the variables described is considerable. Hochbaum studied more than one thousand adults in an attempt to identify factors underlying the decision to obtain a chest X-ray for the detection of tuberculosis.[13] He tapped beliefs in susceptibility to tuberculosis and beliefs in the benefits of early detection. Perceived susceptibility to tuberculosis contained two elements, the respondent's beliefs about the real possibility of tuberculosis in his case, and the extent of his accepting the fact that one may have tuberculosis in the absence of all symptoms. In the group of persons that exhibited both beliefs (that is, beliefs in their own susceptibility to tuberculosis and in the overall benefits accruing from early detection), 82 percent had had at least one voluntary chest X-ray during a specified period preceding the interview. In the group exhibiting neither of these beliefs, only 21 percent had obtained a voluntary X-ray during the criterion period. It appears that a particular action is a function of the two interacting variables—perceived susceptibility and perceived benefits.

The belief in one's susceptibility to tuberculosis appeared to be the more powerful variable. For the individuals who exhibited this belief without accepting the benefits of early detection, 64 percent had obtained prior voluntary X-rays. Of the individuals accepting the benefits of early detection without accepting their susceptibility to the disease, only 29 percent had had prior voluntary X-rays. Hochbaum failed to show that perceived severity plays a role in the decision-making process. This may be due to the fact that his measures of severity proved not to be sensitive, thus precluding the possibility of obtaining definitive data.

Another study dealt with the conditions under which members of a prepaid dental care plan maintain preventive dental checkups or prophylaxis in the absence of symptoms. [14] While the findings generally support the importance of the model variables, an unusually large loss in the sample limits the general applicability of the study. Within the major limitations implied by a small sample, it was found that with successive increases in the number of beliefs exhibited by respondents from none to all three, the frequency of making preventive dental visits also increased. The actual findings show that (1) of three persons who were low on all three variables none made such preventive visits; (2) 61 percent of 18 who were high on any one variable but low on the other two made such visits; (3) 66 percent of 38 persons high on two beliefs and low on one, made preventive visits; and, finally, (4) 78 percent of 18 persons who were high on all three variables made preventive dental visits.

While none of the studies reviewed provides convincing confirmation for all of the variables, each has produced consistent findings in the predicted direction which, when taken together, provide strong support for the model. The interpretations are based on an assumption. The hypothesis that behavior is determined by a particular constellation of beliefs can only be adequately tested where it is established that the beliefs existed prior to the behavior that they are supposed to determine. However, the studies reviewed have been undertaken in situations that necessitated identifying the beliefs and behavior at the same point in time. The dangers of this approach have always been clear.

Work on cognitive dissonance supported these suspicions and suggested that the decision to accept or reject a health service may in itself modify the individual's perceptions in areas relevant to that health action. [15] Obviously, a two-phase study was needed in which beliefs would be identified at one point in time and behavior measured later.

Such a study was undertaken in the fall of 1957 on the impact of Asian influenza on American community life. [16] Its design called for the first interview to be made before most people had the opportunity to seek vaccination or take other preventive action, and before much influenza-like illness had occurred in the communities; the second interview was to be made after all available evidence indicated that the epidemic had subsided. In fact, only partial success was achieved in satisfying these conditions because community vaccination programs as well as the spread of the epidemic moved much faster than had been anticipated. For these reasons the sample on which the test could be made was reduced to 86. This sample had, at the time of initial interview, neither taken preventive action relative to influenza nor had they experienced influenza-like illness in themselves or in other members of their families. Of the twelve respondents who scored relatively high on a combination of beliefs in their own susceptibility to influenza and the severity of the disease, 5 subsequently made preventive preparations relative to influenza. On the other hand, of the remaining 74 persons (who were unmotivated in the sense of rejecting either their own susceptibility to the disease or its severity, or both), only 8 subsequently made preparations relative to influenza. The data thus suggest that prior beliefs are instrumental in determining subsequent action.

A second prospective study tried to determine whether the beliefs identified during the original study were associated with behavior during the subsequent three-year period. [17] It found that neither perceptions of seriousness, whether considered independently or together with other variables, nor perceptions of benefits, taken alone, were related to subsequent behavior. However, the perception of susceptibility did show a correlation with making subsequent preventive dental visits. Fifty-eight percent of those who had earlier seen themselves as susceptible made subsequent preventive dental visits, but only 42 percent of those who had not accepted their susceptibility made such visits. When beliefs about susceptibility and benefits were combined, a more accurate prediction was possible. Considering only those who scored high on susceptibility, and cross-tabulating against beliefs in benefits, 67 percent of those high on both beliefs made subsequent preventive visits while only 38 percent low in benefits made such visits. The combination of susceptibility and benefits is demonstrably important in predicting behavior.

The results of the studies cited above lend support to the importance of several variables in the model as explanatory or predictive variables. However, another major investigation conflicts in most respects with the findings of earlier studies. [18] This study analyzes the beliefs and behavior of a probability sample of nearly 1,500 American adults studied in 1963 and the subsequent behavior of a 40 percent sub-sample studied fifteen months later. Perceived susceptibility and severity, whether taken singly or in combination, did not account for a major portion of the variance in subsequent preventive and diagnostic behavior, although predictions based on the belief in benefits (and barriers) taken alone was significant. The findings did not disclose any explanation for the failure to obtain results similar to those of the earlier studies, but the national study was conducted in a setting which distinguished it from all the other reported studies. In the earlier studies the settings had been such that the population in each case had been offered opportunity to take action through directed messages and circumstances that could have served as cues to stimulate action. In contrast, no such condition obtained for the national sample. With respect to the several health problems covered in the study, neither the sample nor the United States adult population which it represents had been uniformly exposed to intensive information campaigns about available services.

It is unreasonable to assume that preventive and diagnostic services were equally available to all. It may well be that the absence of clear-cut cues to stimulate action as well as unequal opportunity to act may account in large measure for the failure to replicate the earlier results. However, those possibilities must be treated as hypotheses that need to be tested in new research.

Two recent studies lend further support to the general explanatory model of health behavior although its specific variables have been treated more innovatively than in earlier research. Haefner and Kirscht attempted experimentally to increase people's readiness to follow preventive health practices. Their samples were provided with messages about selected health problems that were intended to increase both their motivation to behave in a professionally recommended manner and their beliefs in the efficacy of such behavior. [19] Significantly more persons exposed to such messages visited a physician for a checkup in the eight months following the experimental manipulation than in a control group not exposed to the messages. This significant difference held only for visits made in the absence of symptoms, i.e., preventive health behavior. For individuals reporting actual symptoms during the interval, the rate of physician visits was the same in the experimental and control group. While income as such was not treated, the sample represented a population of nonacademic university employees, a group above the poverty level but, in general, far from affluent. This study provides evidence that it is possible to modify the perceived threat of disease, that is, the combination of perceived susceptibility to and severity of diseases, as well as the perceived efficacy of professional intervention, and that such modification leads to predictable changes in health behavior.

Becker and his associates have shown that the explanatory model of health behavior, in somewhat modified form, can provide an explanation of illness and sick role behavior. [20] The population studied was a poor, primarily black, group of mothers enrolled in a Children and Youth project serving a large urban ghetto. The subject of study was adherence to a ten-day regimen of oral penicillin prescribed for their sick children. It was noted, first, that a substantial proportion (51 percent) failed to continue the penicillin medication for as long as five days, as detected by urinalysis, but those mothers who exhibited each of the beliefs described earlier were more likely to follow the regimen than those who did not accept the beliefs. Mothers were more likely to follow the regimen of penicillin if they believed that their children were susceptible to reinfection, that the current disease was serious, that medical intervention could reduce disease susceptibility and severity, and if they exhibited a generalized concern for their children's health. Mothers accepting each of these beliefs to a lesser degree were significantly less likely to follow the prescribed regimen.

It seems fair to conclude that while the explanatory model does not provide a complete explanation of health behavior, its elements do help to understand such behavior. Where the applied constellation of beliefs exists, the presence of a situational cue, trigger, or critical incident is likely to trip off the desired response. [21] Where such cues are not present, the individual is presumed to be in a state of readiness without necessarily engaging in the appropriate behavior.

HEALTH BELIEFS AND INCOME

It is appropriate now to turn to the question of the relationship between health beliefs and demographic factors. One study investigated the relationships among the use of Papanicolaou tests, demographic factors, and beliefs in the benefits of early detection of cancer. [22] Beliefs in benefits were measured by responses to questions on the perceived importance of early versus delayed treatment for cancer and on opinions as to whether medical check-ups or tests could detect cancer before the appearance of symptoms. The findings disclosed that personal characteristics and beliefs are highly correlated, with each of them making independent contributions to the understanding of behavior. Tests were much more likely to have been taken by women of higher income, who were relatively young, white, married, well educated, and of higher occupational levels. It was also shown that acceptance of the benefits of early professional detection and treatment was highly associated with having taken the test. However, it is the joint analysis that is of most interest. Within every demographic grouping, those who held a belief in benefits were much more likely to have taken the test than those not holding that belief. Similarly, within each of the categories of belief, those with the appropriate demographic characteristics were much more likely to have taken the action than those who did not. It is clear that the joint effect of the beliefs and the personal characteristics is much greater than the effects of either alone.

Hochbaum's earlier study obtained similar findings. Socioeconomic status (education and income) and the combination of beliefs in susceptibility and benefits were associated independently with having taken voluntary chest X-rays in the absence of symptoms. Within each socioeconomic category, however, those who scored high on the combination of beliefs were much more likely to have taken the X-ray than those scoring low.

An interpretation of the two studies suggests that certain beliefs may be necessary for taking preventive or screening tests, but that they are unevenly distributed in the population and tend to be more prevalent among the higher-income females, the whites, the better educated, and the relatively young. It would thus appear that part of the association between income and the use of free preventive health actions is accounted for by an association between health beliefs and taking health actions. In short, poor people tend to exhibit the necessary constellation of beliefs far less often than people of higher income. Little evidence is available to indicate why this should be so, although a number of variables seem particularly relevant to any effort to account for the findings.

The taking of a preventive or presymptomatic health action on a voluntary, health-motivated basis presumes both knowledge of disease processes and a value for, and interest in, planning for the future. To what extent are these characteristics related to differences in income? It has generally been shown that those with low income possess less information about health and disease than those with high income.[23] Even when educational attainment is controlled, a marked association has been found between income and the possession of correct information about health effects of insect and plant sprays, radioactive fallout, and fatty foods.[24]

Studies of the mass communication media have long demonstrated that those lower on the economic scale fail to obtain health and science information from the mass media to the same extent as do those of higher income, although in terms of exposure the poor attend to health information transmitted via radio and television to about the same extent as the financially better off.[25] The previously established relationships, however, hold for exposure to the print media.[26] In short, nearly all available evidence supports the proposition that knowledge of health matters and exposure to health information is associated with income even when educational attainment is controlled.

There is some evidence that health is more salient to individuals of higher social status than those of lower socioeconomic status. For example, when presented with a list of seventeen medically recognized danger signals, more than three quarters of the highest-class respondents checked all but two as requiring the attention of a doctor, while the lowest socioeconomic group displayed a marked indifference to most signals, with 50 percent checking only three.[27]

Two points warrant attention. First, the salience of health is quite different in the several socioeconomic groups, and, second, the scale of values reflected in the findings may be quite functional. For people at subsistence levels the expenditure of money to ward off disease or check on symptoms that are not disabling may be a luxury that must be foregone in preference to providing food, clothing, and shelter. It cannot be surprising that many people who reported being unable to go to a dentist also owned television sets. Kadushin and Levine question whether health is less salient for the poor than for the rich, but the bulk of evidence supports the conclusion that middle and higher economic groups value health more than those in the lower economic groups.[28]

It has been noted that persons of lower status accord greater priorities to immediate rewards than to the achievement of long-range goals. [29] Yet the system of health beliefs described earlier requires an orientation toward the future, toward planning, and toward deferment of immediate gratification in the interest of long-range goals.

The date concerning salience of health and subjective time horizons are associated with the well-known finding of a high correlation between income and the extent of hospital and surgical insurance coverage. [30] Even with education held constant, the marked correlation between income and insurance status holds; those who need insurance the most, possess it to the least extent. Once again one may ask whether that finding reflects a rather rational assessment on the part of those who must choose between the necessities of today and the contingencies of tomorrow.

The poor are also distinguished from the economically more advantaged by their feelings of helplessness and their psychological inability to cope with a hostile environment. Such feelings tend to characterize the lower-economic group's response to local government and to social welfare.[31]

We do not yet know whether and to what extent the concept of anomie carries over into one's responses to health matters, but it would seem reasonable to expect such a relationship.

A consideration of the institutional settings in which most health actions are taken may throw further light on the association of income and preventive action. It is clear that most preventive actions require the individual to enter into a professional health system. Yet, it has been noted that those lower on the socioeconomic scale are more prone to use a lay referral system than a professional referral system, at least in the early stages of symptomatology.[32] If those of low income who experience symptoms are less likely to go to the physician than to friends and family, and will enter into the professional referral system only when they have exhausted lay remedies, they must be even more reluctant to enter the professional referral system when they are feeling reasonably well.

It would be well to recognize that the professional referral and care systems are middle-class institutions conceived by middle-class planners, oriented toward rationality in health matters, generally staffed by representatives of the middle class and, in the United States at least, involving a system of financial arrangements that are more feasible for the middle class to manage than for the lower classes. It does not seem surprising that members of the non-middle class may be reluctant to enter this foreign world.

Research on health behavior supports the conclusion that a culture of poverty helps to explain the health behavior of the poor. The culture of poverty may originally have been based on a history of economic deprivation, but it seems to be a culture exhibiting its own rationale, and structure, and reflecting a way of life that is transmitted to new generations. It is therefore suggested that while financial costs may serve as barriers to obtaining health services, their removal would probably not have the effect of creating widespread changes in the health behavior of the poor, at least not in the forseeable future. The values for knowledge and for health exhibited by the poor, their tendency to use a shorter time horizon as a framework for planning, their reluctance to use professional referral and service systems, perhaps guided by a general feeling of powerlessness in the face of a hostile environment, all suggest that the problem of altering their behavior will prove to be highly complex and not susceptible of simple remedy.

HEALTH SUPERVISION VISITS

It has been suggested that the rate of health supervision visits, that is, visits to practitioners in the absence of symptoms, is increasing.[33] A question may be raised whether such increases, if indeed they are occurring, show the typical social class gradient, with those of higher income accounting for most of the increase. There are no definitive data on the subject but inferences can be drawn from a combination of findings from several sources. Herman notes, as have many others, that while higher rates of disease and mortality still persist among those with very low incomes, their frequency of visiting the physician is considerably lower than for the more affluent, healthier group. [34] Bergner and Yerby note that even when immunizations are free, higher-income families show a much better rate of protection than do poorer families.[35] It has also been noted that while ambulatory services show a lower utilization rate by lower-income households, poor people are overrepresented among hospital patients; their hospitalization rates are as high as, or higher than, those of upper income levels and their length of stay is longer on the average.[36] This probably reflects their failure to receive treatment at earlier stages of disease and disability.

Moreover, the National Health Survey shows that reported willingness to come to a health examination, if the time and place are convenient, is associated with a variety of demographic characteristics.[37] The lowest and highest income groups express somewhat less willingness to come for an examination than those in the middle-income groups (between $2,000 and $6,699 per year). However, the same study also shows that those with chronic conditions are substantially more likely to indicate willingness than those without such conditions, and it has already been shown that the poor are more likely to have such chronic conditions. Therefore, the reluctance of the group with incomes under $2,000 to come for examinations is probably underestimated by the grouped data.

There is also a sharp income gradient in the number of visits mothers make to physicians in the twelve months prior to birth—progressively higher percentages making such visits with increasing income.[38] The same sort of gradient appears when visits to dentists are considered, a common indicator of preventive health behavior. While some of these data are not as recent as one would like, there seems to be no reason for concluding that the poor, as yet, are showing any marked increase in their likelihood of seeking early health care relative either to their prior behavior, or to the behavior of the more affluent. This is not to say that the removal of economic and social barriers will not increase the use of health services; indeed, they may well do so. In an experiment reported by Alpert et al. it was shown that after exposure to comprehensive, personalized health care, low-income families (i.e., median income of $4,100) became more satisfied with the services received, reported an increased likelihood of using a family doctor or pediatrician for selected medical problems of children and reported a greater likelihood of using the telephone as a first contact.[39] Nevertheless, it is still questionable whether such attitudinal changes will result in patterns of use of health services that are like those of the more affluent.

A report of Colombo et al. appears at first glance to conflict with the major conclusion drawn thus far.[40] In 1967 a poverty group, supported by the Office of Economic Opportunity, was admitted into the Portland Region of the Kaiser Foundation. During a period of nearly a year of observation their use of medical services (3.9 encounters per person) was remarkably close to that of a sample of the overall health plan membership (4.1 encounters per person) and, with minor exceptions, the nature of the visits was quite similar, as indicated by the most frequent diagnoses made by physicians. The authors conclude that a strong emphasis on preventive care exists both in the general health plan population and in the OEO population. The basis for this important conclusion warrants detailed examination.

A close examination of both the methods of selecting the poor families into the plan and the mode of analysis casts some doubt on the conclusion that the poor do in fact exhibit a strong emphasis on preventive care. The target area specified "was composed of neighborhoods that had a majority of families who were not defined as poor. These areas contained approximately 4,000 poor families." In short, the poor population selected represented a minority of the residents of the neighborhoods from which they were drawn. The authors also indicate that since many of the neighbors of the poor families selected were already members of the Kaiser Foundation the program was already familiar to the indigent residents. We do not know whether the desire for, and utilization of, health services by poor, urban people living in predominantly non-poor neighborhoods are typical of the nation's poverty population. No information is available on the prior utilization rates of the poor families.

Furthermore, since only 1,200 of the 4,000 identified poor families could be served, a number of selection priorities were imposed of which the two most important were (1) large families with small children; and (2) families with known acute health problems but with no existing medical care source. One wonders whether these selection priorities did not almost guarantee greater utilization of services than had all 4,000 poor families been included.

Selection priorities to include those in greatest need are quite sensible in terms of health need, but the procedure casts doubt on the comparability of the OEO group with a random sample of the total health plan membership. If the random sample of health plan membership included persons less in need, then their slight superiority over the OEO population in total patient encounters masks a tendency for the general population to seek preventive services much more frequently than the poverty population. It is reasonable to believe that this is so when one views comparative national figures on patient encounters. The National Health Survey for 1966-67 shows that children under six years of age in households having incomes of below $5,000 made an average of 4.2 visits to a physician per year while in households with $5,000 or more annual income, the number of visits was 5.9.[41] In the Portland Kaiser study, children under six, from OEO families, had 4.2 encounters with physicians while in the general membership the number of such encounters was 6.1. Colombo et al. report a utilization rate of well-baby and child care of 235.1 per thousand for the OEO population and only 159.3 per thousand for the general health plan membership. These figures, however, are misleading: there were nearly twice as many children under six in the OEO population as in the general health plan membership. Taking this discrepancy into account, one might have anticipated a utilization rate in the OEO population for well-child care of more than 300 per thousand.

The authors also present data on utilization of immuniza-tions which apparently shows substantially more utilization by the OEO population than by the health plan member-ship. Once again these conclusions are derived from total patient encounters without allowing for the overweighting of children in the OEO group. Since the four immunizations reported are primarily intended for those under six years of age, the data were recomputed not in terms of total en-counters but using as the denominator the total number of children under age six in each of the two groups. When that is done, the immunization experience of the two groups is virtually identical. However, since it is reasonable to believe that the OEO population had received insufficient medical care prior to their enrollment in the Kaiser plan, if finances and organization were all important one might have ex-pected a much higher rate of immunization among the poverty group than in the health plan membership whose children had been seen more or less regularly during the period preceding the study.

It should also be noted that the Kaiser organization, initially anticipating that preventive medical care utilization in the young age groups would not be readily generated in this population, developed a staff of neighborhood health coordinators whose task was to stimulate the OEO group to bring their children in for care. Despite this activity, which was regarded as successful, the OEO group probably did not make such preventive visits as frequently as the more af-fluent, when differences in the numbers of children are taken into account and when the apparently greater need in the OEO population is considered.

In summary, the one detailed report that purports to show that utilization rates of health services by poor people increases to the levels of the non-poor under proper organi-zational and prepayment patterns, is unconvincing. In fact, reexamination and reinterpretation of the data and the sampling procedures lead to the conclusion that improved delivery and payment mechanisms—however desirable and necessary they may be for the poor—do not result in the extent of preventive health behavior exhibited by the more affluent.

SOME GENERAL CONSIDERATIONS

It would be too simple to conclude that increasing the utilization of health services by the sick poor would not affect their use of preventive health services. Each time the physician, the nurse, or other practitioner meets with a client, whatever the presenting complaints may be, an opportunity for primary or secondary prevention is offered. A return visit by a child who has been treated for otitis media may provide an opportunity for bringing his immunizations up to date. The treatment of an acute condition in an adult may provide the opportunity for a more comprehensive assessment of his health status. Once the client enters the delivery system, if treated with respect and dignity, he is susceptible to preventive and assessment procedures for which he would not have presented himself in the absence of the symptom.

The main burden of this chapter is not, therefore, to deny the important role played by the financial and organizational arrangements for health services delivery but rather to emphasize that even under the most ideal circumstances such arrangements cannot be expected to influence directly the motivation to take action to ward off future disease or to detect asymptomatic disease.

There is much knowledge about the health behavior of the poor and the non-poor that can be stated with confidence and there is much that is still unknown. Among those items that may now be regarded as factual are the following:

1. There is a marked association between income level and the proportion of persons seeking preventive or diagnostic health services in the absence of symptoms.

2. The observed association remains statistically significant, although it is much less marked in connection with toothbrushing, an action that is both relatively inexpensive and can be undertaken without entry into a professional referral system.

3. There is a marked association between income and the possession of correct knowledge about a wide variety of health-related matters.

4. There is a marked association between income and the extent of beliefs in the efficacy of alternative procedures for preventing or controlling various health conditions.

5. Behavior of the poor may be in part attributable to their beliefs about their susceptibility to, and the severity of, various health conditions and the perceived benefits of taking associated professional health action.

6. The associations between income and behavior and between income and knowledge are related to but are not wholly explained by educational attainment.

7. The professional referral and health system tends to be used relatively infrequently by those low on the economic scale for prevention and health maintenance; the preference seems to be for a lay referral system.

8. The removal of financial and organizational barriers to health care probably increases the use of health services by the poor, but the mere removal of such barriers probably does not create widespread changes in the orientation and behavior of the poor regarding prevention and early detection of illness.

Evidence supports the concept of a culture of poverty with its own structure, rationale, and values. However, any effort to explain the dimensions of the culture of poverty as it relates to health matters must currently be based on less certain knowledge than that demonstrating the existence of such a culture. Even more hypothetical must be any explanation of why that culture contains specific characteristics and how an intervention may modify it in a professionally desired direction. Among the issues that need to be resolved are those concerning the extent to which health behavior, knowledge, and attitude are explainable by such factors as subjective time horizons, values for rationality and planning, feelings of powerlessness, salience of health, and the extent to which such factors overlap.

VI. The Help-Seeking Behavior of the Poor

by John B. McKinlay

The literature on poverty, illness, and medical care is replete with examples of the "established" inverse relationship between social class (or various related indicators of socioeconomic status) and indices of health status. This inverse relationship is held to apply to almost the entire range of medical pathology—whether chronic or acute illness, mental disorders, accidents, or infant and maternal morbidity.[1] A comparable situation is thought to exist when one considers social pathology such as marital instability, unemployment, overcrowding, delinquency, and other social problems. The more intensively one investigates the relatively deprived, or any other social category for that matter, the higher the apparent prevalence of seriously debilitating and often uncared for medical and social pathology. To make a sharp distinction between medical and social pathologies is misleading, since in terms of the etiology and perpetuation of a problem, one may sustain the other. In order to intervene effectively in any particular problem, therefore, it may be necessary to intervene simultaneously on several other causally related fronts.

The seriousness of the present situation of the poor is

John B. McKinlay is Associate Professor, Department of Sociology, College of Liberal Arts, Boston University.

well documented by a recent study of welfare recipients in New York City.[2] This longitudinal investigation in the Yorkville welfare district revealed a phenomenal prevalence of organic disease among the adults studied (five diagnoses per project patient)—a far higher rate than had been found in other surveys of similar populations. An especially high rate of psychiatric illness was also reported. Furthermore, two thirds of the children were found to have health problems at the time of entry to the project. Interestingly, it was found that those studied were unlikely to see a doctor when feeling unwell and tended not to visit a doctor unnecessarily. It is suggested that the same kind of clinical profile or "illness iceberg" would be uncovered in a similar study of a comparable group in other cities in the United States, and indeed in other Western countries. There are no grounds in either the design or analysis of this study to suggest that these results are bizarre or atypical, although the high estimated rates of morbidity may be attributed to either the use of more refined, and therefore more sensitive measures, or to the possibility that the health status of the poor is deteriorating. Both explanations are equally plausible. In a useful study of 1,450 white male applicants for Social Security disability benefits from three regions of the United States, McBroom concluded that there was no evidence to indicate that individuals in this sample, characterized as of lowest socioeconomic status, either experience higher illness levels, as rated by physicians, or report greater functional or social limitations because of their disorders. [3]

The nature of the relationship of socioeconomic status to health has recently been further explored by Pratt in a careful survey study of a New Jersey city.[4] She was concerned to investigate *how* socioeconomic position affects health, particularly the mechanism by which poverty may adversely influence health status, and concluded that one adverse mechanism is a deficient pattern of personal health care, which includes deficiencies in personal health maintenance practices, use of medical services, health knowledge, and health supportive equipment in the home. It was in the use of specialized and preventive medical services that the low-income women were especially deficient when compared to women of higher income. No clear or consistent relationship was found between socioeconomic status and the use of medical services for illness. The studies by McBroom and Pratt represent noteworthy attempts to move beyond the restatement of, and debate on, what can be reasonably regarded as the "established" relationship between poverty and illness.

To date there have been few attempts to specify in any detail the various processes, stages, and types of decisions made by the poor while seeking some form of medical care.[5] Zola suggests that the few studies available in this area suffer from several major limitations. Individuals who do or do not make particular decisions are described, not *how* health decisions are made, and this description is usually retrospective, concerning people who have already judged themselves in need of some form of care and have undergone treatment. Furthermore, presenting symptomatology is usually taken as given, and attention is not directed at the variations that are known to exist in their perception and tolerance.[6] These rather specific criticisms draw attention to two more general limitations. First, much of the work in this area appears concerned with *individual* decision making, ignoring the important influence of social structural factors like, for example, the structure and composition of the decision maker's kin and friendship networks. Second, researchers tend to concentrate on *the decision* to seek care, rather than on the *process of seeking* care.

The notion of a career, which has proven useful in other areas may overcome some of these limitations.[7] This approach orders material in a natural sequence corresponding to the various stages that may be typically passed through by individuals experiencing a sickness episode. Against a backdrop of the distribution and definition of health, illness, and medical care in society, the individual may typically pass through a process of symptom recognition, lay referral, self-medication, and adoption of the sick role to what can be loosely termed "formal" therapeutic encounters. Such a career approach forms the underlying framework for this chapter, and appears to hold considerable potential for understanding the help-seeking behavior of the poor, although it still requires conceptual refinement and, at many points, further empirical investigation.

Before proceeding further, an important distinction should be drawn between levels of health status and utilization behavior. It is often assumed, implicitly or explicitly, that utilization behavior is a fairly accurate reflection of the nature and distribution of pathology in a community. This stems from the naive view of man which suggests that people, in the area of health at least, nearly always act on the basis of self-recognized, role-impairing symptoms. Accordingly, any general increase in utilization must result from some increase in morbidity in the community, and any decrease is a consequence of some overall improvement in health status. Such simplistic associations serve to disguise the complexities of the real situation. Here, four general situations will be considered:

1. The case where there is *no* alteration in health status but *some* alteration in utilization behavior.

2. The case where there is *some* alteration in health status but *no* alteration in utilization behavior.

3. The case where there is *no* alteration in health status and *no* alteration in utilization behavior.

4. The case where there is *some* alteration in health status and *some* alteration in utilization behavior.*

If, as appears to be the case, the poor do experience lower levels of health status than other groups occupying different positions in the social structure, why do they appear to underutilize or misuse certain services to which they are supposedly entitled? Or, to put it another way, why do health status and utilization behavior seem to be unrelated for the poor?

HOW IMPORTANT ARE SYMPTOMS?

Researchers are unsure about the importance of symptoms in the process of seeking help. Some hold that most people act on the basis of any symptom, and that the more serious and visible the symptom, the more probable that some form of utilization will result. Mechanic, for example, has suggested that "much of the behavior of sick persons is a *direct* product of the specific symptoms they experience; their intensity, the quality of discomfort they cause, their persistence and the like." Elsewhere, he asserts "that probably the most important determinant of care seeking is the character of the symptoms themselves."[8]

A body of data appears to support this view that symptoms are primary determinants of help-seeking behavior. For example, Suchman's study of the health behavior of persons in the Washington Heights community of New York provides some evidence of the apparent influence of symptomatology.[9] He selected a subsample of 137 adults

---

*The term *alteration* is used here to denote either improvement or deterioration in the case of health status, and either some increase or decrease in the case of utilization behavior.

(2.5 percent of his initial sample of 5,340) who had, within the two months prior to the interview, experienced some relatively serious illness that had required more than three visits to a doctor and had either incapacitated or hospitalized the person. Pain was found to be the most important signal that something was wrong, and was referred to by two thirds of the subsample. Fever and chills (reported by 17 percent) and shortness of breath (10 percent) appeared less important. A clear majority located the cause of the symptoms in some illness. There can be no doubt that many symptoms leave the afflicted person with little alternative but to recognize that he or she is ill, and that some formal medical care is required. Of course, the examples that Mechanic cites (temperature of 105 degrees, fractured leg, broken back, *severe* heart attack, *extreme* psychosis) could hardly be overlooked and the requisite help-seeking behavior avoided.[10] However, the proportion of symptoms of this severity is small—possibly 5 percent at the very most. Many people, probably the majority, never experience any of these life-endangering events, but they do experience many nondisabling illnesses and symptomatic episodes.* It is to these that attention should be primarily directed; while it may be true that social factors are less important in the infrequent, *extreme* situations, they may not be in the case of nondisabling symptomatology.

An alternative view of the importance of symptoms in

---

*It has been estimated, for example, that the average lower-middle-class male between the ages of twenty and forty-five experiences over a twenty-year period approximately one life-endangering illness, twenty disabling illnesses, two hundred nondisabling illnesses and one thousand symptomatic episodes. These total 1,221 episodes over 7305 days, or one new episode every six days. See L. E. Hinkle, Jr. et al., "An Examination of the Relation between Symptoms, Disibility and Serious Illness in Two Homogeneous Groups of Men and Women," *American Journal of Public Health,* 50 (September 1960), 1327-1336, cited by I. K. Zola, "Culture and Symptoms: An Analysis of Patients Presenting Complaints," *American Sociological Review,* 31 (October 1966), 615-630.

seeking help emphasizes the role of certain mediating factors—events and situations that intervene between the symptoms and help-seeking behavior. These events and situations may also constitute the context within which symptoms arise, and may determine the relative importance, the visibility, and the anticipated consequences of the symptoms. Such issues, rather than the symptom itself, determine if and when some help-seeking action should be taken.

Many studies support this latter interpretation. The now famous "Peckham Experiment" provides an illustrative example of both the pervasiveness and frequent meaninglessness of symptoms for many people.[11] Calling illness "the presence of clinical entities," as determined by a professional diagnostician, it was found on a sample of roughly 4,000 adults and children that 91 percent had come physiological defect or aberration. Additionally, of those who had a diagnosed disorder and also spoke of discomfort with it, only 50 percent were under formal medical care. Neither the nature of the disorder nor its seriousness determined who was under treatment. Every type and seriousness of illness was uncovered in the group—composed entirely of people who were unaware of or disregarded their symptoms. In another equally well-known study, Koos demonstrated wide social class variations in the recognition of symptoms requiring medical attention.[12] The differences in the proportions recognizing symptoms between the higher social classes (I and II) and the lower class (III) have been described in many places.

Starting with the premise (supported by a survey of the literature) that most people have symptoms constantly and contunuously that might be interpreted by health professionals as relevant to disease, Zola suggests that the particular symptoms group, that are acted upon by any person are those defined by his culture, ethnic group, or reference group as relevant for action.[13] In comparison of sixty-three Italian and eighty-one Irish patients who presented themselves at clinics at the Massachusetts General Hospital, he found that four times as many complaints from the Irish population concerned the eye, ear, nose, or throat than all other parts of the body combined, compared with only half of the complaints from the Italian population. Further, only one third of the Irish patients indicated pain as part of their presenting symptoms, in contrast to over half of the Italian patients. About 60 percent of the Irish patients presented problems of a specific nature, while 70 percent of the problems presented by the Italian group were quite diffuse. Zola further attempted to delineate five "triggers," or mediating factors in the patients' decisions to seek medical care.[14] He found, for example, that "interpersonal crisis" and "social interference" were used more often by Italians, while "sanctioning" was the predominant trigger for the Irish. The Anglo-Saxon group, he reports, responded most frequently to the "nature and quality of their symptoms."

This thesis that situational and/or cultural mediatory factors determine the influence that symptoms have on seeking help gains additional support from studies in the area of mental illness. The study by Eaton and Weil of the tolerance of deviance within Hutterite communities provides a useful illustration.[15] Prior to the study it was thought that the prevalence of mental illness was lower in the Hutterite subculture than among comparable groups of non-Hutterites. It was subsequently found, however, that the actual prevalence of mental disorder was, in fact, no different from that in comparable groups, but that its visibility to outsiders was masked by mediating factors in the Hutterite subculture. Other studies of mental illness have also demonstrated this tendency, to normalize neurotic and psychotic symptoms.[16]

A recent study by Ludwig and Gibson of the self-perception of sickness and the seeking of medical care further reinforces the view that the importance of symptoms in seeking help may be situationally or culturally specific.[17] It was shown that the failure to seek care was associated with difficult situational factors, such as low income, experience with welfare, and lack of faith in the medical care system, rather than with symptoms, as used in the study. The authors conclude that: "Particular symptoms, combinations of symptoms and number of symptoms were not found to be related to the seeking of care, but the situational factors remained so regardless of number of symptoms."[18]

The relative importance of symptoms and social factors can be illustrated from a research experience among pregnant, lower-working-class women in Aberdeen, Scotland.[19] For example, for a woman to take some action on a real or potential symptom, she must not only feel threatened by the symptom, but also see at least one course open to her which she thinks may remove it, or reduce the likelihood of its occurence. Both of these dimensions, however, require knowledge which, in the case of many women of low socioeconomic status (who are known to be at higher risk to pregnancy wastage), is unlikely to be available. Furthermore, it is quite possible that it is not the absence of motives which causes the underutilization of services by the poor, but the presence of more patent or salient motives which result in deflected behavior. For example, there is now a considerable amount of evidence showing that, in low socioeconomic groups, motivation arises predominantly from the need to merely exist, and current life crises tend to override any consideration of future health or welfare.[20] This point will be returned to and discussed in greater detail below. Many women seem to display "satisfactory" health behavior, even when health-related motives and worrisome symptoms are not in existence as far as they are concerned.

Evidence from Aberdeen suggests that some lower-working-class parturient women attend for prenatal care only in order to reserve a bed for confinement or to receive various maternity benefits. Sometimes these women, after receiving certain benefits (or the necessary forms for application), are not seen again until they are admitted to the hospital in labor. It is suggested that such behavior indicates a defective understanding of, and/or a lack of sympathy with, the rationale behind preventive prenatal preparation.

In general, therefore, symptoms appear as neither necessary nor sufficient conditions for help-seeking behavior. When we say a symptom acts as a *necessary condition* for help seeking, we do not intend that there is a "necessary connection" between symptoms and help seeking, although we sometimes say that for people to seek some form of care, symptoms must be experienced. For example, in the absence of certain symptoms or states, help seeking may not be relevant (in the absence of a pregnancy one cannot obtain an abortion). The presence of a symptom or condition, however, can in no sense be regarded as a *logically necessary condition* for help seeking; indeed, extensive research has shown that other factors may precipitate help seeking in the apparent absence of symptoms. Symptoms may be regarded as sufficient conditions for the occurrence of help seeking if, invariably, whenever symptoms arise, help seeking results. However, symptoms or conditions may be regarded as sufficient conditions only in those relatively few extreme circumstances cited by Mechanic.

MEDIATORY FACTORS

A Hierarchy of Needs

Some needs and symptoms are not universally obvious and immediate, and behavior often emerges out of a conflict among motives and alternative courses of action. The need to cope with symptoms, even though recognized, may be overriden by more pressing issues. This notion of a hierarchy of competing needs enables us to distinguish between the help seeking of the affluent and of the poor. It seems that much of the social life of the former concerns needs that are perceived as below issues of health and illness on a hierarchy of need. Should some morbid episode present itself, it assumes a priority position which eclipses most other needs for action. In contrast, much of the social life of the poor concerns needs that are perceived as being above most issues of health and illness on the need hierarchy (e.g., unemployment, homelessness, marital disruption, lack of amenities). Should some episode present itself, it assumes a position of relatively low priority and is eclipsed, perhaps indefinitely, by basic subsistence needs. This notion of a need hierarchy makes the well-known statement of one of Koos's respondents more intelligible:

> I wish I could get it fixed up [prolapsed uterus] but we've just got some other things that are more important first. Our car's a wreck, and we're going to get another one. We need a radio, too, and some other things . . . But it's got to wait for now—there's always something more important.[21]

Interference with Routine

A second mediatory factor is the extent to which presenting symptoms interfere with meaningful social life. In a study of how people define illness, Apple has shown that interference with everyday activities was one of the major criteria used by laymen to define illness.[22] Generally speaking, symptoms that are socially disruptive are more likely to be defined as worthy of some kind of lay or professional attention. Here it is the social disruption caused by the symptoms, and not the symptoms themselves, that precipitate social action. Moreover, certain symptoms or conditions are likely to be differentially disruptive in different social categories. Among professional people, for example, psychiatric symptoms (e.g., verbal incapacity, inability to conceptualize, lack of concentration, memory difficulties) are likely to be immediately detected by both the afflicted and their peers since much of professional life requires a high level of functioning in these areas. Generally speaking, such functioning does not appear as important in the everyday life of those in lower socioeconomic categories; symptoms in these areas may therefore be overlooked, or disregarded, since they are unlikely to be as disruptive in their consequences. Among manual workers, certain physical symptoms, conditions or accidents (e.g., backache, sprained arm, laceration, etc.) may be more disruptive of social life, especially employment, than among nonmanual office workers.

The importance of presenting symptoms may vary according to the life styles, occupational activities, and social expectations associated with different social categories. What is regarded as serious and debilitating in one category may be only minor and bothersome in another. Moreover, the ability to "explain" the presence of some symptom or condition probably varies among different social categories. People who undertake heavy physical work requiring lifting and carrying are more likely to interpret backache as merely a result of their job than as a possibly serious illness. By contrast, clerical workers, by perhaps being unable to "explain" the presence of backache in terms of everyday social activity, may become more fearful of the symptom, and respond quite differently.

Accessibility of Medical Care

The nature and accessibility of the medical care system in different societies is a third mediatory factor. There is evidence, for example, that physicians vary in their recognition of what symptoms are appropriate for their professional attention.[23] Presumably, they make their individual preferences known to patients—especially to the poor, who may be seen as presenting disproportionately more so-called trivia—with certain consequences for subsequent help-seeking behavior. Koos has observed that there is a fairly strong feeling on the part of poor people that physicians do not want them as patients. [24] It seems that general practitioners in Great Britain retain their patients for a longer period of time, and probably socialize their patients to some extent into not presenting certain complaints. In the United States, by contrast, where patients generally consult a physician for a shorter period of time, such socialization may not occur. Of course, the role of professionals in regulating the presentation of symptoms is probably also counterbalanced by the nationalized system that exists in Great Britain and the predominant fee-for-service arrangements in the United States. Mechanic has stated that a high proportion of his sample of British general practitioners reported "having too many patients who present trivial or inappropriate complaints."[25] One wonders whether a comparable situation exists in the United States, where patients usually have to pay for any services rendered. In general, it would appear that whether or not symptoms are acted upon is also dependent both on the system of medical care and payment arrangements that exist, and on the behavior of physicians in relation to patients.

It is often difficult for the poor in particular to evaluate the possible danger of certain symptoms and conditions, and consequently, in an effort to reduce the probability of danger, they decide in favor of a professional consultation with certain results for subsequent physician-patient interaction.[26] The operation of this process is rather vividly portrayed in the following extract from an interview conducted with a father on welfare in Great Britain:

> I phoned him [physician] at ten to six. He says "take the child up," well it was a cold night. I said, "I'm not taken him out on a night like this, you'd better come down and see the kid," I says. "He's awfully sick or I wouldn't phone you" ... Ten minutes to twelve he comes into the house. Takes his dog for a piss and comes into the house. His first words, he went over to the bed, "This is gettin' beyond a bloody joke!" He says, "You told me the baby was seriously ill and needs medical attention." "I'm not a doctor, I don't know what's wrong. I phoned you because I thought it was an emergency, otherwise I wouldn't have phoned you." He yattered away a lot about medical stuff and all that patter, big long doctor words ... He looked at me and said, "It's the last time I come to this house."[27]

Changing Patterns of Health Problems

There has clearly been a dramatic decline in the incidence of acute illnesses with their attendant, relatively clear-cut symptomatology. With such illnesses, certain symptoms (e.g., congestion, fever,) may, in the past, have constituted sufficient conditions for help-seeking behavior. These illnesses have now been or are being superseded by predominantly chronic conditions with a slow insidious onset, whose symptoms are generally neither clear-cut, dramatic, nor even visible. While symptoms probably played some role in the past with the relatively clear-cut acute episodes, their role in the future may be of a quite different order. For the reasons discussed above, the poor in particular tend to overlook or appear to disregard quite serious symptoms of acute disease, even while sometimes verbalizing discomfort. It is possible that even greater difficulties will be experienced by physicians and health educators in the future when they request the poor to "look for" the less obvious symptoms of chronic illness—symptoms of which the poor are unaware.

LAY REFERRAL AND SELF-MEDICATION

Once the presence of symptoms or a need for some form of care is acknowledged, several courses of action are possible, some of which may be pursued almost simultaneously. A person may resort to home remedies of proven success in the past, discuss the symptom with relatives and/or friends who may have experienced comparable problems, consult some formally recognized professional, or refrain from any overt social action in the hope that the symptom or condition will either disappear or perhaps make itself more apparent (and publicly understandable). It is at this point, that one appears to "negotiate" with significant others over what possible label should be applied, how severe the episode is, what form of help-seeking behavior may be appropriate, and at what point it should be taken. It may also be at this point, before the possible adoption of a sick role, that one is most receptive to information from health educators and the interventive efforts of health agencies. During this phase of informal negotiation people with role-impairing symptoms are probably most receptive to suggestions regarding culturally appropriate alternatives of action. Once some specific course of action has been decided upon, or, in Becker's terms, a "commitment" has been made and validated by and with others in the lay referral system, it may be some time before an alternative course can be seriously entertained. [28]

The process of lay referral and acts of self-medicating are

seldom separate and do not necessarily occur in the order in which they have been described. While Freidson, Mechanic, and Coe, among others, appear to give primacy to self-medication in the career of seeking formal care, it is doubtful that they would wish to suggest that this sequence is ever the immutable order of events.[29] The precise sequence presumably varies with the situation, and is affected by such factors as the experiential background of the person or category of people involved, the proximity of informal lay resources, and the perceived nature and severity of the symptoms. It is quite possible that several courses of action may be pursued almost simultaneously, with different effects on subsequent utilization behavior

The known tendency for people in poverty to resort to self-medication may in part be due to lack of "knowledge" (that is, medically accepted knowledge), a general alienation from official health agencies and professionals, and, in some countries, the high and ever-increasing costs of medical care.[30] It may be part of the traditional subculture of the poor to use lay resources and to self-medicate at the beginning of an illness. Another explanation may lie in the tendency for lower-class individuals to think of and describe their illness experience with somewhat antiquated and simple mechanistic notions of the body, which are the subject of exploitation by patent medicine advertisements. Certainly, the poor do appear to entertain a conception of the body as a kind of elaborate plumbing system, to be occasionally "flushed out," "unblocked," or "cleansed" as the need arises.[31] This conception is probably reflected in the use of patent laxatives, liver and kidney tablets, and the so-called blood cleaners. Rosenblatt and Suchman have suggested that for the poor:

The body can be seen as simply another class of objects to be worn out but not repaired. It is as though the white collar class think of the body as a machine to be preserved and kept in perfect functioning condition, whether through prosthetic devices, rehabilitation, cosmetic surgery, or perpetual treatment, whereas blue collar groups think of the body as having a limited span of utility; to be enjoyed in youth and then to suffer with and to endure stoically with age and decrepitude.[32]

Such conceptions, and the self-treatment they foster in the lower socioeconomic groups, seemingly contribute to the delay in the presentation of symptoms for formal treatment, with perhaps the consequence that they are eventually declared in some more advanced and often nonreversible form.

The fragmented, inaccessible, and relatively expensive system of medical care in this country is another possible reason for self-medication among the poor. Such people tend to seek alternative lay forms of care, or prescribe for themselves, with a reasonable probability of success. Under a nationalized ("free") medical care system, such as that in Great Britain and New Zealand, there is thought to be more accessibility to professional advice; thus, one would expect a corresponding decrease in the consumption of patent medicines. A survey in Britain has established that, under the National Health Service, self-medication is not, on the whole, used as an alternative to consulting a physician. [33] One wonders whether, after a period of time, such a situation would arise in the United States, following some radical reorganization of the structure and financing of medical care, since in this country self-medication probably does constitute an alternative to "formal" medical care, particularly in the early stages of an illness.

Members of one's kin and friendship networks exert a

considerable influence on the social visibility of some illnesses, as well as on the process of deciding on what and when care should be sought. Various investigators have found that people with visible health and welfare needs, and their significant others, are often reluctant to recognize symptoms or conditions as pathology and instead invoke "normalizing" explanations to account for the problem. [34] In his study in New York City, Suchman found that three quarters of his respondents reported discussing their symptoms with some other person (most often a relative) before seeking formal medical care. Zola has included the influence of others ("the presence of sanctioning") as a key trigger in a person's decision to seek medical care.[35]

Further evidence suggests that the influence of the lay referral system may be more important among the poor than among any other social category.[36] It has been suggested that this influence is intensified by the network cohesiveness of the poor and by a strongly localized character—kin and friends living together, often for several decades in a local area, with little experience of the outside world.[37] Freidson comments: "Dependent for advice on a localized, fairly cohesive group, the lower class sufferer is unlikely to be encouraged or aided in the seeking of types of professional care that are unfamiliar to that group."[38] Given the general lack of financial and other external resources among the poor, relatives and friends may be especially important as a kind of informal "mutual insurance system."[39] The apparent importance of relatives and friends for the poor probably results in greater dependence on them in time of need (which, by definition, is most likely to be most of the time) and perhaps, as a consequence, some delay in using formal resources or agencies outside the immediate social network.

While it may be truistic to emphasize the influence of the

family and its kinship and friendship network on the help-seeking careers of the poor, there have been remarkably few attempts to specify or investigate empirically the nature of this influence. Freidson has provided some of the most systematic descriptions of the importance of the diagnostic resources of relatives, friends, neighbors, and workmates, while seeking some form of care. He argues that

> "the whole process of seeking help involves a network of potential consultants from the intimate and informal confines of the nuclear family through successively more select distant and authoritative laymen until the 'professional' is reached. This network of consultants, which is part of the structure of the local lay community, and which imposes form on the seeking of help, might be called the 'lay referral structure.' Taken together with the cultural understandings involved in the process we may speak of it as the 'lay referral system.'"[40]

Freidson goes on to descriptively classify lay referral systems using two characteristics, and it is at this point that his conceptualization appears clearly relevant to this discussion of the help-seeking behavior of the poor. The two variables are (1) the *degree of congruence* between the culture of the clientele and that of the "formal" healer (the author would prefer to employ the concept "subculture" in the first context); and (2) the *relative number of lay consultants* who are interposed between the first perception of symptoms or need, and the decision to see a "formal" healer. Cultural considerations affect the relevance of the diagnosis and prescriptions to the client, as well as the kind of consultants he considers authoritative. The extensiveness of the lay referral structure is relevant to the channeling and reinforcement of lay culture, and to the salience of "outside" communication.

These two variables—the content and the structure of the system—are used to create a typology of lay referral systems that may predict the rates of utilization of professional services.[41] Freidson conceives of the process of lay referral as a hierarchical information-seeking process through which one moves from the less to the more informed and experienced, and beyond that to the formal medical care system.

Despite Freidson's attempts to clarify the structures and processes that serve to structure and regulate help-seeking behavior, very little reliable empirical work has been conducted in this area. A number of unanswered and often unformulated questions arise when attention is turned to the possible role of the family and associated social networks in the use of health and social welfare services by the poor. Is it possible to detect intrafamily patterns of utilization behavior? Are there certain conditions or episodes in which social-network members play a more important role in defining, consulting, and referring, while other conditions involve noticeably fewer members? Does the geographical proximity of the family, as well as related kin and friends, affect the nature of its influence on utilization behavior? Are kin and friends more important determinants of service utilization than other variables like social class, religion, ethnic group, or even geographic location? Do social network factors play a more influential role in utilization behavior when only certain age groups are involved, or at different points in the family cycle? Is family involvement in any way related to the particular type of agency being utilized? Does the family in any way affect the efficacy of care after a service has been utilized? Does the age structure of the family and its associated networks influence the quality and content of the advice received?

A recent study of the organization of health and social welfare services and their use by lower-working-class families in Aberdeen, Scotland, included an attempt to delineate the apparent role of the family and its kin and friendship networks in the seeking of maternity care. A sample of eighty-seven women, divided into two subgroups according to their utilization of prenatal services, displayed noteworthy differences between utilizers and underutilizers. [42] More underutilizers had relatives and older "family" friends living in the same house and, when their presence was controlled for, underutilizers still had more relatives and friends living close, geographically. Furthermore, it appeared that the utilizers—whether multiparous or primiparous—visited with relatives less frequently than did the underutilizers. When they did interact with relatives, they tended to do so at the relative's house, not their own. The primiparous utilizers, despite the fact that they lived so close to relatives as their underutilizing counterparts, more frequently visited contemporary friends who lived at a considerable distance. The multiparous utilizers lived further away from their family of origin, and close to their friends who were of comparable age. It is possible that such factors as distance and frequency of contact were partly a function of the housing situation, but they may also have reflected an independence from their relatives on the part of utilizers, particularly for the primiparae. Further, it was possible that in some instances the mother (the relative most often visited) was less available because either she, the respondent, or both, were working— a factor that perhaps also indicated independence.

Interesting differences also emerged from questions relating to lay consultation and lay referral for various hypothetical but commonly occurring problem situations. It appeared that utilizers made greater use of friends and husbands and less use of mothers or other relatives and tended to consult a narrower range of lay consultants. These findings appeared consistent with, and perhaps reinforce, the differences in network structure already noted. Underutilizers appeared to rely more on a variety of readily available relatives and friends as lay consultants. In other words, it was possible that there was only one large interlocking network within which underutilizing respondents obtained the greater part of their advice. Utilizers, on the other hand, appeared to have separate or differentiated kin and friendship networks. This suggested a lack of reliance on relatives on the part of the utilizers, but there was no evidence in the data that kin lay consultation was replaced to any large extent by friendship lay consultation. Utilizers appeared to be relatively independent of both kin and friends, and frequently took no prior lay advice at all from the members of their networks, or consulted only their husbands.

To return to Freidson's formulation, it would appear that the underutilizers, with readily available relatives and friends and interlocking network sectors, could be regarded as located within an indigenous, extended lay referral system. On the other hand, utilizers, with relatively inaccessible or unavailable kin (and sometimes friends) and with clearly differentiated social networks, could be regarded as located within an indigenous truncated lay referral system. In a study of the social networks of some London families, Bott reports:

When many of the people a person knows interact with one another—that is, when the person's social network is *closeknit*—the members of his network tend to reach consensus on norms, and they exert consistent informal pressure on one another to conform to the norms, to keep in touch with one another, and if need be, to help one another . . . but when most of the people a person knows do not interact with one another, that is, when his network is *looseknit,* more variation on norms is likely to develop in the network and social control and mutual assistance will be more fragmented and less consistent.[43]

This statement, clearly relevant to the present discussion, suggests that individuals with proximous, close-knit and interlocking social networks (often the case with the poor) will be likely to display greater conformity with the behavior and prescriptions of their significant others than will individuals with relatively inaccessible, loose-knit, differentiated social networks who may display conformity with, or take a positive orientation to, nonmembership groups and employ them as a frame of reference. This may also imply that the latter group would be more amenable to health education programs and professional intervention.

The findings of the Aberdeen study are manifestly important with regard to the influence of social networks as agencies of social control. First, if underutilizers belong to interlocking kin and friendship networks, then they are likely to be confronted with similar values, norms, and attitudes from both, because members of both will be likely to interact independently of the individual's presence. Utilizers, on the other hand, with differentiated networks (the members of which do not interact independently of the individual's presence) will receive varying advice from different sectors—advice open to rejection or acceptance. In general, therefore, it seems that the structure of social networks and the availability of relatives and friends are differentially important in terms of social control and the ability to negotiate over possible alternatives of action.[44]

The relative importance of social networks as agencies of social control is also likely to differ among the poor depending upon their particular social circumstances. The under-utilizers in the Aberdeen study were frequently economically dependent through the desertion or imprisonment of a husband, relied on relatives for child-minding, or were dependent on relatives or friends to provide accommodation. [45] In these circumstances some norm of reciprocity may have been in operation whereby these respondents felt obligated to conform in certain respects to the expectations of the members of their networks.[46] Utilizers, in contrast, having their own council house or private, self-contained accommodation, a stable employment pattern, and an intact marriage, did not appear to be (at least overtly) under the same obligation to relatives and friends and were perhaps freer to pursue a somewhat independent existence regarding lay advice and decisions.

What, then, are the consequences for the help-seeking behavior of the poor of having an extended lay referral system readily available either in the same house or in the immediate neighborhood? First, lay consultation for them may be immediate, and this availability may encourage protracted lay referral (being referred from one lay consultant to another), whereas a somewhat attenuated lay referral structure could encourage a bypassing of lay consultants because of the greater efforts involved in seeking their advice.

A second consequence of the availability of a lay referral system may be an obligation to remain well and not claim exemptions provided by a sick or patient role.[47] Some researchers have suggested that the households of those in poverty are often understaffed because of, among other things, overcrowded accommodation, large numbers of young children, and the tendency to take in elderly parents.[48] It may be that understaffing, combined with the various obligations associated with subletting, child-minding and economic dependence, causes many in poverty to think twice before consulting (either lay or professional) on some presenting problem, and thereby setting off a train of events that could result in the inconvenient legitimation of a sick or patient role.

A third consequence of having an available lay referral system may be that a presenting problem is likely to be evaluated in relation to a wide range of problems being experienced by others in the household or in the immediate neighborhood. The imposing problems of readily available others may result in the relegation of certain personal problems to a position of low priority.

At a number of points in the preceding discussion of the Aberdeen study, attention was drawn to differences in *who* respondents thought they would consult in their lay referral system if some fairly commonplace problem arose. These differences may be of considerable importance insofar as they affect the nature and quality of the advice obtained. Of course, as has been observed, who one consults is largely determined by the nature and severity of presenting problems. Nevertheless, different lay consultants are likely to perceive problems differently and, as a consequence, give divergent advice. For example, it is reasonable to assume that a young woman's mother will more likely have had previous experience of the problem in question, or will at least have heard of others who have experienced it. This problem will, therefore, most probably have its place in an unconscious hierarchy of problems, experienced by the mother, and will be evaluated against this knowledge. Consequently, the importance of the presenting problem or condition may be devalued, or perhaps attention may be drawn to some other problem unrecognized by the daughter. In this way, the consulting of relatively experienced mothers may result in delayed service utilization. On the other hand, husbands, if consulted, may advise immediate action because, having no experience on which to base a judgment, they may inflate the likelihood of danger.[49]

A factor that must be considered in relation to who is consulted is the age structure of the lay referral system, since the age of lay consultants may exert some influence independent of who is consulted, assuming that knowledge of the alternatives of action will vary with age. Older lay consultants may not be aware of the current alternatives, unavailable when they experienced the same or a comparable problem in their youth. Because, in the absence of such an alternative they may have consulted a pharmacist or some other semiprofessional, they may, in their unawareness of presently available alternatives, recommend a similar but outmoded action, resulting either in delay or inadequate care.

Deciding when "formal" consultation should take place may also be affected by the structure and accessibility of the lay referral system. It may be that people of high socioeconomic status, having a less extensive lay referral structure, present problems to professionals and agencies earlier than do the poor, who may typically have a more extensive indigenous lay referral system. This prompt consultation may be supported by both subcultural congruence with professionals, a lower need hierarchy, and a greater sensitivity to the "scientific meaning" of presenting symptoms and conditions. The delay by the poor in seeking help may be partly a result of subcultural disparity with professionals, the presence of more imposing problems, and the extensiveness of their lay referral system.

Lay consultation and self-medication do not necessarily occur in a unidirectional sense (i.e., *before* formal utilization). Freidson in one sense allows for this possibility when he reports that a person "passes through the referral structure not only on his way to the physician but also on his way back: discussing the doctor's behavior, diagnosis and prescription with his fellows with the possible consequence that he may never go back."[50]

HOW THE POOR USE SERVICES

So far the utilization of lay resources by the poor has been discussed, with particular attention to such aspects of the prepatient career as the importance of presenting symptomatology, self-medication, and the process of lay referral and lay consultation. Selected aspects of the utilization of formal medical care and social welfare resources will now be considered.

There is extensive debate over how the poor actually use organized medical facilities. Some observers maintain that they overuse these services and are therefore unfairly subsidized by the rest of the community. Still others suggest that the utilization behavior of the poor is little different from that of other social groups. A majority claim that those categorized as "in poverty" consistently underutilize services, never receiving the full benefits to which they are entitled. Despite the plethora of work in this area, there have been remarkably few attempts to coordinate findings, or to attempt to account for apparent disparities. These inconsistencies are due partly to varying methodologies, partly to differing medical care systems, partly to the different time periods under study, and partly to the rhetorics of interpretation. These research limitations should be highlighted briefly before proceeding further. Of course, it is not suggested that every study of the utilization behavior of the poor contains at least one of the limitations to be discussed, or that any one study contains all of them. The problems to be outlined simply occur with high frequency, in most of the studies to date.

One serious limitation of much of the empirical work relates to the manner in which the population studied is first sampled. A common strategy has been to investigate the characteristics of residents of a particular area or city in relation to some utilization behavior. More frequently, studies are only concerned with behavior in relation to selected agencies, such as general practitioner services, hospitals or emergency rooms, prenatal care clinics, or family planning facilities. Little is gained, however, from the practice of identifying certain groups who seemingly underutilize one particular agency, and comparing them with groups who appear to utilize the one under immediate investigation while ignoring the utilization behavior of these groups with respect to other services. From such studies inference is severely restricted by either the specificity of the population itself, the service selected for investigation, or both. Although it is well known that people in poverty tend to underutilize (or even overutilize) some specific medical and social welfare services, these findings are extrapolated to embrace the whole spectrum of service-orientated facilities. With a naive disregard for variations in the perception and organization of services, some researchers persist in generalizing findings from one service (or a subset of services) to the entire range.

A second difficulty with past studies stems from the fact that they are nearly always retrospective, and focus on the behavior of people and groups who have already initiated formal medical care, have utilized a particular service, and have undergone treatment or received some benefit. In such emotionally charged areas as health and welfare one would think it difficult for respondents to recall accurately minute aspects of their behavior over relatively lengthy periods of time. Further, the distortion that may result from such cross-sectional data is implied in a finding of the longitudinal New York study referred to earlier which showed that, in a cohort of cases newly accepted on welfare, less than half would be on welfare continuously.[51]

A third methodological limitation relates to the sources of the data usually employed in utilization studies. It is common for definitions and measurements to be specific to certain types of data. Most utilization data are derived from use of the following three principal sources: physicians' records, hospital, clinic or insurance records, and direct personal interviews or questionnaires in social surveys. Each source has its own unique advantages and limitations, and some of these have been recently reviewed by Fink.[52] Whatever the source of the data, it is important to distinguish between the true nonutilizers and those classified as nonutilizers because there is no record of medical service. Too often we are likely to find so-called underutilizers using medical services outside the formal health care system or, in the case of insurance records, receiving services for which no claim is made or required. For example, seldom is information provided on the consulting of medical practitioners by telephone; yet these contacts for physicians in the United States have been estimated to equal in number all physician contacts in the hospital.[53] Official statistics and physician records are, of course, more vulnerable to errors of ommission than are sample surveys. Samples focus attention on the patient and not on the health facility or practitioner, and therefore may probe utilization behavior outside the formal medical care system.[54] Certainly it is important that future studies of utilization behavior be related to the total population having access to a system or facility, and not only to the actual users of the system or facility.

An illustration of several of the different types of technical shortcomings found in many studies of utilization behavior is provided in a recent report by Rein, not primarily concerned with the utilization behavior of the poor, but with demonstrating that under the British National Health Service the poor receive care comparable to that received by the rest of the British population.[55]

To this end, the author considered simple rates of utilization (number of visits or discharges) of general practitioner and inpatient hospital services only. Findings were then extrapolated to the full range of services provided under the National Health Service (including prenatal and postnatal maternity, family planning, outpatient, emergency, and dental services, as well as child care clinics). No real attention was given to the reasons for utilization beyond brief mention of the different types of diagnoses made by the general practitioner, for different social classes, and the longer average hospital stay for the poor in Scotland. Furthermore, little attempt was made to offer possible explanations of class differences in the use of the general practitioner by children, or for the class differences in mental hospital admission rates, both of which were mentioned. Finally, the author used apparently contradictory findings on the rates of inpatient hospital discharges by social class (for different populations in time and space) to infer that (1) the poor appear to be increasingly overusing hospital services; and (2) there is no discrimination against the poor in the use or quality of hospital services. In other words, very limited data from a variety of temporally and spacially different populations, employing gross measurement, have provided the basis for general, far-reaching, and logically unacceptable inferences. From such an inadequate study it is as incautious for Rein to assert no relationship between social class and the use of health services as Mechanic claims it is for Kadushin to hold that there is no relationship between social class and illness.

There are several disquieting limitations in much of the available literature. These are not so much strictly methodological or technical deficiencies, as they are. . . .questionable value orientations for supposedly objective scientists. For a long time now, sociologists and psychologists who have been interested in utilization behavior have ascribed culpability for underutilization or overutilization, whatever those terms denote, to the poor. Such people have been labeled "neglectful," "irresponsible," "parochial," "distrustful," and "downright ignorant." Some accumulating evidence suggests that researchers may be moving away from this individualism, and a new set of terms (or refurbished old ones) have been filtering into the utilization literature to characterize underutilizers: "The new poor," "multi-problem families," the "new working class," "unstable families," "the culture of poverty," "indigent," the "culturally deprived." All such terms imply that something more than income is lacking in a nonutilizing group and that these groups are somehow culpable. By adopting such a perspective, researchers have tended to deemphasize the social structural determinants of help seeking, such as the organization and availability of services and cost (emotional and financial), and have disproportionately highlighted the personal and/or social pathologies of the poor. It is possible to argue that, as a consequence, social scientists have played the role of midwife during the birth of much of the present-day punitive welfare legislation. While they have not actually designed and administered this legislation, they have, through certain findings and concepts, facilitated its delivery. Coser has shown how researchers often unwillingly espouse a status quo ideology and fail to consider the unanticipated consequences of their "liberal" theorizing.[56]

Perhaps it is understandable that policymakers and health administrators, among others, ascribe culpability to potential consumers for the failure of programs. Unfortunately, blaming "unmotivated clients," "unreachables," or "the indigent" does not take one very far. Perhaps it does more harm than good. Tannenbaum, Cressey, Kitsuse, Erikson, and Becker, working in the area of the sociology of deviance, have all suggested that the process of labeling an offender and making him conscious of himself as a deviant may evoke the very behavior that is thought to be inappropriate.[57] Merton, although concerned with a different type of problem, has described such a process as a "self-fulfilling prophecy." Lemert has coined the phrase "secondary deviation" to draw attention to the possibility that an offender may act in an even more extreme fashion as a consequence of the definition and labeling of his behavior. Such subsequent behavior, according to labeling or societal reaction theorists, may be substantially similar to the original primary deviance, but has as its source the actor's revised self-conception, as well as the revised conception of him in the community.[58]

At present, the concept of a culture of poverty is enjoying popularity as both an explanation of behavior and as a description of the life styles of the poor. Considering the increasing ubiquity of its application, there have been few attempts to examine the logical status of the concept and some of the problems posed when it is employed.[59] Sociologists subscribe to two explanations of the way subcultures, or cultures of poverty, emerge in any social system. Some use the concept to refer to a process of intergenerational transmission—a system of values and norms that existed prior to and is external to individuals—through which life styles are passed on during socialization. Others view the emergence of subcultures in more structural terms and use the concept to refer to current behavioral responses to situational expediencies.

Although the issue forming the basis of these divergent perspectives may appear at first glance somewhat recondite, this is not so. As Valentine points out, both the social philosophy and the strategy of intervention to help a so-called problem subculture become radically different depending on whether their behavior is seen as subculturally transmitted, or whether it is viewed as a response to current situational factors.[60] In the first instance, the problem becomes one of attempting to modify the behavior of the people associated with the subculture; in the second, the solution must be sought in a basic reform of existing structural arrangements, perhaps of society as a whole. Jaffe and Polgar in a provocative paper have questioned the intergenerational transmission view on the grounds that it dominates the thinking of many professionals and is employed by them to rationalize slow progress. [61]

Given the worrisome trends in the provision of services for the poor, especially in the United States, and the use of social science concepts either to perpetuate the status quo or justify lack of intervention or inactivity, it surely must be timely for researchers to reappraise the effects of their involvement. Specifically, it may now be prudent for concerned researchers to consider seriously Becker's question: "Whose side are we on?"[62] Even by assuming (or claiming) neutrality, we may be reinforcing the very inequalities and injustices whose bases we seek to uncover.

In general, researchers appear to have been preoccupied with only identifying and labeling individual characteristics, revealing the traditional preoccupation of the planners and administrators of services (and perhaps of society in general) with the personal pathologies of underutilizers and showing very little concern with the organizational characteristics of the services which people under- or overutilize. In the light of developments in organization theory, these are important omissions, since it is now clear that *organizational phenomena may be as highly related to utilization behavior as the personal characteristics of users.*[63] A number of factors have fostered this growing concern with organizational impedimenta to utilization. They include (1) a growing body of theoretical knowledge regarding organizational structure and processes; (2) evidence from independent studies regarding life styles of the poor and the ways in which they influence utilization behavior; (3) an awareness, mainly through the failure of intervention projects and health education campaigns, of the resilience of, and the difficulties in changing, the knowledge, attitudes, and modes of behavior of the poor; (4) recognition of the fact that far from being random or idiosyncratic, the knowledge, attitudes and life styles of the poor can be viewed as consistent and understandable responses to problems associated with their position in the social structure and life chances.[64] Recognition of this last factor has fostered the view that attempts to alter life styles without also altering social structure and life chances may do more harm than good. Schneiderman makes this point well when he suggests that: "resistance to the influence of middle class professionals is, in such a context, a sign of health, an effort to protect personal integrity by people who may sense a future no different from their present or their past, and who feel their life style and hence their survival, to be threatened by helpers who invite them to adopt a completely irrelevant, nonfunctional, middle class life style."[65] Schneiderman is suggesting that the underutilization of certain services by a subgroup of society, say the poor, may be "healthy" behavior for members of that social category.

No one can doubt that we have witnessed over the last

twenty years a considerable expansion and improvement of health and welfare services. Some of these advances are manifest in the often dramatic annual improvements in some mortality and morbidity statistics. Almost without exception, however, these improvements have involved increased bureaucratization, the erosion of an individualistic, person-oriented service, and have necessitated much more knowledge and organizational sophistication if one is to obtain the medical care to which one is entitled.

More emphasis is being given to the efficient use of outpatient or ambulatory services; an increased proportion of mothers are discouraged from domiciliary confinements and are hospitalized for delivery; the beginnings of the rationalization of primary medical care services is evident in the widespread movement into partnerships and group practices. The vigorous, usually well-intentioned and influential neighborhood and community health center crusade, when viewed in relation to organizational developments in other services, can be seen as a logical extension of postwar developments in medical provision. Various preventive services are growing alongside and reinforcing the predominantly curative facilities. Almost all of these recently developed services, from family planning clinics and mass radiography campaigns to cervical cytology screening, and well-baby or child health and welfare clinics, are organized in a more or less bureaucratic fashion.

Bureaucratization in the field of health and welfare is, of course, not developing in a vacuum. It is occurring alongside, and is probably being reinforced by a more general trend toward impersonality and formalism in the political, occupational, educational, and economic spheres. No one would argue that there are not good administrative reasons for bureaucratizing medical and social welfare care. Some observers suggest that these developments are a natural concomitant of professional differentiation and specialization. Others maintain that these trends are desirable on the grounds of cost efficiency and manpower savings. One may also argue for the preferability of these developments, either on the grounds of greater availability of high-cost technical equipment and specialized personnel, or the possibility of shifting rapidly from one treatment situation to another. Without in any way deprecating the importance of these arguments, and perhaps despite them, one may still ask if this has to be the "natural order of things," or if it has to be the only way in which health and welfare services can be organized.

Researchers studying lower-class life styles and certain aspects of formal organizations have produced a body of evidence suggesting that not all subgroups of society have an equal facility with, and the requisite expertise for performing effectively in, various types of formal organizations.[66] As yet, however, hardly any of this material (some over a decade old) appears to be used in social planning and service administration. It is now clear that the middle class has a not inconsiderable advantage over the poor in the fields of medical care and social welfare, as long as services are presented in an almost uniform and exclusively bureaucratic fashion. Several reasons have been given for the relatively advantaged position of the middle class:

1. The basic assumptions underlying the structure of health and welfare services (e.g. rationality, future orientation) are often reported as being congruent with the values and life styles of the middle class. There is, therefore, only a very slight gap between the cultural and organizational rationale of the health and welfare system, and the culture of its middle-class recipients.[67]

2. Because health and welfare service employees are generally middle class in origin, there is only minimal

status-sensitivity during an encounter between them and middle-class recipients.[68] Moreover, middle-class personnel are best able to understand those problems which are peculiar to the middle class.[69]

3. Middle-class socialization patterns provide individuals with a role repertoire which enables them quite easily to adopt the role of listener, to understand and tolerate the object orientation of officials, and to nullify the effects of any status distance during an encounter.[70]

4. Such socialization, combined with middle-class educational advantages, provides a general facility with form-filling and fosters the ability to verbalize feelings, attitudes, and "need." [71]

5. The middle class is more likely to respond to health education campaigns and intervention programs which, it is often claimed, tend to be biased in their favor.[72]

The poor, feeling estranged from and apparently lacking the requisite expertise in bureaucratic settings, tend to opt for the more personal and individualistic forms of medical care discussed earlier. They seek and apparently prefer the more personal, continuous and noncoercive care of kin and friends, corner druggists and semiprofessionals. It is quite possible that the use of lay health resources by the poor is, to some extent, also a reaction against bureaucratic developments in formal health and welfare resources. This reaction, of course, while serving to insulate the poor from impersonalization and frustration, would further widen and reinforce their alienation from the very care to which they are entitled.

Not only has there been an emerging emphasis on the manner in which organizational factors can influence the utilization behavior of the poor, but increasingly attention is being focused on the role of the professions in shaping health and welfare policy and practice.[73] Some view professional associations, particularly those of the medical profession, as responsible bodies concerned about improvements in the provision of services for those in need. Others, however, regard them as obscurantist-entrepreneurial elites, impeding major social reform by acting so as to enhance the social position of their members. It has recently been argued, without evidence, that one reason members of the medical profession view with concern much of the proposed health insurance legislation is that, under such a system, the power of the profession would be diminished, and their activities somewhat curtailed.[74]

Increasingly, clients are challenging the autonomy and competence of professionals in the fields of health and welfare, and in other areas of social life. Referring to what they term "the revolt of the client," Haug and Sussman discuss some of the ways in which this challenge is occurring.[75] They, along with others, point out that one of the characteristics of a profession is autonomy (the right to determine work activity on the basis of professional judgment) and that this is challenged by clients on one or more of the following four grounds:

1. The expertise of practitioners is thought to be inadequate.

2. Their claims of altruism are thought to be unfounded.

3. The organizational delivery system supporting their authority is thought to be defective and insufficient.

4. The system is thought, in a sense, to be too efficient and exceeds the appropriate bounds of its power.

The "client revolt" is against the delivery systems, as controlled by the professionals, and against the encroachment of professional authority into areas unreleated to their claimed expertise, rather than against the professionals themselves. Without in any way deprecating the importance or perceptivity of Haug and Sussman's case, their work seems to apply more to health and welfare in the future than to the present situation.

Types of Services and Utilization Behavior

It was pointed out earlier that researchers tend either to reach contradictory conclusions by studying different services, without always recognizing the differences, or to generalize findings from one service. By taking into consideration the differing types or predominant orientation of services one may begin to plot a "utilization" profile for the poor from the results of a number of separate studies. From such a review it appears that this social category tends to utilize services with a selectivity that is primarily a function of the need (or needs) fulfilled by a particular service. Such findings, in both Great Britain and the United States, have led to the development of a continuum of service orientation, to facilitate a classification of health and welfare services.

The three main types of service evolved are survival (emergency), curative (treatment), and preventive.* The first category includes such services as emergency rooms and welfare facilities. The second includes such primary medical care services as general practice and dental facilities. The third embraces immunization and screening programs as well as maternity care (pre- and postnatal), well-baby or child welfare clinics, and family planning services. It is recognized, of course, in making this broad classification, that some of these services can be classified under different

---

*It is, of course, recognized that this distinction is similar to the traditional distinction in social medicine between preventive, curative, and rehabilitation services. The distinction presented in this chapter appears to the author to facilitate more subtle differentiation and affords a general framework for the subsequent discussion. In the interest of clarity in the present discussion, rehabilitation services have been omitted. In terms of the typology to be presented, they may be regarded as an extension of those services with a predominantly curative orientation.

headings in particular situations. This applies particularly to a number of the curative services, which can be regarded as in transition between the extremes of emergency and prevention. In Great Britain, for example, general practitioners may be consulted both in an emergency and with respect to immunization or family planning. The present categorization, however, is based on the predominant function of the service, or its principal orientation, in the belief that this will provide a meaningful baseline for understanding the utilization behavior of the poor.

There is, of course, a close relationship between the above classification of services and the immediacy of the need (whether real or perceived to be so) for which the service is designed to cater. Furthermore, it is suggested that the presence or absence of such a need will largely determine utilization behavior. For example, while the majority of those in poverty never attend for or receive taxation rebates, one cannot automatically maintain that such a group is underutilizing taxation or internal revenue departments. As is well known, most in this social category are either chronically unemployed, or underemployed, and therefore do not or seldom qualify for taxation rebates. In contrast, the same chronically unemployed or underemployed groups will, of economic necessity, probably utilize welfare departments in the United States, whereas another, more stable and fully employed group will underutilize the same services through absence of any need to do so. Using the same argument, if someone breaks a leg, or experiences a severe heart attack, he or she would most probably utilize an emergency (survival) service, given such an immediate and obvious need to do so. The same individual, however, may or may not perceive the need for either a regular medical checkup or immunization.

Some needs, however, are not so universally obvious and immediate. Many needs are differentially perceived and may be given varying priority, depending on situational and cultural factors. For example, some may perceive a chronic cough as needing attention, while others may consider it as a hazard of living, not worthy of any medical attention at all. Another possibility, dependent on the acknowledgment of an actual or perceived need, is that utilization behavior could be affected by the manner in which services are delivered to clients and the appropriateness or "goodness of fit" between services and the values, norms, beliefs, and life styles of the subgroups of society for which they cater. Some needs, perceived or actual, may be recognized as important enough for attention from, say, a social welfare service, and yet the form in which that service is presented may be perceived as so abhorrent or debilitating that it is underutilized. Or, where there exists a choice of services catering for the same need, one service may be preferred above others because of the form in which this particular service is delivered.

Chart VI-1 represents an attempt to highlight the need and service specificity of the utilization behavior of the poor. The poor are typically high utilizers of survival or emergency services, that they use curative services secondarily, and seldom encounter preventive services. The thickness of the arrows is intended to depict these patterns. By contrast, the middle class, for example, would be typically high utilizers of curative services, secondarily utilizers of preventive services, and seldom encounter emergency or survival services.*

*Evidence is accumulating that the poor in the United States are increasingly using emergency rooms for a variety of conditions, not all of which are regarded as emergencies. This tendency may be partly attributable to the inadequacy of primary medical care facilities (curative) in the United States as well as to features of some health insurance which inadequately covers this kind of accessibility under the National Health Service, the poor are more frequent utilizers of these curative services. See J. S. Roth, "Utilization of the Hospital Emergency Department," *Journal of Health and Social Behavior,* 12 (December 1971) 312-320.

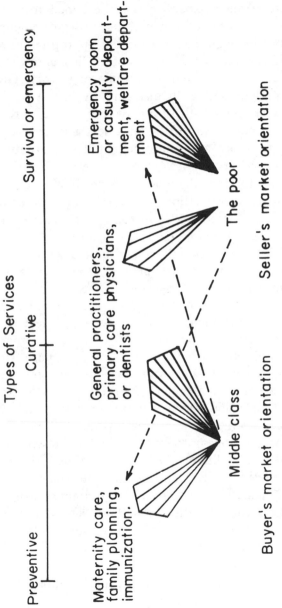

Chart VI-1. Predominant service orientations and the typical utilization pattern of two social categories

An interesting perspective may be added to this discussion of needs, types of services, and utilization behavior by examining, in economic terms, the appropriateness or inappropriateness of certain forms of medical and welfare care organization for selected subgroups of society. Given the relative neglect and even disregard by health and welfare professionals and institutions of the needs, wishes, and demands of potential health consumers who are poor, one is tempted to draw an economic parallel and define some health and welfare services as operative in a seller's market. In such a situation, demand exceeds supply and it is the seller who is in a position to determine prices, conditions, and services. This contrasts with a buyer's market, in which supply exceeds demand and sellers have to be consumer-oriented in order to sell to consumers who are able to choose between many similar types of services being offered. Since health and welfare services appear to operate mainly in a seller's market, they are primarily oriented toward the fulfillment of some need, medical or social, often irrespective of the consumer's demand. Perhaps planners and administrators could borrow a page from the marketing textbooks and seek to determine the extent to which a seller's or a buyer's market obtains in particular areas of health and social welfare. In particular, attention should be given to the increasing number of preventive services which appear to operate at the present time predominantly in a buyer's market. Obviously, in a buyer's market, considerable attention must be paid to techniques for encouraging people to purchase an item and/or to retain loyalty to it. Most health and welfare "needs" can eventually be established by some objective criteria, but if the need is not translated into a "demand" for services, the "sale" has not very much chance of being made. Market researchers are known to be very astute in mobilizing clients, or generating previously unrecognized demands for goods and services, and, with suitable caution, some of their techniques may be worthy of emulation.

Past research on the utilization of services has clearly left many important questions unanswered. For example: Do so-called underutilizers underutilize the whole spectrum of health and welfare services, or, as it has been suggested, only selected services? If the latter is the case, which services are these, and under what circumstances are they utilized and/or underutilized? Is a differential rate of utilization of certain services by the poor linked with the differential presence or absence of some need, actual or perceived? When (or if) the same need is presented to other social categories, do they show a pattern of use similar to that of poor? When the poor make use of a predominantly preventive service, is it for the same reasons as other social categories? It can be hypothesized that only when the primary, immediate problems of survival are under control—housing, income, marriage, and son on—is there an opportunity to consider future needs and to use preventive services accordingly.

In the recent Aberdeen study, repeated interviews of respondents concerning their use of a range of services, divided into the three predominant service orientations (survival, curative, preventive), attempted to shed some light on these questions. In terms of actual utilization behavior, there were clear differences between the two study groups in the use of preventive services other than the originally sampled prenatal care. A clear majority of the utilizers (94 percent) attended for their postnatal checkup and took the baby promptly and regularly to the well-baby clinic (or an equivalent). Only a small proportion of the underutilizers (24 percent) attended for a postnatal checkup, however, and the women of this group tended to take the baby for routine care later, and less regularly, a sizable proportion (36 percent) not taking the baby for a checkup at all. The reasons given for this behavior were, naturally, quite different between the two study groups, but remarkably similar for the different services. The utilizers generally felt that there were benefits to be gained in the use of these preventive services, but were unable to articulate them clearly. The underutilizers expressed either indifference—perceiving no real need to use the service—or were negative in their attitude, feeling that use of the service might result in more harm than good.

With regard to the somewhat transitional curative services, the differences were not so marked. The facilities considered were the Ministry of Social Security (which administered a variety of routine benefits), dentists, and general practitioners. Regarding the first of these services, 31 percent of the underutilizers had attended more than three times in the preceding year, compared with only 14 percent of utilizers. The reasons for using this service underlined this difference: more underutilizers attended regularly for sickness benefits while utilizers attended only periodically for child or maternity benefits, which were not so urgently needed.

A marked difference was observed in the use of dentists. Fifty-three percent of the underutilizers had never visited a dentist, compared with only 8 percent of the utilizers. Of those who had seen a dentist, the last visit was for a routine checkup in only 18 percent of the former group and 33 percent of the latter. The remainder in both groups required mainly urgent treatment. The overriding reason for nonattendance—even when the respondents perceived that treatment was required—was given as fear. There was no apparent difference between the groups in the frequency of use of the general practitioner. However, the *reasons* for use showed considerable disparity. Sixty-six percent of the underutilizers last consulted their doctor concerning some acute or chronic illness, while 48 percent of the utilizers went last for a preventive check-up, only 30 percent consulting for acute or chronic illness. The attitudes toward this service were also quite different. Underutilizers viewed the doctor almost exclusively as a curative service—and then only when the need was urgent, while over 40 percent of the utilizers viewed the doctor as a potential preventive service.

The use of survival or emergency services, at the other extreme of the continuum, again showed marked differences between the two groups. The Supplementary Benefits Commission (which dispenses basic public assistance) was used within the preceding three months by a third of the underutilizers and only one utilizer. Moreover, a clear majority of the latter group had never been (72 percent), compared with only 17 percent of underutilizers. An almost identical pattern of use was apparent for the use of the Employment Exchange (at which unemployment benefits were collected.) Both services are designed to meet immediate financial need.

The underutilizers represent, as described elsewhere in detail, the really poor families of Aberdeen City.[76] They live a *crisis* existence, with ever-present major problems of housing, finance, marriage, and sickness. This is reflected in their almost exclusive use of urgently needed curative and/or survival services. In comparison, the need for preventive services is perceived as negligible, or nonexistent, and is clearly outweighed by needs for survival. In other words, it can be hypothesized that, only when the primary, immediate problems of survival are under control—when housing, income, and marriage are stable—is there an opportunity to consider future needs and to use preventive services accordingly.

Discussion in this final section has so far been concerned with organizational developments in the provision of medical care and social welfare, and with the emergence of an associated, relatively new perspective in the explanation of utilization behavior. The poor, perhaps more than any other category, are likely to be relatively deprived or disadvantaged by the presence of a highly bureaucratized system. The question immediately arises: Does it really matter whether the poor are estranged from, and underutilize, many of the formal health and welfare services to which they are entitled?

Recently, sociological research—mainly within a political context—has been concerned with the development of a theory of mass society. Very briefly, this theory holds that the destruction of the old community has separated the individual from binding social ties and that his isolation produces a sense of powerlessness that can be both personally devastating and destructive of democratic processes. The theory consists of a historically oriented account of contemporary social structure; a set of statements about the present and emerging alienative effects of that structure; and derived predictions about some possible behavioral consequences. One of the major protagonists of this viewpoint, Kornhauser, claims that "meaningful and effective participation in the larger society requires a structure of groups intermediate between the family and the nation. Without such groups the individual cannot readily perceive himself 'as having the capacity to determine his life and to effect the lives of others.[77] Understandably, this hypothesis concerning the functions of organizations has received some criticism. It has been charged with romanticizing the free industrial order; with underemphasising the emancipating features of the supposed new order; with falsifying the extent of contemporary isolation; and with disguising an ideology about society as a description of it. In a recent empirical study of this organizational mediation hypothesis it was stated that these criticisms have not damaged the alienative notion embodied in the theory, because they have not examined directly the presumed alienative consequences of the lack of organizations, serving as the "dependable structure for mobilizing political opinion and action."[78]

It is clear that there is still considerable debate over the thesis of a mass society, and the plausibility of some of its assumptions and implications. Some theorists subscribe to the view that, far from functioning as mediating forces allowing individual expression and control, giant organizations are simply agencies for further alienation. C. Wright Mills espoused this view when, of one type of organization he wrote: "Voluntary associations . . . have lost their grip on the individual. As more people are drawn into the political arena, these associations become mass in scale, and as the power of the individual becomes more dependent upon such mass associations, they are less accessible to the individual's influence."[79]

While the debate on the viability of the mass society thesis proceeds, some evidence has emerged that lends support to the view that membership in a work-based organization is associated with a relatively strong sense of control over events, and that the higher powerlessness of the un-organized worker is not simply a function of his socio-economic status.[80] Although the findings of this study appear relatively conclusive, attention is drawn to the problem of causal imputation. One would like to know whether participation in organizations reduces alienation or whether only the nonalienated participate in organizations whose sssential purpose is to exercise control over certain spheres of life. If the former interpretation is correct, then it becomes clear that the estrangement of the poor from formal organizations can be regarded as a serious disadvantage. The trend toward increasing bureaucratization, not only in health and welfare but also in the economic, occupational, and educational spheres, must result in further systematic exclusion and alienation of those in poverty from the mainstream of social life. These statements are perhaps a little extreme for some, but their plausibility is often argued by social political theorists. Of course, their viability depends in part on the plausibility of the mass society thesis. As yet, insufficient empirical evidence has been gathered with which to make a judgment.

Perhaps in a utopian sense it is possible to maintain that the necessity to utilize particular services will decrease as medical knowledge and technology expand and general living standards improve. Maybe it is true that changing patterns of disease and social pathology will eventually mean that fewer people in poverty will require medical and social welfare care in the future, and that the services which have already been established will increasingly be directed to ever-diminishing residual problems. Set against this possibility, however, increasing industrialization and automation may continue to reduce the availability of adequate employment for the poor, who are without the requisite skills. Changes in family structure, stemming from rising divorce, separation, and desertion, and illegitmacy rates may result (if present trends continue) in more families headed by women, who have generally lower incomes than father-supported families. Accelerated residential mobility and migration from rural to urban areas may add to this general social disorganization. It is suggested that these and perhaps other interrelated trends may increasingly affect large numbers of families, who will, as a consequence, become more dependent on routinely provided health and welfare facilities. Certainly, at the very least, it cannot be assumed that the poor will become either smaller in number, or less dependent on health and welfare services.

VII. The Treatment of the Sick *

by Julius A. Roth

The kind of medical care available to the poor and the way they obtain medical care must be examined in the light of one overriding fact: the private physician-patient relationship on a fee-for-service basis is a basic condition of American medical practice. This assumption is held by the majority of the country's physicians and by their voluntary associations. Certainly, traditional forms of medical practice are undergoing change. A substantial amount of medical care, for example, is delivered by full-time salaried physicians working mainly in government and academic settings. The profession, however, often regards this care as contrary to the ideal patient-doctor relationship and except for leading medical schools—institutions providing it tend to suffer in their recruiting from the resistance and criticism of the rest of the medical world.[1] The private doctor and the fee-for-service principle have also patterned the major part of the mechanisms of health care delivery in government programs such as Medicare and Medicaid as well as the major private medical insurance plans.

This chapter will examine the differences in medical

Julius A. Roth is Professor, Department of Sociology, University of California at Davis.

*The criticism by Dorothy J. Douglas of an earlier draft of this chapter was particularly helpful.

treatment experienced by persons of differing socio-economic levels, particularly the differences between the poor and the more affluent segments of the population. Methods of paying for medical services will not be dealt with directly. Clearly, the assumption of the private fee-for-service model by practitioners, administrators, and government and insurance agencies affects the way doctors and medical institutions treat people of differing socioeconomic levels, and this must be kept in mind.

USING PRIVATE PHYSICIANS

It is an oversimplification to say that two distinct kinds of medical service exist in the United States: the middle class uses physicians in private practice and the low-income classes use the public clinics.[2] The use of a single family doctor over a period of years is probably not as standard a middle-class pattern as is commonly believed. Emergency ward interviews suggest that many people use a number of different private doctors at different times and for different purposes. The doctor in general practice may give total or partial care to one or all members of the family in all combinations—care for acute illnesses only or for chronic illnesses only, general practice care only or with surgical, pediatric, or obstetrical care. He may have a paramount or a subordinate role compared to various specialists that the family uses simultaneously. But, in any case, the use of a family doctor or doctors usually means a more stable relationship to the medical profession than does the use of public clinics. Also, a family doctor is more likely to conceive of himself as the patient's agent in certain areas of conflict.

The use of a family doctor is a function of income. In one study, when 4,320 families with children in the pedi-

Table VII–1. Relationship between income
and having a physician

Family income	Number of families	Percent of families having a physician who usually looks after the children
Welfare	621	16
less than $3,000	333	24
$3,000–$4,500	1369	38
$4,500–$6,000	1009	55
$6,000–$7,500	452	62
$7,500–$10,000	191	63
More than $10,000	75	85

Source: Joel J. Alpert et al., "Types of Families that Use an Emergency Clinic," *Medical Care* 7 (January–February 1969) 57.

atric age group were asked whether they had a doctor who usually looked after the children, the proportion of affirmative answers increased dramatically from the lowest to the highest income group (see Table VII-1). Only 16 percent of the families on welfare had a doctor; 85 percent of the families with an income of more than $10,000 did. In the steady increase of the percentages, two points of break should be noted: only a minority of the families with incomes under $4,500 had a usual physician; beyond that income, the majority of them had a family physician. Above an income of $10,000 practically all families had a family doctor.

The other indices of socioeconomic status (occupation and education) show a similar, although weaker, correlation with the frequency of having a "usual physician." Race and rural or urban residence also leave their mark. Negroes at any income and occupational level are less likely to have a continuing relationship with a physician than whites of the same income and occupational level.[3] Several explanations may account for this finding. The use of a family doctor may depend on cultural traits such as patterns of consumption and spending in which the white and Negro populations are known to differ. Again, it may depend on the somewhat elusive psychological factor of social distance: the Negroes at any income level may feel more distant from the white, upper-class physician than the white of the same income level; hence, Negroes tend to avoid the offices of physicians in private practice and prefer the public clinics where the institutional setting works to protect against the feeling of social distance. A study of physicians' knowledge of their patients supports this explanation. It is found that, in addition to the frequency of contacts, the social class and race of the patient were factors and that the physicians seemed to know lower-class Negro patients the least.[4]

Most of the studies on medical care have been conducted in urban areas, and relatively little is known about the delivery of such care in rural America. There is every reason to believe, however, that because of the relative absence of physicians in rural areas any segment of the rural population is less likely to have a family physician than a comparable segment of the urban population. Physicians tend to settle in urban areas, and this trend has been increasing since World War II. In addition, it is often noted that within urban areas physicians tend to move into the suburbs and other high-income areas, and their number is decreasing in the low-income neighborhoods of the core cities, especially in the ethnic ghettos.[5]

The availability of physicians in private practice in the cities, even to the poor, is favorable when compared to their presence in the rural areas. In spite of many national and local campaigns, the rural areas have not been able to attract sufficient numbers of practicing physicians, and many of those who have been drawn to rural practice are foreign-trained physicians who are more likely to take the less desirable positions avoided by their American-trained colleagues.[6] Moreover, the location of physicians in the commercial centers of the urban areas makes any access to them difficult for those residing in the remote parts, and makes access extremely difficult for the rural poor who do not have cars. A study of the ambulance services in North Carolina concluded that ambulances are used in a disproportionate degree to transport the poor, mainly Negro and aged, to hospitals and physicians' offices for routine treatment not involving an emergency.[7]

For the rural population the accessibility of the physician is further hampered by the relative lack of health insurance that would help to pay for the medical expenses. The most popular health insurance plans recruit the participants at their places of employment and labor unions, and such an arrangement puts the farming population at a disadvantage. A study carried out in North Carolina found that coverage by health insurance was more common among urban people, white families, and those with higher incomes and education than among their rural counterparts; moreover, it found that those who had dropped their insurance and had not re-enrolled had the greatest unmet medical needs. Another study put the conclusions in more general terms: "Subscription to health insurance is more a function of ability to pay than of health needs.[8]

USING PUBLIC CLINICS

Those who do not use pribate practitioners must turn to the public clinics, and public clinics represent the common sources of medical care for the country's poor. In every group, as income decreases more families use the public clinics, and they use them more frequently (see Table VII-1). When more than 4,000 families who used the Boston Children's Hospital Emergency Clinic were followed up for a period of six months, the welfare patients were most likely to return for one or more visits to the same clinic, while the group with the highest income was least likely to do so (see Table VII-2). The proportionally greatest decline by income groups appeared for those making two or more repeat visits to the clinic, suggesting that the low-income groups are more likely than the high-income groups to rely on the services of the emergency clinic. They tend to return to the same clinic with another complaint or use the clinic for the treatment of prolonged and perhaps chronic ailments.

The middle-class family tends to use the public clinic occasionally, for accidents and for other emergencies at times when the family doctor is not available or as a checkup in times when the family is not fully satisfied with the usual doctor. In addition, the middle-class family is

Table VII–2. Repeated utilization of a pediatric emergency clinic during a six-month period

Family income	Number of families	Percent with no repeat visits	Percent with one repeat visit	Percent with two or more repeat visits
Welfare	601	71	21	8
less than $4,500	1705	79	16	5
$4,500–$7,500	1439	86	12	2
More than $7,500	263	91	8	—

Source: Personal communication from John Kosa, based on the Harvard Study of Health Care Among Low-Income Families.

likely to take to a selected public clinic certain chronic diseases requiring prolonged treatment. The low-income family, on the other hand, relies on the public clinic as the main source of care. This does not mean that the low-income family receives its total care from public clinics, let alone from one clinic. One study found that 57 percent of clinic users also had a private physician and for certain disorders they would contact their regular physician or arrange for an office visit with a recommended doctor, but in other situations they would consider the clinic as the best source of care.[9]

A more detailed study actually distinguishes four typical utilization patterns:

1. A stable relationship with a physician in private practice implies that such a physician is used for total primary care and that the public clinic is visited only at the recommendation of the usual physician or when the latter is unavailable.

2. An unstable relationship with a physician in private practice implies that such a physician is named and from time to time is used as the regular physician, but on other occasions the family freely uses the public clinics without contacting the regular physician.

3. A stable relationship with a clinic implies that the family uses one public clinic at least for one kind of service and approaches other sources of medical care only occasionally or rarely.

4. Finally, the unstable relationship with a clinic implies that the family uses several public clinics, presumably in accordance with the momentary convenience.

The four typical utilization patterns are conspicuously differentiated by the socioeconomic status of the users. The group having stable relationships with a private physician is characterized by the highest socioeconomic status. The status of the group decreases for each following type and reaches the lowest level among those who have unstable relationships with a clinic. In the Boston sample studied, more than half of the Negro families and families with Spanish surnames (mainly Puerto Ricans) belonged to the fourth type.[10]

A comparison of the middle-class pattern care through private practice with the lower-class pattern of public clinic use often raises questions about differences in the quality of care. Popular statements on this issue are numerous, and even medical authorities are wont to issue impressionistic judgments under the claim of general validity. Objective assessments of the issue are not available, largely because there is no simple over-all index to measure the quality of health care that would compare one complex system of care to another that is vastly different but equally complex. As for the complexity of the system, it is useful to realize that there are numerous public clinics in this country which differ not only in their organization, affiliation, program and policies, but also in their quality of care. It is difficult to find a compelling reason for calling any category of clinic the "best" although medical writers (usually affiliated with medical schools) often assume that medical school clinics and hospitals represent the finest that medical practice has to offer.

Private practice primary care holds forth the promise of offering the individual client or the family total care by a single physician or small group of physicians.[11] In contrast, public clinics are typically organized to provide episodic treatment for specific ailments with a minimization of the development of a personal relationship between physician and patient. The very structure of public clinics militates against the treatment of problems that do not fall into a clearly defined diagnostic category. However, there is no good evidence to show that private community medical practices usually fare any better in uncovering the more subtle and complex aspects of the patients' complaints, so this difference is not so great as may first appear. In reading the literature that compares private practice to public clinics, one must be careful not to be taken in by medical authorities and their social science protagonists who like to compare an idealized (and largely unsubstantiated) picture of the relationship of the private practitioner to his patient with a stereotypical picture of patients caught in the mesh of a giant impersonal clinic bureaucracy. This is not to deny that important differences exist, but rather that they are almost certainly exaggerated, that they have not been carefully investigated, and that they are almost always discussed in sweeping terms rather than closely analyzed.

Among the various reform movements, the comprehensive care programs appear to be most promising in providing more personalized, nonfragmented, and systematic care to the users of public clinics.[12] One experimental study has furnished evidence that a properly conducted comprehensive care program is able to overcome the usual shortcomings of the public clinics and provide a system of care for a low-income population that is near to the care given in ideal forms of the private practice of medicine. In the sample receiving comprehensive care the rate of hospitalization and operations became lower and the rate of health visits became higher than in the control group. The rates of more than twenty categories of morbidity were about the same for both groups, but the mothers receiving comprehensive care judged the general health of their families in more favorable terms than the mothers in the control group.[13]

It is questionable, however, whether the methods used in the small population of the demonstration project can be applied to the masses of poor in the urban centers, let alone the rural areas. It might very well be that the idea of comprehensive care is a luxury that the country as a whole cannot afford. Efforts are being made to incorporate some of the practices of comprehensive care programs in neighborhood health centers located in urban poverty areas. Often they have proved difficult to staff with professional medical personnel, and they typically perform a task little different from that of the traditional public hospital clinics, although they may be somewhat more conveniently located for the target population. Their success may depend in large part on the degree to which they can escape the complete dependence on highly trained professional personnel and make greater use of "indigenous" staff with brief training in more limited skills. There has not been sufficient experience with such efforts to make an evaluation possible. At the moment, it looks as if the dual medical care system—private practice and public clinics—will serve the mass of the population for many years into the future.

THE CASE OF THE POOR PATIENT

The use of a family doctor may encompass a variety of utilization patterns, and over several years many families receive care from a number of general practitioners and/or internists and pediatricians as well as from many other specialists. Such families may call upon any one of these physicians in an emergency (that is, a complaint they believe cannot wait until the regular office hours), depending on their conception of the current medical need, the availability of physicians, and the personal preferences of the family.[14] Families that commonly use a private practitioner, and can pay his fees either directly or through insurance coverage, can usually call upon a private physician, but the impoverished family, having made no recent use of private practitioners, finds it difficult to obtain private services and, very often, does not even try to obtain them.

It is difficult for an indigent person to come to a physician's office and ask to be treated for a routine illness. The older practice of differential charges according to ability to pay and the carrying of some "charity cases" by each doctor has largely disappeared.[15] Some poor patients are on government programs (federal Medicare or state Medicaid) or on the Blue Cross-Blue Shield minimum payment provision, in which case the established fee schedules limit the charges, and the physician is likely to collect less from such persons than from the regular patients. The physician tends to classify such persons as less desirable patients, whom he may refuse to accept entirely; more often, however, he tries to pass them on to a colleague with a less thriving practice.

Apart from the ability to pay, people coming from a recognizable poverty subculture are likely to have less access to private physicians. They are considered the least desirable patients. The doctor has probably dealt with "their kind" during his years as a student and resident in outpatient and emergency clinics, and he has concluded that they are often dirty, follow poor health practices, fail to observe directions or keep appointments, and live in a situation that makes it impossible to establish appropriate health regimens. As one resident put it, this offers "a less pleasurable way to practice medicine."[16]

The major point of contact with the orthodox medical world for the urban poor has been through the outpatient clinic. In such settings there is typically no continuity of care, although it is commonly assumed that continuity of care by the same physician is desirable and that the care given in outpatient and emergency clinics is inferior. But a few data from observations on emergency wards suggest that from the viewpoint of the patient, continuity is not always the desired form of care. [17] Some patients prefer to use medical professionals on an episodic basis and to dispense with their help, and with their potential control as well, between these episodes. This is particularly clear in cases of patients who have been involved in fights, suspicious accidents, and of women who have attempted abortion. In addition, some patients who do not have such obviously compelling reasons prefer to present themselves to a new physician each time; they would just as soon not have somebody reconstructing their past history from a cumulative chart and basing the treatment on what went before, rather than on the story the patient is presenting at the moment.

In public hospital outpatient clinics there is no question about admitting the poor. The care these clinics provide has commonly been labeled as inferior by private medical practice, although for expert attention private practitioners may refer their patients to clinics associated with medical schools. The care is provided largely by the staff of house officers-in-training. The equipment for diagnosis and treatment is usually more readily available in a clinic than in a private doctor's office, as some patients point out when claiming that they receive better treatment at outpatient clinics than in doctor's offices.

From the staff's viewpoint, outpatient clinics represent medical Siberia. House officers tend to dislike the kind of people they meet in the clinics. The clientele is often seen as desirable only insofar as the doctors-in-training can learn more about medicine by treating them.[18] With medical students and interns the patient is likely to receive careful (and often slow) attention with a risk that mistakes will be made because of the student's inexperience. The more advanced resident, having seen many cases of the common conditions, will be interested in the less common disorders of his area of specialization. Patients falling into the right categories will be treated as "interesting cases" and will receive exceptional attention.

The rejection of the poverty-level patient by private practice medicine has its origin in part in the experience of interns and residents in the public outpatient department. Here the neophyte doctor learns that these people have characteristics which he finds irritating and on which he (often with the prompting of more experienced colleagues) makes negative moral judgements. His later decisions about where to practice and what kind of practice to establish are influenced by his desire to escape a clinic-like population. This same motivation has made it difficult to staff poverty-area clinics even when the positions offer salaries equivalent to average incomes of established private practitioners in that region as well as medical school clinic appointments. The typical young doctor approves of spending public money for the medical care of the poor, but *he* himself does not want to participate in the program.[19]

Of course, this "typical" response may change with the growing radicalization of students in many medical schools, especially with the increasing numbers of blacks, Chicanos, women, and other minority group members now moving through their medical education. Members of this new breed of students are saying that they do not want a traditional medical career and that they are interested in direct community service and the participation of the client population in health care. Because of the slow pace of medical education, it will be a decade or more before current student "radicals" are likely to have a major impact on the organization of health care. If they mesh their philosphy with the growing movement for consumer control of medical care, the result may well be a substantial change in the forms of health care available to us, a change from which the poor should benefit.

With the present system, however, people who are blocked in their access to private physicians tend to visit other healers. Limited evidence indicates that osteopaths, chiropractors, and naturopaths are used to a progressively greater degree as one moves down from the socioeconomic scale, especially by persons of certain racial or ethnic backgrounds. Calling on the advice of druggists and using patent medicines also seems to be more common at the lower socioeconomic levels. Such treatment is not only less costly but the lower-class person is less likely to feel rejected by a druggist and is more likely to be given the treatment he wants than if he were to visit a physician.[20]

THE SOCIAL ATMOSPHERE OF THE EMERGENCY CLINICS

In city and county hospitals the emergency ward serves to a large extent as an unscheduled clinic for the poor. But it also serves a smaller clientele with a more varied background for accidents and sudden acute illnesses, or persons who cannot obtain medical service elsewhere during off hours.[21] It is a rule of public hospital emergency clinics that everyone should be seen by a doctor, and everyone is if he waits it out. The nature of the medical service provided is, in some ways, similar to that of the outpatient clinics, although more episodic. Usually there is no follow-up and at each visit a different physician treats the patient.

The workers on emergency wards with large slum-area clienteles develop a negative conception of their patients. They seek to establish a defensive position against the lower depths of society. They often exchange stories demonstrating how unintelligent, untrustworthy, and immoral the patients are. New clerks, aides, nurses, and doctors are instructed by the older hands not to tolerate any abuse or disobedience from the clientele, not to accede to their demands, or do burdensome favors for them. Of course, such talk does not closely represent the actual behavior of the personnel—the clerk who states categorically that most patients are "garbage," in fact treats most of them with a fair degree of politeness, but the patient entering an emergency clinic is not likely to find himself in a friendly, comforting atmosphere. He will often wait until employees get around to him, be made to stand while questioned even if ill or aged, notified peremptorily about the rules and procedures ("Sit down over there"; "Put out the cigarette": "You can't go back there")and subjected to questioning which would be considered impertinent by middle-class people ("Are you on welfare?"; "Is there a father in the home?"; "Are you able to pay for this visit?").

The regulars—patients who receive much of their care at the emergency ward—expect long waits and little concern for their comfort or self-respect. They "roll with the punches" more than the newcomer. They are not entirely helpless in the hands of the hospital personnel and have their techniques for obtaining prompt and effective treatment. They know the best times to come; they know when to remain silent and when to assert themselves in order to be assigned to an appropriate treatment area; they know what symptoms to dramatize to get priority, and what persons to approach for the needed information.

Of course, the staff does not treat all patients the same way. Some patients are seen as urgent emergencies who deserve all the assistance that the personnel can give them ("That's what we are really set up to do"). Other patients are clearly respectable middle-class persons or fall into some favored category (for example, city employees, policemen, friends of staff members), and are treated with special consideration. The common stance of emergency personnel is, however, that a patient is a "welfare case" unless there is evidence to the contrary.

Certain categories receive the brunt of staff hostility, and these tend to come from the impoverished and disreputable segments of our society. There is an almost universal hatred of drunks. If they have to be transported, they will be treated like baggage. Their stories are not believed, and they are frequently insulted or treated with a deriding jocularity. They are kept for a long time without examination and then given only cursory attention even when they have sustained an obvious injury. Serious disorders producing neurological malfunction (epilepsy, diabetic coma) are sometimes missed because of the assumption that a dirty ragged man smelling of alcohol is "just a drunk."

Abdominal pain among unmarried young women is often labeled "pelvic inflammatory disease" (PID) before examination and is often associated with a dissolute sex life or attempted abortion. Patients with suspected venereal disease are occasionally rejected by clerks and even physicians who establish their own moral barriers. Psychiatric cases are commonly regarded as nuisances, and the tendency is to get rid of them quickly, either to the psychiatric ward or to the outside world. (However, psychiatric patients and children who cause trouble often get quick treatment because they are considered uncontrollable.)

A patient who does not like the way he is treated can always leave (except for a small number of police holds), and in fact, "elopement" is common, running as high as 5 to 10 percent in some emergency clinics. If a person has a private physician, he can contact him; the private-doctor system and the public-clinic system can be used interchangeably. However, precisely those who are treated with hostility by the clinic personnel are least likely to have ready access to a private physician. Their rejection of clinic care may mean that they deprive themselves of all possibilities of care, although in large cities a patient may move from one clinic to the other.

In city, county, and medical center emergency wards a common question is repeatedly raised: Is it really an emergency? A frequent conclusion is that the majority of people seeking care there do not have an emergency and are simply "abusing" the emergency room. There are a number of standard atrocity stories that one hears in various parts of the country all stemming from the common notion of abuse by the clientele. There is, for example, the person who has been suffering from a sore throat for the last two weeks without seeing a physician and finally shows up in the hospital emergency room on Sunday at 3:00 a.m. demanding immediate treatment. The "welfare case" is more likely to be denigrated in such circumstances than the person who can pay his way or who has a private physician. The matter becomes one of moral stigma. "They're getting free care, so they think they can take up the valuable time of doctors and nurses any time they damn please." Thus, if the patient (especially if he is on welfare) has no problem which is a "real emergency" by definition of the staff, he is more likely to be given short shrift, superficial diagnosis, and careless treatment if any at all. If the patient reacts to such treatment by complaints or abusive language, he will be threatened with ejection and perhaps refused service entirely.

Smaller private hospitals without training programs will usually have no house staff and operate limited emergency services. Their standard way of dealing with emergencies is to have one physician on call (with members of the staff taking turns in rotation), who must be summoned from his home or office by a nurse after assessing the situation, collecting information, and deciding what should be done. A number of hospitals are experimenting with a contract physician plan which has a doctor in the hospital available for emergency care. In practice, this service is limited by an adherence to the norms of the private medical system. Thus, it requires that each patient first declare his private physician and that the private physician should be contacted before referring the case to the contract physician. Nurses often insist on notifying the patient's family doctor even when the patient would prefer the doctor on call. Patients who persist in trying to bypass their own doctor are told that "the system doesn't work that way." And indeed it does not. In such a case, the patient can gain his preference only by denying that he has a family doctor. Poor persons without private physicians are even less welcome in such hospitals than in public institutions.

The clerks or nurses ask the patient about insurance, employment, responsibility for payment, and other matters of bill collection. Obviously the poor are at a severe disadvantage since the picture they present of themselves does not make them readily acceptable to the hospital. It is noteworthy that in presenting one's ability to pay, a good insurance policy is frequently better than income and wealth, unless the latter are so conspicuous that they are matters of public knowledge. However, an offer to pay cash is not likely to be refused and may even be encouraged. If the patient is on a state or local medical aid program, he is tabbed as "welfare," with the discriminatory behavior that goes with the label. He is likely to get relatively superficial treatment and discouraged from becoming a regular patient.

INPATIENT CARE

Almost everyone receives some medical attention on an emergency ward, but when it comes to inpatient service, the private hospitals are restrictive. The hospital administration wants payment guaranteed before admission, and sometimes a deposit is required for as much as one week's room and board. The question of finances may occupy the major attention of the nurses and doctors considering a clinic admission. The usual way of handling the indigent person who requires admission is to transfer him to the appropriate city or county hospital. The introduction of Medicare has modified this practice in the case of the aged, since patients whose payment is guaranteed by the government are desirable from the viewpoint of the hospital administrator. Medicaid, on the other hand, has had much less impact in most states because it has been underfinanced and often fails to make payment on claims.

Duff and Hollingshead show how private and semiprivate accommodations are available at a teaching hospital only to those patients who have given evidence of ability to pay. Admissions officers refuse "too high" a level of accommodation if they doubt this ability—a judgment sometimes made in part on the basis of appearance, verbal performance, residence, occupation, and other social class indicators.[22]

Because of the complexities of the means tests and residence requirements stipulated by state and local governments for welfare eligibility, a great many patients do not qualify for welfare aid but are unable to meet their medical expenses. These people are the men without a country in the medical world: they are unacceptable to the private medical system and face serious obstacles when trying to obtain care in public hospitals and clinics. The teaching hospitals need indigent patients as teaching material and admit such patients to service wards. Here they are treated by the house officers with the attending physicians supervising. Costs on such wards are held down by having somewhat less nursing coverage, using less floor space per patient, and doing without amenities such as television sets in each room. It is usually more difficult to get admitted to a service ward than to a private room; services wards are more crowded and may specifically exclude patients with given conditions which are not considered sufficiently serious or important to the training program. The indigent patient with a given condition is less likely to be admitted than a private patient with the same condition.[23]

Thus, the poor are taken out of the private medical-care system and relegated to the care of public hospitals. In New York City in the early 1960s, for example, about 90 percent of the patients in municipal hospitals were public charges.[24] The municipal hospitals of New York have substantially larger proportions of poor, old, and minority-group patients, as well as long-stay patients, than the service wards of the voluntary hospitals, although in recent years Medicare has probably reduced the proportion of the elderly in municipal hospitals.

In the medical center studied by Duff and Hollingshead, patients admitted to the wards were heavy users of outpatient clinics, while those admitted to private and semiprivate rooms had made little or no use of thse clinics.[25] Thus, the hospital route for the poor is from outpatient clinic or emergency room to inpatient ward. For the more affluent, the route is from family doctor or private practice specialist to private or semiprivate room (though a few will come through the emergency room in cases of accident or sudden acute illness).

Some of the government medical care programs have been aimed at changing the categories of indigents to groups of deserving people and encouraging private doctors and hospitals to accept them. Thus, Medicare makes an effort to define its beneficiaries as similar to those who have acquired a Blue Cross-Blue Shield contract or some commercial insurance plan. It is still too early to tell just how this attempt at redefinition will work, but the present information available indicates only very partial success. One hospital, for example, had an old geriatric building with large open wards containing no partitions except pull curtains. Since the local Medicare administration required units with no more than four beds to qualify for payment, the hospital administration erected partitions within the large wards of the geriatric building and divided the open units into four-bed cubicles; the building was then assigned to Medicare patients. Whether this meant that Medicare patients would be treated in the way the old welfare cases had been treated we do not know; but it certainly suggests that the Medicare program has not led the hospital administrators to abandon the old welfare category.

Another private hospital changed the label "Ward Service" to "Chief of Medicine Service" (or "Chief of Surgery Service"), but in other respects seemed to leave the operation of these floors unchanged. Altogether the innovations in these hospitals seemed to be purely nominal. The fact is that many elderly people under the Medicare program are not able to afford the co-insurance part (Medicare pays only 80 percent of the costs over a deductible of $50) and they must apply for welfare to cover the rest of the costs. This labels them as welfare cases.

CHRONIC PATIENTS

Chronic diseases requiring long-term care give the poor person a greater claim on public treatment facilities than acute disorders. If the chronic ailment poses danger or inconvenience to the public, special facilities are likely to be provided (tuberculosis or mental hospital, nursing home,

home for crippled and disabled, school for the mentally retarded).

Long-term treatment institutions are largely government operated and publicly financed by default. The private medical system has shown little interest in populations that are difficult to treat in the medical as well as the social sense and are also in a very poor financial state; it has been quite willing to leave such institutions to public medicine. It is instructive to consider why public chronic-disease institutions have populations that are heavily overrepresented at the lower socioeconomic levels.

Studies of tubercular patients have repeatedly concluded that the income and occupational levels are relatively low in the tubercular population, with single (unmarried) status, separation and divorce, transient life, unemployment before hospitalization, and drinking or alcoholism more common than in the general population. A sizable portion of the tuberculars are on welfare. However, a study of tuberculosis clinics found considerable evidence that many tuberculosis patients were unknown to public health authorities because they were being treated by private physicians.[26] There is no way of getting accurate data on the size of this group but their numbers are a significant ratio of those hospitalized for tuberculosis treatment in the same area. Such nonreporting has been recognized as a serious problem by the National Tuberculosis Association.[27] These patients have never been included in the tuberculosis populations on which the reports of social characteristics have been based. There is every reason to believe that patients who have private doctors and thus manage to avoid public hospitals and clinics are of a higher socioeconomic status and are likely to have a stable family life and stable employment. This throws considerable doubt on the reports of the common social characteristics of tuberculosis populations and makes one wonder whether there are similar biases among other patient populations.

Now that effective drug treatment for tuberculosis is available, a poor person usually has no difficulty getting into a hospital. His problem is more likely to be one of getting out or having some choice in entering or leaving a hospital.[28] The patient of higher social status, receiving treatment from a private physician, never becomes entangled with public health officials. If he does enter a hospital, he is likely to get out earlier than others because he is trusted to take care of himself. The poor patient, especially with a history of being transient, unemployed, or alcoholic, tends to be regarded by the medical staff as irresponsible and requiring additional hospitalization "to be on the safe side." Many hospitals keep those labeled as alcoholic substantially longer than other patients in the same condition. In one hospital Negroes were explicitly kept longer (and also more often given chest surgery) on the grounds that they led a "harder life" on the outside and required more treatment.

A patient may leave against advice. In tuberculosis hospitals this happens frequently; in some hospitals 50 percent or more of the discharges may be against medical advice. The hospital staff has ways of discouraging discharge against advice and applies these methods primarily to those in a weak social position. If the latter leave the hospital, they may be harassed by the representatives of the health department and may be threatened with eviction from their living quarters, loss of jobs, or with having their welfare aid discontinued. Frequently the public agencies within an area establish a blacklist of patients who have left one facility against advice and make sure that the patient does not receive treatment during a certain period of time.

Some communities enforce laws against patients who

leave against advice or refuse hospitalization. The laws are backed by the argument that tuberculosis is an infectious disease and patients must be isolated to protect others. There is a considerable disagreement among medical authorities concerning the virtue of this argument. It is clear, however, that these laws are applied differentially by social status. Persons prosecuted and jailed (or placed in a locked ward) are almost entirely those of unmistakably lower socioeconomic status—largely transients, alcoholics, and persons with limited education and without influential allies. In one area where incarceration for tuberculosis has a long history, I once inquired whether anybody from the middle classes had ever been placed in the locked ward. Three different persons interviewed told the story of the same dentist who had consistently refused treatment even though he had positive sputum, and who was finally locked up under court order for violating the health code. It was the only example they had. As it turned out, this dentist had received special consideration and was given repeated chances to institute private treatment on his own, but continued to practice his profession for months in spite of warnings about the danger to his clientele. When action was finally taken against him, his lawyer got him released within three months, while other patients spent six to twelve months in the locked unit before being released.

In mental disorders a similar picture exists on a larger scale. Persons of low socioeconomic status are less likely to be able to put up an effective defense in commitment procedures.[29] They are much more likely to end up on the wards of a state mental hospital rather than at a private hospital or with a private practitioner; they are more likely to be institutionalized in a home for the retarded than kept at home; they are more likely to be treated in public clinics than in private clinics. They are more likely to be given custodial care than therapy, organic therapy rather than psychotherapy, and directive psychotherapy rather than analytic psychotherapy. Even when financial ability is not directly concerned, such as in free public clinics, their treatment is more likely to be relegated to medical students and social workers, while those of higher status receive the services of established psychiatrists.[30]

If the tuberculosis patient finds it difficult to leave the hospital, the difficulties are compounded for the mental patient whose admission is often tied to legal commitment and whose release is subject to reviews and hearings. In other cases it is a lack of suitable living arrangements after hospitalization that keeps many patients institutionalized for an unduly long time, and the arrangements for suitable living are closely associated with the patient's socioeconomic status. Altogether, it is generally recognized that patients of low socioeconomic status find it more difficult to leave a treatment institution, and they stay institutionalized longer than patients of higher socioeconomic status.[31]

The differential treatment of the chronically ill is best illustrated by the large chronic-disease hospitals that are becoming increasingly common features of metropolitan areas.[32] Their many inmates have some specific chronic ailment or disability, but so have many people on the outside who manage to keep out of public institutions. Indeed, these chronic-disease hospitals, instead of being primary treatment institutions, serve mainly as the dumping grounds for the unwanted, especially the aged. Most of their patients have no families or friends or are not wanted by them. Most of them were economically marginal before entering the institution, and the welfare policy of seizing all their assets in payment for hospitalization destroys whatever financial independence they had. The practice of stripping patients of their assets and blocking them from any income while hospitalized (even Social Security checks are seized by the welfare agencies) tends to perpetuate their residential and economic dependency. Their indigency becomes a sentence of enforced institutionalization.

Such patients are forced to depend on institutions although not all of them spend the rest of their lives there. Some are able to take advantage of the treatment services offered and gain release, and those with family ties, with money, or outside support are more likely to escape. In a sample of sixty cases, it was found that only one fourth of those who had been impoverished when entering the hospital returned to community living; about one third of those whose income was markedly reduced during hospitalization returned to the community; but all those who continued to be financially independent left the hospital. In this selective process the financial ability to live outside the hospital appears to be more important than the actual physical condition.

The mental hospitals, chronic disease hospitals, homes for the mentally retarded, nursing homes, or training schools serve ostensibly different purposes; yet, any description of their operation makes it sufficiently clear that they fulfill the same function in our society. They are intended to remove those who have proved to be a nuisance to others in more advantageous social positions. Their mere existence retards efforts to find viable ways of accommodating the aged, the disabled, the poor, and the other unwanted.

The latest government support programs have had the unfortunate effect of increasing the establishment of dumping grounds for the unwanted. Medicare has made nursing homes and "convalescent hospitals" (often the same thing with a more grandiose label) far more profitable than before, and private enterprise has leapt at the opportunity. Families who previously did now know what to do with its aged members or with a seriously disabled person are now likely to have a chain of nursing homes or hospitals nearby to take on the burden. Perhaps things are not bad in many cases, but considering the past problems and conditions of many nursing homes, it would have been preferable had this solution to the problem of society's unwanted been experimented with and more carefully thought out. The new insurance programs have only contributed to the multiplication of what are apparently more of the same dreary places.

THE UNDESERVING POOR

The definition of what constitutes a deserving applicant for medical care has changed and presumably will continue to change; Medicare is a recent example of organized official effort to change definitions. The Medicare program was intended to be not only a means of paying medical bills, but also a way of placing a category of persons, the aged, into the "deserving" class, much the same way as Social Security, retirement pay, and the Blue Cross refund are regarded as deserved compensations rather than doles.

It is clear, however, that the state medical aid programs have not succeeded in defining their beneficiaries as deserving. Our society is so lacking in clear-cut indicators of one's station of life that it is often difficult to tell the deserving from the undeserving. The Medicare system applies without discrimination to an ascriptive class and does not provide categorical indicators within that class. The state aid programs provide an indicator, the means test; by virtue of being on a state program, a person has placed himself in the class of indigency or poor risk. He becomes classified as a welfare case, and his unacceptability becomes pronounced if the state aid program is poorly financed and the doctor or hospital is uncertain about receiving payment for services.

Generally speaking, medical care programs have no chance of getting their beneficiaries accepted as deserving unless they are applied in a categorical manner to all persons in an ascriptive class without regard to income or assets or other attributes or conditions. Such a principle, although it would not remove all the differentials among socioeconomic groups in medical care (note the vast difference in the quality of "free" public schooling between city slums and middle-class suburbs) is the basic precondition to a greater acceptance of the poor by the private medical system.

There are other possibilities. Medical school conglomerates are spreading their influence and control over an increasing portion of the medical care structure of the country. Medical school staff are not as directly dependent on the collection of fees as are private practitioners. Thus, there is the possibility of defining the deserving patient in a way less tied to economic status. However, the poor do not fare much better in medical school centers than they do in the private practices.[33] They are less likely to be turned away entirely, but they are more likely to be treated as mere teaching material to be manipulated in terms of their contribution to the training program, their personal wishes ignored, and their challenges to the system met with the threat of being cut off from further care. Although medical school hegemony may raise the quality of medical care in an academic sense, it is doubtful at this point whether there is any improvement in care for the masses of poor people.

Still another approach would place more medical care resources in publicly operated organizations under conditions that would attract physicians. Such a move would make publicly sponsored health care the norm rather than the deviation which it now is. The chances of physician cooperation in such a venture will increase as more and more medical school classes contain substantial proportions

of minority group members and political activists.[34] Publicly sponsored medical care entails more than increased funding from the public treasury. Experience thus far has
demonstrated that pouring more money into the present
form of medical practice simply makes medical care more
expensive without making it any better or correcting the
maldistribution of services. Thus far, government programs
have established no procedures for holding medical practitioners, medical care organizations, or insurance companies
accountable for their actions. If public money is to be spent
for the welfare of the health consumer, that consumer must
be given an effective part in the operation of health care
services.

VIII. Readjustment and Rehabilitation of Patients

by Marvin B. Sussman

We know very little about what happens to patients after they have gone through a general or mental hospital, medical care or rehabilitation institution, and a number of factors have inhibited research in this area. First, not enough investigators have found it sufficiently rewarding to undertake costly longitudinal studies and follow up patients after their discharge from a rehabilitation setting. It is difficult to deal with the problems related to the design of such studies in view of the limitations of current methodological techniques, the persistence, motivation, and longevity of investigators and subjects, the cost of such studies, and, finally, the inherent biases in studying institutional populations.[1]

A second inhibitor has been the posture of the institutional system regarding follow-up studies and evaluations of service. Most of these institutions require a form of evaluation indicating that the services offered have beneficial consequences for the patient population and promote convalescence, recovery, and eventual restoration as a working member of the community. The very nature of the institu-

Dr. Marvin Sussman is Selah Chamberlain Professor of Sociology and Director of the Institute of Family and Bureaucratic Society, Department of Sociology, Case Western Reserve University, Cleveland, Ohio.

tional system requires that it produce successful cases in order to obtain funds from the public or government. A number of investigators have pointed out that any agency must justify its existence by translating the services it performs quantitatively in terms of dollars per person served.[2] The agency is forced to function with a marketplace ideology while espousing humanitarian concerns. In the case of rehabilitation, success is measured by the expected contribution the handicapped person will make to the gross national product after he is restored to the community. This type of orientation, attempting to satisfy the demands of other institutional systems upon which health systems are dependent, requires a biased evaluation. It begins with the selection of cases that are "good" from the standpoint of the consequences of treatment, and this selection usually takes place when the patient is admitted. Institutional systems, being evaluated by lay boards and other groups that furnish financial support, tend to select clients who will optimize their success rates in terms of client economic productivity after treatment.[3]

The staff of institutions, especially the professionals, constitute a third constraining factor for investigators. They may view an investigation as a challenge to their expertise and control of the work situation. Such alarm is not without foundation since the traditional model of superordination-subordination in health care is increasingly questioned.[4] Research may exacerbate an already volatile situation. Current client movements are seeking more equal relationships with experts and are questioning and in some instances rejecting the traditional posture of wisdom, superior knowledge, and authority.[5] Currently being threatened is the essential ideology of most professions: "We know what is best for the patient or client" and good medical care is synonymous with patient conformity.[6]

A fourth inhibiting factor has been the lack of conceptual clarity concerning such terms as illness, disease, social class, and the deployment of social class in studies regarding differential morbidity. It is obvious that each of these phenomena requires different structures, mechanisms, and processes for proper handling; yet they are treated as being identical, and the consequence is terminological confusion. The spirited debate between Kadushin and Antonovsky makes it clear that, in the development of concepts such as social class in relation to illness, we have tended to ignore the meaning of illness, the setting in which it occurs, and the relationship of illness to other problems the individual must learn to handle.[7]

REHABILITATIVE HOSPITALIZATION AMONG THE POOR

One may speculate whether the need for rehabilitative treatment is more pressing among the poor than among the non-poor, but, in any case, the availability and utility of such treatments show conspicuous variations by income classes. Getting into a hospital or other rehabilitative institution poses different problems for members of different classes because there is more than one path to medical care. Individuals of different economic levels enter at various stages of illness and vary in their experiences with medical care systems, particularly with their discharge from a hospital or rehabilitation setting. There appears to be an interrelationship between gaining entrance to, and obtaining discharge from, a medical care institution.

In the field of mental health, studies indicate an underutilization of medical facilities by the poor because of their negative attitudes toward mental illness, the middle-class character of mental health rehabilitation, and their limited knowledge of the routes to medical care systems. The poor as a rule "get in" when they come to the attention of social and welfare agencies.

Most lower-class individuals view mental illness as the opposite of normality, and they equate mental disease with one of the severest forms of disorder, namely, being "crazy."[8] They avoid voluntary hospitalization and regard any institutional treatment as involuntary. Those in control of mental care institutions look at this orientation as being basically primitive and backward but accept it; as a consequence, lower-class individuals with disturbed behavior are not only institutionalized but, unless they respond quickly to treatment, are relegated to custodial care. As a result, as one study found, within the surviving population of a state hospital, 93 percent of the lowest income group were still in the state hospital ten years later, while almost all patients in the middle- and upper-income groups had been released.[9] According to another study, the functionally psychotic individuals of the lowest socioeconomic group stay in the hospital longer than other groups.[10]

Social marginality appears to lead to a prolonged stay in mental hospitals. Aged, divorced, or single patients, those in unskilled occupations and of low education and social class have the longest hospital stay.[11] Such indicators of social conditions evidently enter into the hospital staff's decision to discharge or retain a patient. The lack of family pressures for discharge, the absence of an appropriate home for the patient after discharge, difficulty in obtaining work, marital status, race, and many related factors lower the probability of a discharge and tend to produce the residue population that fills the back wards of our mental hospitals.

A study of an experimental home care program of schizophrenics reported that better educated and higher status persons were more successful in home treatment than lower status persons.[12] This study was not measuring specifically posthospital performance but was concerned with the consequences of treating schizophrenia in the hospital or in the community. Nevertheless, its finding substantiates the notion that less educated and lower status persons do less well in handling their illnesses at home, while higher success rates in maintaining rehabilitation gains are positively related to social class status.[13]

SOCIOECONOMIC LEVELS AND TREATMENT:
A MYSTIQUE

Over the past twenty-five years a plethora of mental health researchers has indicated that socioeconomic variables are determinative of psychiatric diagnosis; type, duration, and source of treatment; presumably who receives attention in the hospital and with what concern; the responsiveness of the family to the hospitalization; and posthospitalization follow-up and care of discharged patients. Yet few of these reports explain why this relationship exists if, in fact, it does. Is it due to the variable responsiveness of patients to the hospital staff and professional personnel or visa versa? Does patient culture have any effect? Are persons of higher socioeconomic level more apt to organize an "in-group" and use the system more effectively?

The credibility of the social class/treatment hypothesis stems from early observations by Dunham and Meltzer of some relationship between duration of hospitalization and the patient's economic status and level of education.[14] Hollingshead and Redlich a few years later demonstrated a similar relationship with schizophrenics among their psychotic group; the lower the social class of the patient, the higher the proportion of long-term treatment cases.[15] Hardt and Feinhandler in 1959 reviewed the research on this hypothesis and found that reported data from various studies were inconclusive in prognosticating duration of hospitalization according to social class membership.[16] Their own study indicated, however, substantiation of the Hollingshead thesis that the risk of long-term hospitalization is inversely related to the social class level of the patient. A cohort of male schizophrenics was used and clinical characteristics of the patients, class differences in admission procedures, and mental health status at the time of discharge were not significantly related to duration of hospitalization. Puzzled by these findings the authors close with a somewhat prophetic statement of research needs, "Deserving more careful exploration are the relative contributions to the discharge decision made by behavioral changes in the patient, differences in the pattern of family support and intervention, and staff variations in defining such phenomena as 'discharge readiness' and 'overcrowding.' Studies of contrasts in the natural history of hospitalization as experienced by patients from markedly different class levels could be useful in leading to the specification of those conditions responsible for different outcomes."[17]

It is strange that health investigators over the years did not go beyond establishing this "demographic" relationship of differential treatment according to position in the social structure by undertaking basic studies on causation. Even the proffered explanations are based on imageries and stereotypes of class behavior, inferred rather than observed. Consequently only a few approaches to the study of this issue can be offered at this time.

Roth and Eddy in a study of sixty patients in a rehabilitation hospital for the physically disabled discovered that patients who exhibited behavior of overt mental disturbance or incompetence, aggressive nonconformity, or refused to help themselves when they were physically able to, were rapidly removed from the rehabilitation to the psychiatric ward.[18] The patient responses reported in the rehabilitation setting would also relegate the mental hospital client exhibiting them to the custodial wards of that institution unless they fitted the diagnostic categories selected for treatment by the hospital staff. The point is that patients who are difficult to handle, and consequently do not fit the available therapeutic regimens are viewed as losers. Problem patients are considered to be losers. While everyone loses in taking this approach—the family, staff, patient, and society—the institution persists in treating potentially successful cases through careful case selection as a hedge against criticism and loss of support of its benefactors and the public. The requisites of institutional image building and the professional and paraprofessional need to record treatment successes in order to maintain power, and attendant rewards may be key elements of the differential care hypothesis.

The responses evoked by the individual or group perceived to be deviant because of nonacceptance of institutional norms may be critical to the decision to treat a patient, keep him in residence after he has reached "maximum hospital benefits" or to discharge him prematurely. The characteristics of "social marginality" such as age, marital status, education, occupation, social class, race, religion, and admission status are used as salient explanatory variables by Krause in his recent review of "Factors Related to Length of Mental Hospital Stay."[19] He examines findings of cohort studies after operationalizing marginality.[20] Socially marginal persons have a clumping of these characteristics and are treated as outgroup members or strangers by the less marginals and the professional staff.

It has been hoped that the consequences of social marginality could be drastically altered by the advent of the "new careerists" into health care systems. These recruits from the indigenous communities of the marginals by virtue of their selection and opting for uplift training programs are somewhat less marginal than the poor of their communities. However, because of their similar racial and ethnic backgrounds with their future clients' one might expect them to function as links between the client and care systems. [21] They could play significant negotiating and socialization roles and bridging functions for the stigmatized, marginal patient if not coopted by the system by taking on the norms of higher-class career-oriented recruits.

The viability of this notion is still to be ascertained. In one study an insufficient number of new careerists took on the bridging function between client and staff, community and agency, to sustain this perspective.[22] The research involved 812 students, of whom 141 were in a New Careers program, called henceforth "new careerists." Table VIII-1 indicates a "mixed" picture of rehabilitation-oriented new careerists in relation to the bridging function.

The sample is subdivided into new and non-new careerists by interest in a position in the rehabilitation field. Three items— "orientation toward people," "identification with working people/blacks," and "family social class status IV and V," were perceived as characteristics most likely to be those of the linkers. Approximately two thirds of the new careerists who indicated an interest in a rehabilitation career had high orientations toward people and were of class backgrounds similar to those of potential clients; but only one third identified with working people or blacks. This group, in fact, is less identified with potential clients for community-agency linkage than other new careerists not planning for work in rehabilitation.

The difficulties in diagnosing mental illness; the linking of specific diagnostic categories, often catch-all, nonspecified ones such as schizophrenia, with the lower class; and the

Table VIII–1. New career status and rehabilitation career interest, by selected variables indicating potential "bridgers"

Potential bridgers	Rehabilitation Career Interest							
	Present				Absent			
	Non-new careerist		New careerist		Non-new careerist		New careerist	
	Percent	Number	Percent	Number	Percent	Number	Percent	Number
High people-oriented focus (Score 3–5)	53	345	66	95	27	289	45	22
Identifying with working people, blacks	27	361	34	105	31	296	48	25
Family social class IV or V	57	353	68	98	58	285	77	22

Source: Gerald S. Berman, Marie R. Haug, and Marvin B. Sussman, "Bridges and Ladders: A Descriptive Study in New Careers," Institute on the Family and Bureaucratic Society, Case Western Reserve University, November 1971.

transformation of a disability into a social welfare problem may also account for the differential treatment phenomenon. By mid-1972 the disease model of schizophrenia was being questioned; it is viewed as a vague definition whose process of development is not understood but has freely been applied to some 200,000 Americans languishing in hospitals. The treatment still defies an adequate solution and so-called schizophrenics overcome their "characteristic" disturbances and "inappropriate" responses in spite of the treatment.[23] In normal interaction, strangers—those considered as outgroup members and kept at a social distance—easily fall into the schizophrenic category. It is no small wonder that lower class patients are quickly identified as deviants and labeled "schizos" with merciful precision and are given the option to become well in spite of the system.

A related issue is that "lower class" almost by definition portrays an individual or family with problems requiring the assistance of social welfare institutions. A similar imagery is conjured with disability. Scott demonstrates this last point succinctly in his study of the blind. He writes, "when an individual's vision is slightly better than 10 percent of normal, he is regarded as a sighted person who has a severe visual loss. When his visual acuity drops below this arbitrary line, agents of the society begin to treat him as a blind person who possesses residual vision. When his vision exceeds the minimum level specified by the official definition, his seeing problem is treated as the legitimate concern of medicine. When he becomes officially blind, his condition is transformed into a social welfare problem."[24] The relevant point is that often the disabled client or patient is beleaguered with demands that he utilize the social resources now made available, and his ability to respond to these options for bettering himself may determine the medical and rehabilitation treatment he will be offered. The social welfare aspects of his problem are exaggerated in many instances at the expense of needed medical treatment or rehabilitation.

Still another variable seems to obscure the effect of socioeconomic differences upon the length of hospitalization for physical illnesses. A study comparing three hospitals obtained an estimate of the average duration of hospitalization for common operations and found that, regardless of the treatment, patients remained longer in teaching than nonteaching institutions.[25] In addition to this institutional factor, the methods of paying for hospital care—an indicator of socioeconomic status—also displayed considerable differences. Private patients and those with voluntary commercial insurance had slightly shorter hospitalization periods than patients with Blue Cross, while patients who had "other" methods of payment, such as welfare, government funding, or industrial compensation, stayed in hospitals the longest. Another study, concerned with the ability of the patient to maintain rehabilitation gains after discharge from a chronic disease hospital, found that the patient is likely to arrive at his maximum hospital benefits about the same time his hospitalization insurance expires.[26] The underlying logic of this situation is the high cost of medical care: in the hospital concerned, the average cost for care had risen to 105 dollars per day in 1971. As a consequence, great pressure is placed on public officials in the case of welfare patients and on family members in the case of private patients to make arrangements for a discharge about the time the hospitalization benefits expire.

There is other evidence that the economic factor is related to length of stay in the hospital. Investigating the efficacy of the kin network in providing adjunct support and therapy to the disabled individual during and after discharge from the rehabilitation hospital, the patients were categorized according to whether they were in functioning family and kin networks or relatively isolated. These differences were insignificant in receiving financial support from family members to pay for their illness; both groups paid about the same amount of money for their illness and relied largely on nonfamily sources of payment. There were, however, significant differences in the amount of emotional support given to the individual—a support vital for effective rehabilitation. It appeared that chronically ill individuals and their responsible others were willing to accept financial support from established sources such as government pension plans, insurance programs, and prepaid hospital insurance. They accepted a third party for the support of illness, and this had a very specific relationship to the length of stay in the hospital.

REDUCED REHABILITATION POTENTIAL

Social group identification, membership in a family, active work, and social life are important factors in a study concerned with predicting the vocational and economic status of patients after their discharge from a tuberculosis hospital.[27] Three types of patients had markedly reduced rehabilitation potentials, and they were designated as "family isolates," "anomic," and "otherwise ill" (see Table VIII-2). The family isolates, i.e., individuals found to be living alone, were classified in light of the notion that living alone can bring forth by-products of isolation that militate against rehabilitation. Patients classified as anomic not only lived apart from family members but in addition had unstable work records for five years prior to diagnosis of tuberculosis. The "otherwise ill" were those individuals whose tuberculosis was complicated by other medical conditions. It was found that those living alone suffered dispro-

Table VIII–2. Tuberculosis patients with reduced
rehabilitation potentials

Patient sample	Number	Percent
Total medical register sample	384	100
Never hospitalized	79	20
Hospitalized	305	80
Total hospitalized sample	305	100
Normals	115	38
Types with reduced		
rehabilitation potentials[a]	190	62
Family isolates	108	35
Anomics	65	21
Otherwise ill	154	51

Source: Marvin Sussman, Marie R. Haug, and
Marjorie R. Lamport, "Rehabilitation Problems
Among Special Types of Tuberculosis Patients,"
American Review of Respiratory Diseases, 92
(August 1965), 262.

[a]Because of overlapping, patients were
categorized in more than one type. Numbers and
percentages of types add up to more than the total
with reduced rehabilitation potentials.

portionately from other illnesses compared with those living
with family members. Each of these "problem types" was
more likely to suffer medical relapse, fail to find steady
employment, or have economic difficulties than the "normal" group. In short, they were least able to shake off the
effects of the illness.

Concerning the severity of illness at time of diagnosis and
ultimate hospitalization, most patients were already infected with active tuberculosis when originally diagnosed
and were promptly hospitalized. Among the others (N=86),
whose first diagnosis showed a nonactive and noninfectious
state, those whose disease remained in the minimal stage

were compared with those whose disease progressed until hospitalization became necessary. The two groups showed clear differences in family living arrangements. More than two thirds of the family isolates were eventually hospitalized due to exacerbation of the disease, while of those living with family members, two thirds maintained a dormantly stable disease without hospitalization.

The finding that isolation is a condition related to progressing disease supports Kissen's research in Scotland, where he found significant relationships between "broken love links" and the onset or relapse of tuberculosis.[28] Love links are ties that provide identification, security, affection, attention, and other conditions necessary for the individual's psychological well-being. A break in a love link, such as the end of a love affair or marital separation, may create a crisis with such effects that the individual is unable to cope either with long-range problems or those of everyday life. It could be argued that in a medical sense the individual's resistance to disease decreases, the loss of the love link triggers an onset of tuberculosis, and the latent or inactive infection now becomes manifest.

Hospital admittance itself seems to be related to both isolation and socioeconomic status. One might rightly assume that persons living within family networks are subject to family pressures to "take care of themselves" and thus tend to seek medical advice sooner than persons living alone. At the same time, it is generally observed that persons of higher socioeconomic groups are likely to obtain medical help at an earlier stage of illness and thus often manage to avoid hospitalization. In the tuberculosis study just described, the higher-income patients were more apt to receive drug treatment at home or in a general hospital, while patients of the lower socioeconomic level, with their tendency to defer treatment until a severe stage of the illness, were likely to be admitted immediately into a tuberculosis hospital.

REHABILITATION PERFORMANCE AND SOCIAL CLASS

The ways in which the patient with a chronic disease enters a rehabilitation hospital differs markedly from the pattern of hospital entry associated with acute illness. In one rehabilitation center in Maryland, a study of 612 patients with cerebrovascular accidents showed that socioeconomic conditions rather than the desire for rehabilitation appeared to be the major reasons for seeking hospitalization with minimal delay.[29] Patients who were seventy-five years and older, females, nonwhites, and without spouses, showed a short delay, perhaps because such "down and outers" had fewer of those obstacles in their paths to rehabilitation which are presented by anxious family members and physicians. It is probable that patients used to having "troubles" can perceive of rehabilitation as improving their current level of minimal functioning.

A pattern of exchanging noninstitutional for institutional living conditions may be emerging among the disabled poor. Potentially the patient may profit from this exchange because, in long-term medical care, he receives social services and vocational retraining also. Support for this notion comes from the five-year follow-up study of the maintenance of rehabilitation gains after discharge from a rehabilitation hospital.

If hospitals develop systems of following up discharged patients they may be able to capitalize on a "locking-in" phenomenon that is endemic to long-term experience in an institutional setting. The patient is already primed to maintain links to the care system and to accept direct or consultative services to maintain his achieved level of functioning. Support for this notion is based on data from a five-year follow-up study of discharged rehabilitation patients. [30] Table VIII-3 sums up the data on patients discharged over a five-year period who participated in follow-up observations after discharge. It indicates a tendency on the part of the lower-class patients to maintain contact with the hospital personnel and use them as consultants for their problems. For such patients, the long-term experience in the hospital might have created "dependency longings" and a desire to return; thus, they are likely to respond with a willingness to cooperate to the interest shown by the medical staff. Successful posthospital care appears to be the result of hospital personnel interest and the poor patient's needs and longings.

Leaving the hospital against medical advice (AMA) has grave implications for the patient's posthospital functioning and eventual rehospitalization. Reports that every year al-

Table VIII—3. Rehabilitation patients (by social class) failing to participate in follow-up observations

Social Class	Number	Failed to Participate[a]	
		Number	Percent
I	3	0	0
II	5	1	20
III	23	4	17
IV	58	10	17
V	64	5	8
Underclassed	24	1	4

Source: Morris W. Stroud, Ill, *et al.,* "Rehabilitation of the Disabled and the Hospital" (unpublished manuscript).

[a]Includes those who could not be located as well as those who refused to participate.

most half of all tuberculosis patients leave the hospital against the advice of their physicians do not appear to stimulate research in this area.[31] To be sure, such studies might make visible what appears to be an institutional failure.

One study of AMA used a stay-response or quit-response dichotomy among patients of a Veteran's Administration hospital.[32] The probability of the quit-response was highest for the unemployed (.83), followed by the laborers (.64) and other physical workers (.62), while white-collar people scored .51, and students only .27. These data indicate some relationship between economic-work status and use of hospital facilities.

It would be erroneous, however, to assume that poverty in itself increases the incidence of AMA. It is rather the conditions surrounding poverty and the medical resources available to the poor that are more specifically related to AMA. In looking at our rehospitalized group, a marked relationship appeared between rehospitalization and AMA discharges. Over half the patients hospitalized more than once had left against medical advice. The chances were almost two out of three that if the patient left the hospital before the physician considered him ready he would be back for another stay. Most of the AMA cases came from the isolated and anomic groups.[33]

Longitudinal studies on the posthospital performance of patients with severe physical disabilities and from different socioeconomic strata are limited in number. The data of one study, however, indicate that deterioration in activities of daily living or early death in the posthospital period is associated with economic dependence. The economic dependence scale is composed of evaluations in four areas: (1) receiving or not receiving agency support for maintenance; (2) ownership or nonownership of residence; (3) employed

Table VIII–4. Economic dependence and deterioration
of activities among patients with fracture of the hip

Level of economic dependence	Percent deteriorated in activities of daily living or dead		
	One year	Two years	Five years
I (N = 5)	20.0	20.0	20.0
II (N = 52)	46.2	57.7	71.1
III (N = 71)	66.2	71.9	84.5
IV (N = 15)	80.0	93.4	100.0
V (N = 4)	75.0	100.0	100.0

Source: Sidney Katz *et al.,* "Continuing Care Project," unpublished manuscript, Benjamin Rose Institute and Case Western Reserve Medical School.

Table VIII–5. Economic dependence and deterioration of activities among patients with first stroke

Level of economic dependence	Percent deteriorated in activities of daily living or dead		
	One year	Two years	Five years
I (N = 17)	76.4	76.4	82.3
II (N = 54)	68.5	75.9	90.8
III (N = 39)	89.8	92.3	100.0
IV (N = 15)	93.3	80.0	100.0
V (N = 2)	100.0	100.0	100.0

Source: Ibid.

or not employed; and (4) independent living without personal assistance, or living in a protected environment such as a boarding home. The index of Independence in Activities of Daily Living (ADL) is based on an evaluation of the functional independence of patients in bathing, dressing, using toilet, transferring from bed to chair, continence, and feeding.[34] The data show that higher economic dependence is associated with higher rate of ADL deterioration and early death (see Tables VIII-4 and VIII-5). Class I is of low economic dependence and Class V is of high economic dependence. ADL evaluations were made one, two, and five years after discharge from hospital. For both hip fracture and stroke patients the higher economic dependence was associated with a faster rate of deterioration or early death.

The data on posthospital performance and AMA behavior unequivocally indicate a relationship between socio-economic status, morbidity, mortality, and maintenance of rehabilitation gains. Causation between poverty and these factors has not been established, but the correlation is sufficiently high to suggest a need for collective efforts to modify this association and devise new approaches to dispense medical care.

THE MEDICAL CARE SYSTEM
AND THE REHABILITATION OF THE POOR

Contemporary patterns of medical care and the demands placed upon the health institutions mean that follow-up of patients is rarely accomplished by the medical institutions alone and is much more a function of the patient's willingness to maintain a relationship with the health care system. We have to make the assumption that the conditions which lead individuals to seek medical care and to utilize medical care systems at the onset of illness are the same as those which motivate them to use such facilities after parenthood. The few modifying variables would be their experiences with the medical care system as well as their acceptance of, and identification with, the medical care system.

The principal factors in the under-utilization of medical care facilities by the poor are the bureaucratic structure of medical care, the value orientations dominating the medical care system, the differential assessment by health organizations of the desirability of clients, the potential outcome of treatment, the economic costs, and the family responses to discharge.

Medical care systems are bureaucratic structures organized according to specialization of functions. It was found that under-utilization of medical care by New York City blue collar workers was related to the fact that the poor had little contact with professional members of medical care specialties and turned first to a "lay referral network of immediate friends and relatives."[35] They were ignorant of the services available, especially preventive services, and were unprepared to cope with the bureaucratic structure of medical care. Medical care systems operate on principles of scientism and rationality. They believe in performing a service and assume that a person coming to them is willing to have his problem solved and permit the system to operate fully. In other words, they expect the patient to assume the traditional sick role and allow the medical system to work out the solution. In this sense the health enterprises are culture-bound, basically directed by middle-class-oriented technology which severely limits their availability to impoverished individuals.[36]

Bureaucratic health systems consist of specialized professional and occupational systems, each possessing a theoretical stance in regard to illness, treatment, and rehabilitation.

The separate systems are more or less integrated into a complex system of work in which there is constant competition and struggle for status and power. Each occupational system has its own needs, and much of the behavior in an occupational system is found to be consistent with these occupational values and goals.[37] These occupational systems make demands on their co-workers as well as on their patients, and these demands may not be in consonance with the demands of the recipients of medical care.

This last point is illustrated by a study on the expressed satisfactions and dissatisfactions of givers and receivers of outpatient care, namely staff and patients, in a large university hospital.[38] One important finding related to the variability and ambivalence expressed by different occupational groups composing the hospital staff. They differed greatly in value systems, perceptions, and definitions of the ideal and real clinical situation; they varied in satisfactions and especially in their concern for the patient. All stated a concern for good outpatient care, but manifested occupational variations as to whether their primary interest in the patient was for purposes of teaching or research. Members of the paramedical staff indicated a greater concern with deficiencies in patient care, whereas the medical-clinical staff felt that patient care was adequate but deficiencies existed concerning teaching and research.

One can interpolate from these findings that the patient is viewed as a subject who fits into the rest of the institutional system. The patient is confronted with a bureaucratic system that adapts his interests to its own. If there is a happy coincidence of interests, the patient will gain in treatment and care. Patients who do not fit the model, either in terms of diagnosis or the role of the good patient, find the system too formidable to handle, especially for posthospital treatment.

The effects of victimization of the poor client by powerful bureaucratic systems may be mitigated by actions of another and contending bureaucracy, the welfare system. The lengthy stay of poor patients in hospitals, the high cost of therapy and inadequate service in meeting patient needs, may result in tension and hostile action by the welfare system, which is legally required to pay the bills of the indigent. Complaining in order to initiate investigation and organizing indigent groups to support change in institutional policies are two devices increasingly used by the underclassed.

The association of certain types of illnesses with deviance is another factor explaining the small amount of follow-up in the posthospital period.[39] Lower-class patients are more sensitive and defenseless to the public's labeling of their illnesses as deviance. This holds whether or not a stigma (such as the stigma of irresponsibility) is attached to the particular illness. Because of the many psychological and economic losses that may arise as a consequence of a deviant label, the lower-class patient is reluctant to participate in follow-up programs unless they are offered in a discreet, unobtrusive way.[40]

A lower-class patient with a relatively favorable condition, i.e., one that is curable and free from the stigma of irresponsibility can ill afford to participate in follow-up programs because participation implies absence from work and loss of income. While one cannot fully agree with the statement that, "the poor person actually cannot afford to recover from illness," the major point is well stated.[41]

Tuberculosis is a disease that arouses loathing, for which the individual is often held responsible, and which has a prognosis of possibly being improved and controlled but not cured. The public response of fear, disgust, or loathing produces for the individual a barrier to normal social interaction and, as Goffman has indicated, makes him feel isolated.[42] A high percentage of tuberculosis patients, like alcoholics, deny that they have the disease. Streeter, investigating the fantasies of tuberculosis patients, found that one third of them denied that they had the disease or that the disease was caused by tuberculosis bacillus.[43] Even after a lengthy hospitalization and successful treatment, our posthospital study found that many tuberculosis patients refused to be interviewed, claiming that they never had been in the hospital; some of them undertook elaborate steps to avoid the interviewer and refused to be followed.

All treatment control and welfare agencies use diagnostic stereotypes. What may start initially as diagnostic hypotheses usually persist, and all cases are fitted into these stereotyped descriptions. The consequence is a scientific model of diseases relying on the notion of "normal cases with standardized treatment, prognosis and diagnosis."[44] Each practitioner attempts to utilize these diagnostic categories in handling the illnesses of clients and attempts to convince the patient that his stereotype is the correct one. The patient in turn may have his own, but the physician to some degree proselytizes the patient into believing that he has the type of disease that the physician perceives according to the symptoms.[45] The physician "sells" the patient on this diagnosis and the appropriate behavior which will enhance recovery. It is obvious that if the patient does not agree with the physician, he is apt to go elsewhere or disregard the medical regimen. Consequently, if the patient feels that he has been mislabeled, he will avoid involvement in any follow-up program. In case of mental illness, where the lower-class patient is forceably detained in an institution, the chances of his entering and staying in a posthospital treatment program are practically nil. In case of physical illness and disability, the same patient is likely to delay rehospitalization in the hope that he may enter a preferred institution or service that has a diagnostic model closer to his perceived condition.

PAYING FOR HOSPITALIZATION

The economic costs of medical care and convalescence are factors impeding follow-up after discharge from a hospital or rehabilitation center. They deter institutional systems from expending effort in follow-up programs, especially for the poor. At the same time, the lengthy hospitalization with often insignificant improvement in the actual condition leads to some disenchantment, moving many patients to discontinue association with the institution once they leave it. Yet the length of stay in hospitals is not determined by the desire of the patient but rather by the source of his financial support. One study of the cost of hospitalization in a chronic disease institution found that the source of funding appeared to influence the average duration of hospitalization and attempted rehabilitation.[46] A comparison of

Table VIII—6. Length of hospital stay for patients discharged from a rehabilitation hospital, by source of funding

Source of funding	Number of patients	Average stay in days		
		In prior hospital	In rehabil- itation hospital	Total
Private	107	66.9	70.3	115.3
Public	44	48.3	142.7	187.0
Private and public	26	67.1	191.3	240.1

Source: Morris W. Stroud, III, et al., "Rehabilitation of the Disabled and the Hospital", (unpublished manuscript).

patients with private and public funding revealed marked differences, and the patients with total or partial public funding had a considerably longer total hospitalization (and an even more markedly longer rehabilitation hospitalization) than patients with private funding (see Table VIII-6).

To understand this difference, a few factors need to be controlled. Disability (such as impairment in activities of daily living and/or mobility existing for six months prior to hospitalization) might prolong treatment and rehabilitation, but such prior disability was more prevalent in the group with private funding than in the group with public funding (29 percent versus 19 percent). An examination of the diagnostic categories did not produce significant differences between the two groups of patients. In view of such background data it may be of interest that, when the improved independence in mobility and ADL status during hospitalization and in the five-year follow-up period was examined, patients with public funding (total or partial) performed somewhat better than patients with private support. Patients with public funding showed slightly more gains in mobility and ADL during hospitalization and the follow-up period (66 percent versus 61 percent) and suffered slightly fewer failures in attempted rehabilitation (33 percent versus 40 percent).

Poor patients are kept, on the whole, almost twice as long in the hospital system than the better-off patients. Such an arrangement may, in part, help to meet some of the teaching and research needs of the institution involved; it may help in a major way to pay for the overhead and related costs of the hospital. At the same time, the data suggest two possible conclusions: either the lower-class patients come to the hospital sicker and more disabled than the higher-class patients, or they are less successful in obtaining release from the hospital. On the basis of available evidence, we are prone to discard the former and accept the latter explanation. The higher rate of previous disability among the privately supported patients as well as the finding of insignificant differences among the hospitalized poor and non-poor for hemiplegia, para- and quadriplegia, hip fracture, amputation, arthritis, and neurological disorders gives little support indeed for the first conclusion. As for the second, it appears that the poor meet the needs of the institutions to have a stable population for income, teaching, and research purposes. Also, the poor are less likely to have family settings to which they can be discharged and have available sufficient nursing homes and financial support for nursing-home care; thus, they stay in the hospital for a longer time. At the same time, the poor person can least afford to be absent from his family, neighborhood, and job, whereas the person of a higher social class, who has a much shorter period of recovery from a serious chronic illness, has more resources for handling the interruption and increased possibilities of resuming normal work and social roles.

Current high costs of hospitalization and rehabilitation suggest a "pricing out of the market" for most families, especially the poor, and the growing expansion of government sponsored and financed medical care systems. Current delivery systems are being re-examined, as are noninstitutionalized settings that may be used as therapeutic milieus. Empirical data from a longitudinal study of disabled patients provide a complete analysis of the economics of rehabilitation for 208 patients, including prior hospitalization costs, the general hospital-bed costs and the charges of extended care and retransfer to the general hospital sections.

The total cost for the 208 persons was $1,033,628 in 1960. The average cost per patient hospitalization was $4,969. In the transferring hospital it was $2,027, and in

Table VIII-7. Costs of hospitalization in 1960 for 177 patients with completed rehabilitation at Lookover Hospital, U.S.A., by principal diagnosis, number, average stay

Principal diagnosis	Number	Average stay in weeks	1960 Average cost ($)[a]	1971 Estimated cost ($)[b]	1971 Corrected costs based on estimated 20% reduction of time in hospital[c]
Rt. hemiplegia	18	30.9	$5,296	$15,888	$12,710
Lt. hemiplegia	23	15.1	3,084	9,252	7,402
Paraplegia	22	42.7	8,884	26,652	21,322
Hip fracture	16	30.8	5,242	15,726	12,581
Amputee	28	49.1	8,015	24,045	19,236
Arthritis	26	19.6	3,512	10,536	8,429
Multiple sclerosis	19	13.3	2,568	7,704	6,163
Other neurological	11	21.7	4,335	13,005	10,404
Other non-neurological	14	32.8	5,933	17,799	15,239

Source: Morris W. Stroud III, et al., "Rehabilitation of the Disabled and the Hospital" (unpublished manuscript).

[a] Costs per week are based on rate schedules of 1959–1962 in Lookover and neighboring facilities.

[b] Hospital costs are estimated to have increased over-all three times, from $33 per day in 1960 to $105 per day in 1971.

[c] There is an inverse correlation between increased hospital costs and shorter hospital stay. We estimate the number of weeks hospitalized to be 20 percent less in 1971 than in 1960.

the chronic disease hospital $3,429. Excluding $192,952, the cost of extended care and retransfer to the general hospital section, the average hospitalization was $4,042 for a stay just under twenty weeks with a $32.90 mean daily bed rate. A more detailed breakdown of the data is found in Table VIII-7. It is estimated that hospital bed rates have increased from $32.90 in 1960 to $105 in 1971. This means that the average cost per hospitalization of patients with one of nine major diagnoses is estimated to be $12,250. This staggering sum suggests that new models of care may be in the offing, since governmental and private sector sources do not have the financial means to continue such costly care.

POSTHOSPITAL PERFORMANCE

Some data support the hypothesis of a direct relationship between the performance levels of patients after discharge from a hospital and the class status of their families. Insofar as mental illness is concerned, there appears to be a higher rate of rehospitalization among middle-class than lower-class patients, largely based upon the fact that families in the lower class have a higher tolerance toward deviant behavior than those in the middle class.[47] The family establishes the norm of tolerance, and although by professional criteria the patient may be sick enough to require rehospitalization, the family does not relinquish him to the institution. If the norm of tolerance persists and the sick person is no economic burden to the family, then a large number of individuals are unhospitalized and are widely scattered in the communities. The community in this sense becomes the therapeutic milieu for many mentally ill patients. One should treat with caution hospital readmission rates as criteria in determining the efficacy of a hospital treatment program.

The meaning and significance that illness has for the maintenance and interaction pattern of the family are determining factors affecting the patient's posthospital performance. A long-term illness and disability is likely to be associated with a rallying among family members at the onset of the illness.[48] Once the illness passes the acute stage, the professional caretakers make an assessment of whether the patient can be returned to his family. Careful consideration is given to the financial capabilities of the family and the potential stresses, frustrations, and other reductions in achieving family and individual goals. These considerations enter into the decisions whether the patient should be kept in the home and influence the attention, empathy, and acceptance that family members can give to a disabled person. This does not mean that family members are devoid of sympathy, and many families function under great deprivation in order to give comfort and economic support to the ill person. Rather, the family as a system has its own needs for maintenance over time, and with the increased development of specialized institutional systems, it can be relieved of major burdens.

An examination of the work status of discharged mental patients points out that those who are gainfully employed have bargaining power, and they can develop new roles or revitalize old roles of high prestige within the family. Those in a dependent (nonworking) situation have only short-term security and are subject to unilateral decisions on matters such as rehospitalization.[49] These findings support the theoretical notion of the family as a unit possessing exchange systems involving bargaining and reciprocities. To a large degree the success of a follow-up program depends upon the potential benefits to be received by the family as well as the patient.

Because of societal specialization and differentiation, health care systems have become centralized and consequently have all the problems that are endemic to bureaucracies. Such systems, while oriented toward the care of the client, still function largely for the benefit of the professional and other workers. Clients who have or develop abilities to confront the superordination of the system may on occasion mollify its demands for conformity and subordination. Middle-class persons are generally more successful because of money, education, and connections in "working" the system than poor lower-class ones.

Related to this centralization is a value system that emphasizes the restoration of the sick or disabled to independence and productive employment in order to add to the gross national product of the society. Furthermore, such care and rehabilitation are done within an economic framework commonly identified as cost/benefit—whereby one considers not only the cost of care in relation to the required treatment but also takes into account the cost of the investment with respect to its potential return. The value system implies that economic self-sufficiency is a necessary condition for a quality of life. Through economic contributions the individual can then enjoy the comforts of family and friends and receive the attendant psychic incomes. It is not within the context of current health care practices to look at the reverse process whereby one focuses on the psychic and sociologic factors as preconditions for restoring the individual into a meaningful place, vis-à-vis economic factors, in the society.

As a consequence of this economic ideology there is little investment in diagnosing the illnesses and disabilities of the poor. The poor are labeled through diagnostic procedures that place them in unclassified categories, and they tend to be held for long periods of time in custodial care if funds are available from welfare or other sources. Part of this phenomenon of keeping poor patients in institutions longer than necessary is a function of the professional's perception that poor discharged patients have no place to go after leaving the institution and will be better off in than out..

Finding an adequate home and support from primary groups is a critical factor in the posthospital maintenance of achieved levels of functioning. A great need exists to explore how one may use family networks and other primary group support systems for the care of the posthospital mentally or physically ill or disabled. New forms of primary group organization may have to be developed, at least on an experimental basis, to handle the poor, desolated, alienated, and often aged patient.

One major question is how can the poor get a "fair shake" out of the existing establishment of health care? There have been a few studies concerned with developing paraprofessional careers for the able-bodied poor in the hope that they could perform linking and bridging functions between the masses of the disenfranchised and the organized human service systems. These have produced mixed results; some who enter this occupational track maintain their identity with those who are deprived but far too many take on professional norms and orientations and soon become co-opted by the system. One possible solution might be the development of systems of advocacy and ombudsmen, which use experts with managerial competence and an array of skills to enable the poor through collective action to negotiate specific contracts for health care services. Such systems of advocacy and ombudsmen are being seriously considered by the Congress in its preparation of new bills to update public laws governing medical care, social security, and rehabilitation services.

These are hopeful developments of the future, but at the present the posthospitalization care of the poor can be generally characterized as a state of medical deprivation.

Considering our knowledge of poverty, one can agree with Edward Suchman that medical deprivation is a special case of overall social and cultural deprivation.[50] An understanding of the problems of the poor in relation to medical care in the period after patienthood can only be obtained by accepting the fact that a large number of social-psychological, economic, and cultural factors produce the conditions of poverty. Medical deprivation, whether it is induced by the institutional system or by the individual himself, is part of an overall condition of deprivation.

IX. Patient Care, the Poor, and Medical Education

by Raymond S. Duff

Caring for the sick is a challenging and complicated technical and personal task. The technical aspects, often called the science of medicine, are concerned with physical or biological problems, while the personal aspects, referred to as the art of medicine, deal with personal and social adjustments to life stresses regardless of physical afflictions. The interactions between the physical and the personal or social aspects of each individual are extensive and complex. In addition, the processes of care take place in a network of social interactions involving family, health professionals, and health institutions—interactions that are influenced by the economy, the illness itself, the family, the role of the sick person within the family, and the availability of care. These realities are presumably reflected in the education and performance of health professionals, yet physicians-in-training are socialized in a setting where the technology of medicine takes precedence over the art of healing. The immediate impact of this divergence from reality is felt most acutely by the sick poor who usually make up the "clinical material" of medical centers. But the resulting flaws in medical education and professional socialization may affect the public as a whole.

Dr. Raymond S. Duff is in the Department of Pediatrics, School of Medicine, Yale University, New Haven, Connecticut.

THE SOURCES OF CLINICAL MATERIAL

The use of the poor as clinical material in a medical center was traced by Duff and Hollingshead to economic, social, and professional considerations.[1] The poor are not attractive clients to medical practitioners in private practice since they have difficulty paying for their care. They are quickly referred to a public clinic or medical center. The near poor who can and do pay for some care are often seen, hastily but at low cost, by private physicians with "mass practices." Sometimes minor or psychosomatic complaints are satisfactorily treated or at least placated by medications or other means. This treatment process and its associated rituals have been described by an experienced clinician and are probably far more prevalent than most people realize.[2] If the symptoms disappear, perhaps of their own accord, coincident with or as a result of the treatment, patients require nothing further. If the symptoms persist, however, or the illness is thought to be complicated, the patient, his family, and the practitioner are prompted to select another course.

Most often, the patient consults with family and friends, who tell him their views of his problem and of his practitioner; they usually suggest he see another doctor or go to the hospital. Earlier, the patient and his family may have reasoned that going to the clinic subjected one to the risk of being used for learning and research. At this point, however, they emphasize the dramatic cures or improvements brought about by young doctors at the medical center, regularly publicized by the public relations departments and relayed through the mass media. Most poor people know of some instances of very satisfactory care received in a medical center. In spite of its drawbacks, the clinic comes to be the preferred source of treatment.

The poor often fail to consult specialists for social as well as economic reasons. They know the cost of consulation is high, and they realize, often after humiliating experiences, that some doctors do not "take welfare." They are uncomfortable in the specialist's office with the better dressed, better educated middle- and upper-class individuals who can afford to be there. In addition, they are rarely referred to a specialist by the mass practitioner because he wishes to maintain harmony with his colleague for those patients who are socially and economically appropriate for such referral. The specialist fears that the presence of poor people in his office may offend his preferred patients, who would then leave his practice to his financial detriment (perhaps a case of Gresham's law applied to medicine).

For professional reasons as well, physicians with a mass practice commonly prefer to send poor patients with difficult physical or psychosocial problems to the hospital: they feel incompetent to deal with their problems. Some practitioners with mass practices refer all personal friends and upper-class patients to other physicians, partly as an efficiency measure to avoid obstructing the rapid flow of patients through their offices and partly to prevent ill will, which might result if these patients were treated like the poor. They also fear that more knowledgeable patients and their families might identify areas of incompetence which, of course, the physicians do not want exposed.

The poor thus have little or no choice in determining their health care. When they become very sick, the choices narrow or disappear, and they enter a new dependent relationship with the faculty of the medical center.

THE INTERESTS OF THE MEDICAL CENTER

Medical centers have become famous in the twentieth century for their contributions to the understanding and treatment of diseases in man, brought about by applications of the expanding knowledge in the physical and biological sciences. As a result of the reforms following the Flexner Report, specialization in medical education and care paralleled that of research into diseases of the respective organ systems of the body; and a major crusade against diseases emerged. Regarding this, Richards wrote: "Every militant crusading philosophy, as this one certainly has been, has two inevitable consequences: the first is to build itself up, the second is to disregard other philosophies; both of which become more apparent as the years move on."[3]

The crusade against disease was initiated by varied interest groups that reflected hopes to eradicate or control specific illnesses such as tuberculosis, heart disease, cancer and venereal diseases. Freidson points out that physicians and leaders in health institutions such as hospitals are to some extent "moral entrepreneurs" who label diseases as bad, and fight against them.[4] They tend to see diseases when others do not; that is their natural bias. Such biases often are shown by voluntary health agencies, most of which are well known for their ostentatious propaganda to gain public support. Success of the health professions and special interest groups in getting such support on a grand scale was described by Drew as a "noble conspiracy."[5]

Medical school faculties have been heavily committed to the crusade against disease. Since World War II they have received increasing support, especially from federal grants, for research. These grants, secured primarily through the efforts of individual faculty members and their respective departments, have increased the power of individual faculty members and their departments while reducing the influence of the medical school administration. If a faculty member were not able to attract funds for his projects, he might not be retained, while surviving faculty became more powerful as they expanded their areas of research and achieved national and international recognition. These developments understandably skewed faculty interest toward research. Although direct support of medical education was not available for political reasons, some benefits for education nonetheless accrued. As Sheps and Seipp pointed out, the National Institutes of Health "clearly, though not publicly" channeled some funds to medical education through research grants.[6]

It is these same faculty members, through their supervision of physicians-in-training, who are responsible for the care of the poor in the teaching services. Since the poor have few vocal advocates, the frequent faculty assertions that the care provided on teaching services is excellent have not often been challenged. There are exceptions, however. Thompson and Glick reported: "While many physicians in academia have said repeatedly that the patients in municipal hospitals are provided with the best medical care, a more careful analysis reveals that this claim is hardly worthy of the scientists making it. For when faced with a choice, how many of those who make such statements would be willing to send a close relative to a municipal hospital for care *anonymously*?"[7]

In contrast to the relatively specific and extensive funding for research projects, the financing of the care of the poor who appear in medical centers in large numbers has always been problematic. Dreary and protracted negotiations over the payment for their care have rarely been satisfactory. At no level of government have the poor, unlike war veterans, been adequately represented by a special interest.[8] Local welfare authorities resist expenditures on the grounds that hospitals are inefficient or are providing more than adequate care to the poor. They contend that part of the cost of teaching and research is reflected in the bills for patient care and that the research and teaching functions of the medical center result in discontinuous, specialty oriented, fragmented care. Faculty members, supported mostly by outside funds, feel free to speak out although their views on these issues may be unpopular locally. They usually believe that the community should be grateful for the benefits they bring to the area and that the least the local administration can do is to provide adequate financing for the care of the poor.

Through their teaching of medical students, house officers, and fellows, medical school faculty influence patient care. The patients receive first-rate technical care, particularly for those diseases that interest the faculty. The poor, however, usually have multiple physical and psychosocial problems of a chronic nature. Care for these problems clearly involves the sustained efforts of professionals with a range of interest as wide as the range of patient problems. Since medical schools and teaching hospitals have little support for such faculty, the majority of patient problems are ignored. Even when such professionals have faculty appointments, they are a minority, and the conflict between those interested in diseases and those concerned with patient care is a distressing problem. The patients seek care offered by the faculty specialists, but they need and want much more, while the faculty of medical schools need diseases to study but they usually do not want to deal with the psychosocial problems of the patients. Undoubtedly, medical students and house staff are affected by these situations, and they in turn surely influence the environment of patient care, medical education, and research.

This environment has been studied in many settings. One study, of internship on the Harvard Medical Unit at Boston City Hospital, reported that faculty have only limited time for teaching and practically none for patient care: "[faculty] contact with interns is limited to conferences, lectures, and occasional consultations on the wards. In their actual work, interns receive little, if any, help from Harvard physicians." Further, "The process of [intern] succession and situational learning allow the [Harvard Medical] Unit to prepare and use interns to provide patient care without unnecessarily interrupting the research and other activities of Harvard physicians."[9]

While the house staff have little control over conditions set by the hospital and the faculty, they do control, within broad limits, the admission, treatment, and discharge of patients. This control becomes theirs whether or not they are ready to cope with the responsibilities thrust upon them. To protect their own interests, they must subscribe to the philosophy of the faculty since these doctors are their mentors and have a major influence upon their futures. Overt disbelievers in the prevailing philosophy of the faculty can be brought into line by positive or negative sanctions. While the house staff and medical students have long reflected faculty sentiment, they are usually aware of the strains resulting from divergence of patient and faculty interests. They often reflect a view that their education "becomes sandwiched between the burden of handling the community sick and the pressures of research."[10] Recognizing these problems, house staffs have attempted to organize nationally as a pressure group. However, since they occupy temporary positions as students in postgraduate medical education and have limited influence in their local situations, they have succeeded only in creating periodic forums for airing grievances.[11] Physicians-in-training usually become heavily occupied with and even overwhelmed by providing a service, support of which either from the hospital (community) or faculty is disarticulated from the level of demand. How do they make choices in the face of conflict between patient interests and their own education? Chaiklin demonstrated that if they have a choice at all they decide in favor of their education, and they complain if the choice forced upon them interferes with their plans.[12]

The role played by physicians-in-training was studied in detail by Duff, Rowe, and Anderson in a pediatric out-patient setting.[13] They found that physicians as well as students did not understand the concerns of children and their families that prompted 75 percent of the visits. Students sought a history and problem formulation that coincided with their ideas, regardless of the fact that the family had different ideas about their problems. Even when the attending pediatricians discovered this divergence, they did not take corrective action. The time they spent with the children and their families was related strongly to the teaching schedules of the clinic, not to the problems at hand. They felt their primary role was to teach the students, not to provide a service to the patient, and they failed to appreciate that not dealing with the child's problem constituted a service deficiency and a training defect.

Thus, while the technical aspects of patient care are taught and applied in medical centers, the provision for and teaching about the personal aspects of patients are neglected. This is a result of faculty emphasis on research, the power of the faculty in deciding medical center policy, and the inability of the poor to influence their own care. The latter point is a consequence of the position of the poor in society. As members of the lowest socio-economic group they are unaccustomed to demand service. They are also often members of a minority group, with a wide social gap between themselves and those usually entrusted with their care. On the adult services they are usually also separated by age from the student physicians who are young and unprepared to counsel the sick, disabled, and dying. In addition, the sick person is often fearful and dependent, if not frankly childlike.

The families of the sick poor are unable to command attention. As laymen, they cannot judge the technical aspects of the patient's problems. They are preoccupied with the tasks of making a living and solving problems other than those associated directly with health. Indeed, health is often given a lower priority than essentials of living such as food and shelter. Further, the discontinuities of the medical training program limit the influence of poor patients and their families in health care. Each patient has to deal with several physicians-in-training who work together to provide services in any one assignment and rotate among services in accordance with their educational schedules. The result is "committee sponsorship" of the patient. There is no recognizable continuing physician-patient relationship by any criterion suggested by the American Medical Association or by the television programs that dramatize illness or patient care. The commonly projected images of the physician's role in dealing with patients and families differ markedly from the actual role.

In summary, physicians-in-training are taught, in effect, to disregard the interests of patients. Technological imperatives in medicine easily override the interests of the sick poor and their families. This was illustrated vividly in a recent interview with a pediatrician who was asked what voice poor families in his medical center were given in deciding the management of children with hopeless prognoses. He said they were given no choice and added: "We go the limit for everyone. The state pays for it. Maybe this isn't always right, but it is justified by the teaching and research we can do this way." While there may be many moderating influences to such extreme positions, the career incentives in training centers favor such positions; the available information indicates the performances of faculty and physicians-in-training reflect these realities.

THE PERFORMANCE OF PHYSICIANS

Mechanic emphasized that "much of the demand for medical care is motivated by people's personal problems, which affect their health and vitality."[14] It was noted by Gardner that individuals with common physical illnesses are more likely to seek care when they suffer from personal and social stresses.[15] Of course, those who are physically sick usually have associated personal problems. An approach to patient care that attempts to deal with these factors was outlined by Lipowski, who emphasized that physicians should exert considerable effort in practicing the art of medicine to solve personal problems.[16] Duff and Hollingshead, however, in a study of 161 patients, found that such efforts were rarely made. Physicians carried out many procedures, sometimes admitted patients unnecessarily, and usually did not explore the personal problems of patients. It was concluded that most physicians had little awareness of the feelings of patients in all categories, not just the poor. They rarely were concerned with patient's views of illnesses and symptoms, or the influence of these upon the personal problems of patients. The problems of patients were not understood adequately and the solutions offered were often illusory.

These observations coincide with several reports that reflect the quality of decision making in health care. The writing of prescriptions is one example. Forsyth and Logan classified the apparent therapeutic intent of 6,288 prescriptions in general practice in England. Less than one third were specific or probably specific, examples being respectively insulin for diabetes and antibiotics for respiratory infections. Approximately two thirds were classified as possibly beneficial, (for example, antihistamines for allergies), hopefully useful (amphetamines for obesity), or placebo.[17] One interpretation of these prescribing habits is that the doctor can appear to be doing something for the suffering patient whatever the nature of the problem. As Balint found, some prescription writing constitutes problem avoidance by patients and physicians.[18]

The growth of prescription writing has been striking. Gosselin reports an approximate doubling in prescription writing in each of the two decades between 1950 and 1970.[19] He attributes this in part to a medical profession "eagerly" awaiting "miracle drugs." By 1969 the volume of prescriptions reached 1.2 billion, or approximately six prescriptions per person per year. By these figures, physicians in active practice on the average wrote in excess of 4,000 prescriptions in that year. Gosselin expects this same exponential growth rate in the next decade.

Prescribing habits have been considered to reflect a style of practice. Wilson, who analyzed his own prescription writing for one year, asked: "How is one to teach (and to learn) the art of non-prescribing?" [20] In the same medical journal, an editorial stated: "Fashions have ever been the bane of medicine. The general practitioner of today is every bit the creature of fashion as any mini-skirted minx." Muller contends that patients, the pharmaceutical industry, and especially doctors account for our "over medicated society."[21] She also reported that high frequency of prescriptions was associated with physicians' limited understanding of patients.

Comparing surgical rates provides another indicator of decision making. Lewis and Bunker found that higher surgical rates were associated with higher surgeon-population ratios and the availability of insurance and hospital beds. [22]

In these studies, the magnitude of difference was highly significant, in some instances being twofold or more. Differences in illness rates and hence "need" for the surgery were not likely explanations of the findings.

In a study of pediatric inpatient care, Duff and associates found that an average of 25 percent of the admissions in four hospitals were unnecessary.[23] Antibiotics were frequently misused, and surgery sometimes was unnecessary. Medical records often indicated that personal and social problems existed; but usually they were ignored.

While the views of patients and families toward the expense of their care is easy to gauge (they don't like it), their role in the decisions about their care invites attention. Duff and Hollingshead found that while patients and families agreed they wanted care for physical illnesses, they felt less keenly about an exploration of those personal or family attributes that accounted for many of their symptoms and more than half of their disabilities.[24] Concerns of the psyche cannot be comprehended, much less dealt with unless the professionals undertake a skillful, sympathetic exploration of both physical and psychological difficulties. This says only that the physician should be prepared to understand the patient's problems in the context of the patient's life. Ironically, however, the patient is often unwilling to reveal himself—what he is, does, and feels—though the roots of his symptoms may be linked so intimately to him. Thus, the patient, especially one with low self-esteem or other unpleasant feelings about himself may be most cooperative with the doctor who is concerned quite exclusively with physical disease. Both doctors and patient then agree upon a limited agenda and a similarly restricted approach to patient care. As in the medical centers, the physician can diagnose and treat physical diseases; and in practice he can be paid well for it. The patient can pursue the relief of symptoms without becoming too involved in unpleasant ways. Regarding this aspect of the doctor-patient relationship, Magraw states, "The fundamental issue be tween patient and doctor at this point is honesty. If the doctor is to understand the patient, he must be willing to use his own honest dedication to his job to force this issue and to insist that the patient 'show his hand' as part of the price for help."[25]

There are indications that doctors and their patients do not clarify the patients' complaints. For example, the recommendations of physicians are often rejected by patients and families. Davis reported that patient noncompliance rates in several studies were from 30 to 50 percent higher than most physicians believed. Francis, Korsch, and Morris found noncompliance related to gaps in communications between physicians and patients or families. Elling found that compliance was related as well to a variety of lay beliefs and practices about health.[26]

Medical recommendations may be rejected by patients or families when the prognosis is poor. Patients may find an early death more acceptable than chronic dialysis or kidney transplant. Death from malignancy may be preferred to a life limited by suffering from disease or by the rigors of treatment.[27] In the case of a child with a very poor prognosis for a meaningful life (as in mongolism or severe meningomyelocele), some parents wonder if their desire to have *any* child may violate the child's possible preference for relief in death.[28] They also question to what extent the limited family resources must be spent for lost causes.

In brief, the prescribing habits of physicians, decisions to hospitalize, differential surgical rates, and the management of persons with a poor prognosis suggest that physicians in practice, just as faculty and physicians in training, have a marked tendency to diagnose and to decide therapy chiefly on technical considerations rather than considering personal and social realities as well. Physicians are usually paid for the performance of selected acts such as surgical or laboratory procedures or an office or hospital consultation. They are not paid for solving either physical or personal problems, and for the latter they may be penalized since such problems require much time for which physicians are not likely to be paid. As a result, physicians probably do many things that are unnecessary and may be harmful. While patients may derive some satisfaction in these situations, they or their families often reject physicians' choices. What proportion of such rejections are respectively fortunate, unfortunate, or of little consequence for the patient and the family is not known. However, it seems evident that two major sources of lay dissatisfaction emerge: high cost, which needs no documentation here; and a disquieting sense of alienation between the seekers of help and the profession of medicine. Commenting on a state of "irritable tension in both patient and doctor," Coleman states that "the most common way the doctor has of dealing with this problem is to attempt to substitute for it an attitude of professional superiority and distance, which is in effect a reproduction of parental attitudes of omnipotence and omniscience. 'I know everything, I can do everything for you. There is nothing that I cannot do. Trust me and everything will be all right.' Such an attitude serves the purpose of denying that the physician is disturbed by the patient's challenge of his competence; at the same time, because it is a defense arising out of feelings of weakness, it does not really have the intended result of reassuring the patient or the doctor. However, since it is the attitude most patients are used to in one form or another, it is allowed to pass as coin of the realm instead of the counterfeit it is."[29]

Medical practitioners tend to view lay contexts of illness

and its management with distant skepticism. As May points out, they usually consider "irregular practitioners" such as Christian Scientists, spiritualists, chiropractors, curanderos, and acupuncturists as quacks;[30] and they discount the important roles often performed by druggists, clergymen and grandmothers as pediatricians. In this light, the reforms that followed the Flexner report might be seen, as May indicates, as "an attempt to limit competition and increase control over the delivery of health care." That control, Gross believes, is pervasive.[31] He finds physicians too often patronizing, sometimes arrogant, father figures who ignore the interests of the sick and their families.

Physicians as high-status technocrats become dominant; patients of lower status and dependent, may "belong" to the doctor.[32] The doctor as technocrat has little reason to take into account those patient "sentiments" which Henderson reported "are likely to be the most important phenomena" in the patient-physician relationship.[33] In the resulting confusion, priorities concerning the personal and social aspects of individual patient care and the relative social importance of different diseases are not likely to be considered. Physicians are reluctant to point out these problems because they fear being misunderstood or attacked by their patients or colleagues. Apparently, as long as illusions are appealing to the public and are rewarding to the professionals, there will be much difficulty in assessing priorities, however important this may be, for rational health care.

Thus, the dependency of the sick upon high-status persons (physicians) creates a special power imbalance not in the patient's favor and often not in his interest. This imbalance is exaggerated by the ways physicians-in-training are socialized into the profession of medicine. For the poor, it is a case of Hobson's choice. And this choice in due course tends to be offered to the majority of the sick.

As to recommendations, two approaches follow from the foregoing analysis. The first, is audit of performance. Lembke traces the course of such developments in the twentieth century.[34] He finds limited success in the medical audit and an early, abortive attempt to relate medical and hospital services to the end results for the patient. Although the management of diseases has changed and usually improved, it seems doubtful that much progress has been made in auditing patient care since 1914 when Codman advocated the systematic examination of the end results for the patient by the medical staff, the hospital administration, and the trustees.[35] Codman seems to have been in advance of *our* time, nearly sixty years later. It appears this will be so until both the public and the profession become responsible allies dedicated to solving health problems. While an elaborate discussion of this subject is beyond the scope of this paper, success in audit probably will depend upon disinterested *professional and lay review* of care. Such review should be applied both in training and in regular practice situations; and it should influence both professional and lay educational policies and practices.

The second approach would break up that unique linkage of medical education to the care of the sick poor. Those who are used as teaching subjects need more protection from the educators and the students; and the latter two need protection from high concentrations of the problems of the poor. Health professionals should be reminded that people are persons first and patients second. Clearly, in the present circumstances the poor cannot perform this function adequately; and even if they could, faculty and physicians in training cannot respond. As a result, major flaws in training are created and are ignored. These flaws appear to be reflected in the care of most persons.

X. The Reorganization of Practice in the Community

by John D. Stoeckle

The care and treatment of the poor have always required special solutions. The history of medical services for the poor is a history of special financing, special treatment-institutions and clinical organization, and even special therapeutic, health-education and human-relations methods.[1] Within this special system, the poor have had medical bills paid by taxes and charity rather than by their own funds, wards rather than private rooms, clinical teams rather than private doctors, school health examinations in place of office checkups, bureaucratic outpatient and public health clinics rather than private offices, and a greater reliance on authoritarian methods of inducing cooperation and education. The poor and their medical needs were thought to be different and to require these special solutions that have been separate from and cheaper than private, solo practice, the major medical care organization. In reorganizing the health services today for everyone, should those for the poor still remain something apart? Hardly so. Our ideals

Dr. John D. Stoeckle is Chief, Medical Clinics, Massachusetts General Hospital, Boston, Massachusetts.

about equity in access, about equality in treatment, and the importance we attach to health for the achievement of the poor and non-poor alike no longer permit special solutions. Moreover, we cannot afford them. The enormous cost of medical technology requires common use.

The pressing medical care needs of the poor today are the same as for everyone: out-of-hospital care. There are already enough, if not too many, hospital beds and services for all. The indices of health status of the poor—more dental caries, more psychological distress and psychiatric disorders, more infant-perinatal deaths, more chronic diseases and longer disability from the same illness than those with higher incomes—are, in fact, problems that require more out-of-hospital care. These health problems are also universal. Further, most of the deficiencies in the treatment of the poor are not in the hospital but in those organizations that provide treatment outside it. And while the poor are handicapped in access to and treatment within community medical practices, so are many others. Finally, while insurance covers hospital costs for nearly everyone, coverage of any kind for out-of-hospital care is limited for those at the bottom and for those in the middle it is hardly comprehensive. Thus, the reorganization of care outside the hospital no longer requires a special solution for the poor alone but a general solution for everyone.

But not everyone will agree about the importance of practice in the community. Many argue that it is not important to change out-of-hospital care as long as the poor continue to be victims of inequalities among hospitals. Sociologists, as participant observers, and physicians, as policy critics, have documented that the long-stay institutions, like the mental and chronic disease hospital, have less for accommodations, staff, and treatment than the modern acute hospital, and that the poor are more handicapped in them. Residents in the "dumping grounds" of long-stay institutions are mostly poor. Others also know about these inequities. Patients going through medical institutions easily recognize them as did John Vaisey in his *Scenes from Institutional Life;* moviegoers can view them on the films at the local cinema; so can visitors on a walking tour through hospitals. Well documented, easily visible, and sometimes dramatic, these differences between long and short-stay hospitals continue to make the hospital the popular focus of reform to the neglect of out-of-hospital care. So often the inequalities of hospitals are muted by giving them more money for accommodations without changing their organization. However, this very conventional and comfortable approach to reform of the hospital is mistaken. Alternatives to and reorganized practices for managing illness in the community can avoid what may seem to be the very necessity of hospital use and the experience that goes with it. Reorganization of practice outside the hospital is a more difficult matter but it is a necessary and a more significant reform.

The poor and others have sought treatment in five types of community medical practices (Table IX-1) and each, in turn, has been a proposed solution to the organization of medical care in the community for everyone. The first two are the traditional older organizations—solo private practices, recently self-regulated as foundations for medical care, and the hospital outpatient department; the third is the somewhat newer, private group practice that is either fee-for-service or prepaid (health maintenance organization); and the fourth and fifth are the newest medical practices—health centers and free clinics. Finally, a national health service should be mentioned, although it does not exist and is rarely discussed as a serious proposal to the solution of medical care in the community.

Table X–1. Out-of-Hospital treatment organizations: health centers, free clinics, outpatient departments, group practice, prepaid group practice plan, medical foundations and solo practices.

Treatment organization	Number	Type of funding	Amount	Patient population or visits (million) estimated
1. Health centers Neighborhood health centers	125	Office of Economic Opportunity, 1966 Health, Education & Welfare Dept., 314	188 million (FY 1972)	1.2 mil. enrolled 5.2 mil. estimated visits
Maternity-infant care projects (neighborhood centers attached to hospitals)	56	Title V Social Security Act 1963	116 million (FY 1972)	660,000 total women (210,000) infants & children (350,000) 2.8 mil. visits estimated
Children and youth projects (50% medical school attached, 50% public health depts.)	60	Title V Social Security Act 1963		

Community mental health centers	349	National Institute of Mental Health Operating Grants	105 million (FY 1972)	.3 mil. visits estimated
2. "Free medical clinics"	170	Voluntary, some from public health depts., e.g. Los Angeles		1.0 mil. visits estimated
3. Outpatient depts., voluntary, municipal, federal hospitals	7,123	Medicare, Medicaid, fees, municipal and federal taxes, insurance		180 mil. visits estimated
4. Prepaid group practice plans, prototype health maintenance organizations	20	Insurance-per capita basis	Federal funds 23 million for planning HMO's (FY 1972); 22 million for operation (FY 1972)	7 mil. enrolled; 30 mil. visits estimated
5. Private group practices	6,371 (40,000 MD's)	Fee for service insurance; prepayment for over 50% income in only 1% of groups	—	130 mil. visits estimated

Treatment organization	Number	Type of funding	Amount	Patient population or visits (million) estimated
6. Solo practices	200,000 MD's	Fee for service and insurance	)	520 mil. visits estimated
7. Medical foundations	40	Insurance, fees	—	?

Sources: Information on health centers was obtained from *Special Analysis K, Federal Health Programs,* Office of Management and Budgets (Washington, D.C.: U.S. Government Printing Office, 1971) and from *Promoting the Health of Mothers and Children* (Washington, D.C.: U.S. Department of Health, Education and Welfare, 1970). Information on Free Clinics was obtained from personal communication, Dr. Jerome L. Schwartz, and from J. Gordon, "The Free Clinic Movement," *National Service Center for Health Service Studies,* 1 (1971). Information on outpatient departments were obtained from Nora Piore, Deborah Lewis, and Lennie Seeliger, *A Statistical Profile of Hospital Outpatient Services in the United States: Present Scope and Potential Role* (New York: Association for Aid to Crippled Children, 1971). Reported here are civilian hospital OPDs that number 5,859: those of federal and special hospitals (veterans and tuberculosis facilities) number 1,264, making a total of 7,123. Actually 80 percent of visits to federal-special OPDs are by civilian beneficiaries. Information on private group practices and solo practices obtained from *Medical Groups with United States—1969* (Chicago: American Medical Association, 1971) and *Reference Data on Socioeconomic Issues of Health,* ed. K. K. Monroe (Chicago: Center for Health Services Research and Development, American Medical Association, 1971). Visits to the different practices were calculated on the basis of 4.3 per person enrolled. Facts on governmental funding of out-of-hospital programs were obtained from *Special Analysis K,* Federal Health Programs.

These organizations or reorganizations of medical practice raise two questions: In which type of practice are the poor likely to receive optimal treatment? Will any or all of these organizations really insure the equitable distribution of health services available and accessible to the poor and everyone else?

SOLO PRACTICE

Most out-of-hospital care in the United States is provided by individual private practitioners; outpatient clinics at hospitals and other settings account for a smaller percentage of such care (Chart X-1). Visits to solo doctors number approximately 520 million (60 percent of all physician visits), while visits to outpatient departments make up only 20 percent (180 million). Public health clinics account for a trifling 1 percent.[2] Even though these latter two sources of care are used proportionately more by low-income individuals, many poor receive much of their care from private practitioners, and many use more than one source of medical aid. These facts can easily be learned from clinical encounters with patients and from published studies documenting the expenditures of public funds to private doctors for ambulatory care. A Chicago study revealed that private practitioners received 29 percent of the payments for office care, while the remainder went to institutions.[3] A survey of sources of medical care used by the outpatient clientele of a voluntary hospital revealed that 57 percent also used private physicians.[4] In a survey of New York municipal hospital outpatients, the private doctor use was 32 percent.[5] The National Health Survey reported that patients with annual incomes under $4,000 had 66.4 percent of their visits in private offices and 19.7 percent in a hospital clinic.[6] The percentages were similar to those with incomes under $2,000. In Massachusetts, 75 percent of the welfare pay-

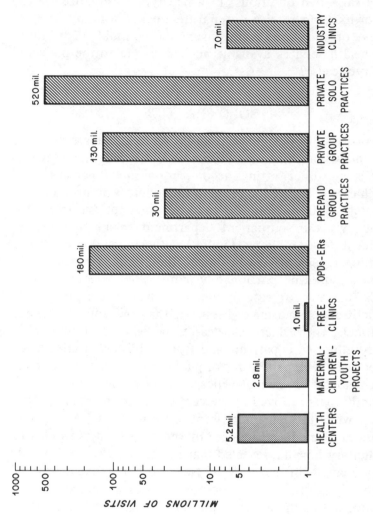

Chart X-1. Treatment organizations and their use (estimated annual visits)

ments for out-of-hospital medical services, namely, out-patient clinics and physicians, went to community private practitioners; the pattern was reversed only in the City of Boston.[7] Of low-income families eligible for OEO health centers, 30 to 60 percent listed the private doctor as their usual source of care.[8] The care of the poor through private practice, although very sizable, is simply less visible than their care in municipal and private hospital clinics; hence, the latter and not the private practice are the usual targets of critics like Roth. Although the private doctor is assumed to be good or better, we actually know less about his care. Certainly, if the care of the poor requires reforms, these will have to include private practices, as well.

Regardless of the type of medical practice—public or private, group or solo—many ambulatory practices available to the poor are thought to have built-in barriers to their use.[9] Because of these barriers, the poor do not use office care with the same frequency as the affluent. The reason for this may not be that care is inconvenient and fragmented but, rather, that it may simply be less available. In areas where the poor live there are, to be sure, fewer solo practitioners. A Chicago survey found that the ratio of physicians to residents was 0.62 per 1000 in poverty areas, compared to 1.26 per 1000 in a nonpoverty area. In Boston the poverty areas have seen a steady decline in the number of doctors practicing there. The number of doctors having offices registered in two of the largest poverty districts of the city has declined by 50 percent and 30 percent respectively within the last twenty years.[10] The South End Medical Club, an organization of general practitioners with offices in that area of Boston, had, in the 1920s, a large active membership engaged in community practice; with the exodus and death of physicians, membership gradually declined so that the organization disbanded in the 1950s. Such findings suggest that the office care available to the poor within their residential areas is limited in quantity. Some practitioners have left without replacement, some have changed their practice from general to special, and others have clustered in other areas of the city. As a result, solo practice care is less available and less accessible to the poor.

THE OUTPATIENT DEPARTMENT (OPD)

Until the advent of health centers and group practices, the Outpatient Department-Emergency Room had been the only alternative to private solo practice. Although an alternative, the OPD is not a distinct and independent form of practice, but a hospital-based organizational accommodation of community private practice. Historically, hospital care was the responsibility of voluntary boards and public authorities, while private medical practitioners had the mandate for care in the community. As a result, in a world where everyone was not a paying patient, some organization was needed for nonpaying patients. Each doctor might view his own office as the best of all possible OPDs to treat a few nonpaying patients, and many did. But for a large number of the "sick poor" the hospital OPD became the administrative and economic mechanism for distributing the "free service" of its staff by separating the management of out-of-hospital practice from professional treatment, a separation that conflicted with the management ideology of individual entrepreneurial medicine. As a practice, the OPD was limited in access and scope. First, its patients were restricted: the OPD was accessible only to those who could not afford a private doctor. The means test, implicit in the voluntary ethic of "free care for the sick poor," controlled access. The part-time work of the private doctor, a morning treatment session each week, limited the scope of services even with the OPD managed by the hospital administration. Thus, the OPD has not been an independent practice but an accommodation of the institution of private practice in the community and at the hospital.

Such historical restrictions on patients and staff have made the OPD a segregated organization, in which all its elements and participants have had but one definition, and each was closely interlocked with the others.[11] Its features have been (1) poor patients or those with limited incomes who "could not afford private care"; (2) a special facility located at the hospital but separate from the community or hospital-based offices of the hospital's private practitioners; (3) a part-time staff made up of both the hospital's private medical staff, volunteering some time for treatment often in exchange for hospital admission privileges for their own patients and, in some instances, a contractual staff of doctors in training assigned for part of their time to work in the OPD while giving most of their attention to hospitalized patients; (4) a clinic or group organization consisting of several physicians supported by nurses, secretaries, and sometimes aides; and (5) a system of fees set at less than cost.

This structure of the OPD as an organized practice with single definitions of buildings, patients, staff, clinical organization, and pricing system all closely interlocked has changed as the hospital has expanded both its ambulatory services and its practices. First, ambulatory facilities or building services at the hospital now provide fixed rental and transient office space for some or all of the hospital staff as well as OPDs. Twenty percent of physicians in private practice (51,000) are now working in hospital-based rented offices—in essence, a private OPD managed by each staff member. Similarly, many hospital emergency rooms—OPD's are simply building services that provide transient office space for doctors to see their own patients at the hospital, or facilities that are managed as treatment concessions by doctors in private practice. Second, outpatient diagnostic services for studies such as X-ray and laboratory examinations are now accessible to private patients of the hospital staff as well as to those of the hospital's outpatient clinics. Finally, fee-charging policies are changing to permit the access of patients of all backgrounds. The tradition of charging less than cost has disappeared as the financing of out-of-hospital care has been expanded so that it is shared, in part, by the patient, by the government (Medicare and Medicaid), and by the insurance subscriber. As full costs are charged, the means test has been removed, so that special treatment services within the OPD such as emergency rooms, walk-in clinics, radiation therapy and special disease clinics have become accessible to and used by all the public. The outpatient department is no longer a segregated institution.

The development of community-based health centers and Medicare-Medicaid for private care were predicted to result in a decreased use of outpatient departments. However, OPD-ER use has continued to increase in the last five years. The 180 million OPD visits of 1970 are 20 percent of the total 860 million physician visits, compared to the 14 percent of 1965 (Table IX-1). Of these 180 million, 134 million visits were at the 5,829 OPD's of the nation's community hospitals, one third were at emergency rooms—a rise from the 20 percent of a decade earlier—and the remaining two thirds were at OPD clinics.[12]

Despite the rise in OPD use, critics will claim that the poor are basically handicapped in treatment at OPD's compared to their treatment at other sources of medical aid. Several characteristics of OPDs have been criticized. First, access remains limited, less so for lack of money since these barriers have been partially removed by Medicaid and Medicare than because of bureaucratic reception and registration. Second, treatment is depersonalized and discontinuous. Treatment organized only around different medical specialties fails to care for the patient and his family as a unit. Staff assignments that are only parttime fail to provide any continuity of care unless it can be supplied by the full-time nursing and social work staff. Third, communication with patients may be limited.[13] Fourth, OPDs have not always been as efficient as other practices in large part because many have both teaching programs and part-time staffs that impose restrictions on efficiency. Finally, facilities may be substandard.

Some of the deficiencies of the outpatient department stem not from its organization but from its support; moreover, its organization can change. Registration and reception can be simplified and personalized. The possibility of full-time medical staff for OPDs, as in health centers, is now possible with new financing. The staffing patterns that result can improve continuity, personalize care, and make it possible to organize some treatment around family care models as this becomes valued. Deficiency in communication has been studied only in OPDs, but indifference may be related as much to the doctor's training and orientation as to the organization of the OPD. If facilities are not standard and supporting services are inefficient, it is because this department has not commanded the resources for improvement or the interest of the hospital trustees, managers, staff, public agencies, volunteers, and segments of the community who hold a different set of priorities than out-of-hospital care. Many of these features are changing as the better financing of out-of-hospital care makes change possible and as traditional professional preferences for the entrepreneurial model of practice changes, permitting a salaried practice arrangement.

HEALTH MAINTENANCE ORGANIZATIONS (HMOs)
OR PREPAID GROUP PRACTICE

The legislation that provided for the establishment of health maintenance organizations (HMOs), Title XI of the Public Health Service Acts of 1971, did not define them precisely, so that even medical foundations might be included in the definition; nonetheless, prepaid group practice is the major model for HMOs, and the intent of the legislation is to convert tax-supported health centers, OPDs, and fee-for-service solo practice into insurance-supported HMOs. Prepaid group practice had its origins in the hospital outpatient department, in the "lodge" and "company" doctor of the late 1800s, in professional efforts to organize specialty medical practices early in the 1900s, and in the continuing efforts of cooperatives and unions since the 1900s to secure care at reasonable cost.[14] Their internal issues have been management, costs, and specialization.

The hospital's administrative invention, the OPD, separated the management of practice from professional care to make the staff available for the care of sick poor; retaining its professional controls, group practice similarly separated management to increase professional productivity. For cost control, the "lodge" doctor was retained for the care of members of fraternal-ethnic organizations by a fixed annual fee assessed to each; similarly, the company doctor for "the working poor," miners and factory workers, was paid an annual capitation fee, the "check off option," to be responsible for their treatment. By capitation payment, the doctors were assured an income and were meant to provide care below the cost if fee-for-service had been charged. They did, although the scope of their services rarely went beyond the immediate medical aid of a dispensary. On the other hand, the group practice of medical specialists had different intentions. Developing around the work of surgeons, group practice was for the coordinated care of patients whose treatment was divided among specialists and for the control of a practice domain big enough to maintain referrals to specialist surgeons without depending entirely on those from diffuse networks of solo practices. The Mayo Clinic is among the earliest and most notable of group practices organized around medical specialization. The Group Health Association of Washington, D.C. (1937), the Kaiser Foundation Health Plan (1938), Group Health Cooperative of Puget Sound (1944), United Mine Workers Health and Retirement Fund (1946) supported clinics, and Health Insurance Plan of Greater New York (1947) are similar examples of group practice based on prepayment. Some twenty prepaid practice plans now cover an estimated seven million persons (Table IX-1).

Today, the intent of the HMO legislation is to provide grants, contracts, loans, and loan guarantees for such prepaid practices, particularly in "medically unserved areas." HMO goals are to provide (1) comprehensive, as distinct from sporadic, care; (2) preventive as well as curative care for a "defined population," namely, those enrolled in the group; and (3) control of costs for such services by financing care on a yearly per capita basis rather than on an individual fee for each service, a payment mechanism that provides incentives for the practices to control their costs.

The major model for the HMO idea have been the Kaiser Foundation Health Plan, Kaiser Foundation Hospitals, and the Permanente Medical Groups.[15] This organizational complex of insurance, facilities, and group practice had its beginnings in 1938 with the care of industrial workers and their families. The basic elements of the Kaiser Medical Care Program have been itemized by Saward as (1) prepayment of medical services, usually by monthly dues; (2) group practice for treatment of patients; (3) facilities of a medical center that includes both hospital and clinic; (4) voluntary enrollment; (5) capitation payment; and (6) comprehensive services.[16] Prepayment does away with fee-for-service and gives all subscribers equal benefits for the same rate. Differential rates, for example, higher ones based on the higher risk of enrolled older groups, are eliminated. The medical group practice is a self-governing, full-time, salaried unit with contractual arrangements with the prepaid insurance plan and is paid by capitation, a fixed sum for each enrollee. All treatment facilities are administratively integrated for both inpatients and outpatients. The group practice is based at the hospital and its clinics, but staff are also available at some "detached" clinics in neighborhoods. Enrollment in the plan is voluntary—the usual three choices for the potential enrollee being the Kaiser Plan, an indemnity policy providing the subscriber a cash benefit for illness, or Blue Cross-Blue Shield insurance providing specified out and in-hospital service using the doctor of the patient's choice. Among various employee groups, prepaid practice is chosen by 20 to 60 percent. With per capita payment, both the physicians and hospital are paid for services they contract to render, producing a predictable income for the planning and provision of services. The comprehensive coverage in this definition means that services are not restricted to one site of care, such as the hospital but include home, outpatient and inpatient care, both within the hospital itself and the posthospital extended care facility, as well as drug coverage and mental health services. It does not, however, refer to the full range of therapeutic services.

A major argument on behalf of prepaid group practices is that costs are reduced, particularly those for hospital care. Perrot's analysis of hospitalization under various plans for federal employees found that those under prepaid group practice were hospitalized about one half as much as those under Blue Cross-Blue Shield and indemnity plans.[17] More ambulatory care at less expense is used by members of prepaid group practice plans compared to persons using other practices.

Some reservations with respect to HMOs should be mentioned. Continued savings from the reduction in hospital use is uncertain. Expansion of HMOs to include more elderly persons and those with higher risks may not sustain the current savings on hospitalization. Comparisons have not been made on how comprehensive and preventive are the services of prepaid practices and how often they are used. While they do offer inpatient and outpatient care and so are comprehensive by site and number of services, care that is comprehensive for such social-medical problems as alcoholism and drug use so prevalent in poverty districts may be limited. Under the Kaiser Plan, for example, contracts cannot exclude treatment of drug abuse and alcoholism, but special programs for these disorders may not be organized. People with such problems are often treated at municipal clinics and outpatient departments. Whether HMOs will devise new services or strategies of access and treatment for the special poverty groups they enroll is uncertain. In offering conventional medical services, different patterns of use among their "poor" subscribers may result, namely, more emergency ward use than scheduled visits, as observed by Kosa and others.[18] The critique by Cohen and Waitzkin of the Harvard Community Health Plan is that its special subsidy and increased premium for low-income groups is based on their expected higher use of services, an expectation not likely from previous studies, at least not unless utilization is stimulated by programs of "out-reach," which add another expense to premium rates.[19] When out-reach and social work services are added, they are not financed, as in OPDs, as part of charges for medical services but are financed separately through government grants, artificially reducing the costs attributed to prepaid practice.

Many of the prepaid group plans—the Health Insurance Plan of New York and the Kaiser Plan to mention two—have enrolled poverty groups under a capitation payment arrangement. The plans might increase utilization among low-income subscribers. Two studies indicate that some increase does occur but it does not yet equal that of higher-income subscribers and follows a pattern of greater emergency ward use.[20] Since some 30 to 40 percent of prepaid subscribers go outside their plan for some services, whether more of the poor will go outside or just will not go is also uncertain. The fiscal pressure of HMOs to contain costs also can increase incentives for underuse. While this possible outcome is a common critique, the most significant concern is not underuse but fewer and limited services.

NEIGHBORHOOD HEALTH CENTERS

Health centers are the most popular organizations in the current reform of out-of-hospital care for the poor.[21] Public concern with distribution, use, quality, and orientation of the whole system of health care is reflected in the aspirations of the health centers, their locations, organization, staff, and treatment strategies. Since 1966 some 125 have been established with federal funds from either the Office of Economic Opportunity or more recently from the Department of Health, Education and Welfare. In addition, a large number of centers have been developed by municipal health departments and private voluntary hospitals with and without some federal financing. In Boston, for example, some twenty-five health centers have opened since 1966.[22]

Another 116 health centers have been funded by the Children's Bureau under Title V of the Social Security Act (Table IX-1), but these are limited to the care of children and mothers.

The idea of the health center as an institution for out-of-hospital care is not new. In the course of its historical development it has come to combine seven characteristics: (1) a common, decentralized facility in the community for doctors, nurses, social workers, health educators, and others concerned with out-of-hospital care and the social welfare of patients; (2) group organization of medical practice, which may range from informal contacts of independent practitioners to a tightly knit staff with specific assigned tasks, roles, and duties that maintain strict interprofessional boundaries; (3) district responsibility for a population or clientele usually restricted to residents of a limited geographic area or to those enrolled for services; (4) services rationally linked to other institutions by formal referral channels and agreement on specific tasks rendered by the center and other institutions; (5) community participation; (6) a program of curative and preventive medicine for individuals and the community; and (7) public financing through grants for facilities and services. The forms of the centers vary and have been shaped not only by public needs for health services but by professional concerns with efficiency, coordination, quality, and effectiveness of health care in the community.

Each of these organizational features is meant to improve care in the community. Decentralized location is meant to insure easy access from the homes of the community's residents. District responsibility, by limiting the area of responsibility, makes the provision of personal and preventive services feasible. Only then can such services be applied to the whole district population and their effects be contin-

uously monitored. The group organization of medical practice is salaried and uses nonphysician health workers in
teams to provide the patient's care and treatment rather
than the doctor alone. Nonphysician health workers extend
the working arm of the doctor in delivering care, and the
team (doctor, nurse, physician assistant, aide, and social
worker), rather than the single therapist provides personal
and family care that is more comprehensive than in the past
and, presumably cheaper than the doctor working alone.
The preventive orientation is accomplished by tactics of
reaching out to the population through aides and family
workers rather than depending on residents alone to initiate
care. Automated health screening may also be used as a
cost-saving technical device for case finding for secondary
prevention. Community participation includes various options for community residents to be involved in management, health center jobs, consumer representation, and governance. The purposes of community participation vary
from those of civic training through consumer representation about appropriate services, to actual community control through governance of the center and its programs,
money and staff, or to social-economic uplift through jobs
in the health center. Public tax money in the form of
federal and municipal grants provides the major financing
for the health center. Medicare and Medicaid receipts from
the center's users make up additional capital for its operation.

So far, few reports are available to judge the effectiveness
of centers in reducing illness and disability. Moreover, results may be quite difficult to get.[23] One experiment in
Chicago found a reduction in infant mortality. Mothers of
fifteen years or less in a maternal care-center program had
an infant death rate of 10.0/1000 compared to 36.0/1000
for mothers not in the program.[24] As might be expected,

utilization data are more readily available. A major impact of the Columbia Point Health Center, in Boston, was to increase physician visits at the health center to the norms of those with higher incomes and to decrease the use its patients made of the hospitals.[25] The emergency ward, a site of out-of-hospital care considered inappropriate for many patient care needs of the poor, had its use reduced by a health center in Rochester, New York. But similar shifts have not occurred in the Bunker Hill Health Center connected with the Massachusetts General Hospital in Boston.[26] This shift, or lack of it, in the patterns of emergency ward use may reflect many factors: the hours centers are open, transportation routes to centers and emergency wards, the referral traditions of practitioners and patients, and the unwillingness of institutions to cooperate. Health centers are opening throughout the country at a time when intracity transportation is at its worst. As a result, the long-term benefits and costs of small, decentralized centers and district coverage are difficult to judge. Looking at other examples of transportation and medical use, the improved transportation under the federal-state highway program has made many of the very small southern hospitals created by the Hill-Burton Hospital Program less necessary since people can so easily get to bigger ones where more can be done. Similarly, better ways of getting about in cities may affect the current health centers' size, location, and use. Looking at community participation as community control or governance, it takes various patterns in centers, and the effects are uncertain and difficult to measure. Most studies are institutional case reports on the problems of simply trying to establish workable relationships between the community and center.[27] Few studies have tried to measure the effects of various degrees and patterns of community control. In one survey that did, high levels of community control did not increase utilization of services and but marginally affected the community's satisfactions and identification with health centers—effects presumed to be derived from participation.[28] Community control will not serve as a substitute for well-run medical services. Despite these reservations about the instrumental effects of participation, those who have been involved in the process would seldom do without it. The press for community participation in health centers may not reflect new values in organization but may only be, as Hollister has observed, a transient interest.[29] Health care has been the first place where poverty groups could gain access to money and jobs when so little was available in other fields such as housing or education. Center financing through grants supplemented by Medicaid and Medicare receipts does offer the poor free services that must still be obtained by tests of eligibility, a chronic barrier to access. And the costs of those services are higher compared to many fee schedules in private practice and comparable to those of outpatient departments.[30] But this is not an unexpected result, since centers provide many nonmedical, social, and mental health services that in private practice might not be provided for poor patients. Unfortunately, this cost differential is used as an argument against the development of the health center as a general model for care in the community without any attention to what services are valued and needed.

Looked at broadly, centers are now important but miniscule efforts to solve the general problem of medical care distribution in poverty areas, examples of special treatment institutions for the poor, new bureaucratic organizations in place of disappearing solo practice, and social-political reform that involve the poor in the workings of a health agency. Because they are costly, the proposed government policy on health maintenance organizations aims to convert health center financing and organization into a prepaid group practice. If so, health centers may become just another organization in the free market of medical practices available to the poor and everyone, but then devoid of some of the treatment services needed for the rehabilitation and maintenance of the low-income patient.

FREE CLINICS

While health centers and HMOs are central to current thinking about a rationalized "health care system," free clinics are not; unplanned, uncoordinated, and under-financed, they are outside the system.[31] With the unpaid work of students and practitioners, ex-patients and private citizens, some 170 free medical clinics have opened since 1967.[32] At the same time, many other nonmedical free clinics opened to provide social-psychological help, making up what is now called "the free clinic movement."

The clinics are not simply new community-based facilities for special people—the youth, the poor minorities, or neighborhood residents who use them—but they are also attempts at organizational reform and political acts meant to influence education, medical care, and treatment.[33] Five elements of free clinics are (1) entitlement to free care, (2) simplified access, (3) treatment for stigmatized patients, (4) peer organization, and (5) self- and group help.

Like regular medical practices, the free clinics intend to provide medical aid, but in ways the "established practices" may not or really cannot do. Even before the enactment of a national health insurance scheme, care is free to everyone. The old voluntary tradition of free care for the poor alone or for those who cannot pay the full amount is rejected. While free care is a natural entitlement to clinic users, it is not without costs, although these are cheap. Because volunteer help is the rule, with but few exceptions for paid secretaries, the visit costs range from 80 cents (Berkeley Free Clinic, Berkeley, California) to $3.50 (Cambridgeport Medical Clinic, Cambridge, Massachusetts). The other donated ingredients of clinics also help to make them "free." Thus, their varied premises (storefronts, houses, traveling vans, unused apartments) may be gifts from interested citizens, universities, medical societies, or public agencies; the supplies and equipment are the leftovers from doctors' offices and hospitals; the medicines may be office samples, bulk drug purchases provided by health departments or contributed samples from "detail men," and laboratory tests are written off at no charge when sent to generous directors of private or hospital laboratories.

The clinics are for those who cannot secure help in the established institutions—the emergency wards, OPDs, health department clinics, private practices, and college health services. Because the free clinics are more willing to deal with problems that are not only medical but social and, for some, "moral"—drug use and its complications, illegitimate pregnancies, birth control, venereal disease, running away—they do attract youth who, uncertain about their reception and treatment, are reluctant to use regular practices, and poor minorities and neighborhood residents who may not even have available help. Medical aid for illnesses common among clinic patients and the fact of free care are the determinants of clinic use.

The free clinics are much less bureaucratic not only because they are smaller than the community-based health centers they may resemble, but because they try very hard to be. Often only an evening walk-in service, they require little but name and address (or nothing at all) to register. Medicine, if needed, may be dispensed at the visit without the client making a separate trip to the drug store. Despite walk-in arrangements that avoid the four to five steps in registration at outpatient departments, waiting queues are not avoided any more than at OPDs, emergency wards, or hospital walk-in clinics. Yet, even if patients do wait two or three hours, they do not complain when asked about it, perhaps because their problems are recognized as among the staff's clinical priorities.

The miniature size of these clinics—seldom more than three to six rooms—and the volunteers they recruit make their staff a more egalitarian, peer organization in which the hierarchial differences among professionals are played down, and clinical work is easily exchanged between nurses, doctors, students, pharmacists, social workers, ex-patients, and local volunteers. The purpose of de-emphasizing professional status are threefold: first, for more personal communication with patients both directly by being less distant with them and indirectly by improving the interchange among the staff (which social studies suggest does improve communication between staff and patients);[34] second, a search for new ways of handling authority, namely, by diffusing it, when clinical work is divided among the helping professionals; and third, for some, the de-emphasized professionalism is political, the beginning within a medical practice of a more socialized and classless society.[35] If bureaucratic registration and depersonalized treatment do turn away the poor, the open access and personal communication may then help them to use and comply in treatment.

Despite the convention that professional help is "always the best," the free clinics also add self-help and group help. Their "rap sessions" run by patients themselves are, in effect, mutual aid societies for youth that may provide all the help that is needed or may lead to more systematic professional counseling. This type of patient participation in actual treatment is quite different from the community participation of health centers. Unlike health centers, few free clinics have formal community participation designed to provide clinic jobs, to promote civic uplift, or to control money, doctors, and services. Some, of course, may have a lay-professional board, as advised by the Los Angeles Council on Free Clinics. Such boards can help raise money and protect the clinic, providing a legitimacy for the police and licensing agencies who often want it removed because of its attraction for "undesirable people." Indeed, some clinics, such as the Young Patriots Organization, Chicago, have been pressed to close because they had no license, but more often, public officials are ambivalent.[36] On one hand, they feel youth and minorities need help; on the other, they feel clinics are "making things too easy for kids," or are subversive cells of belligerent minorities and should therefore not be open. The usual result is to leave them alone. Staff participation in organization can also be important. This takes place in starting these cooperative ventures, in working with minorities and youth to learn from them what help is needed, and then in working at providing what treatment, if any, is possible.

These features of free medical clinics may not be common to all, for both their organization and treatment programs may vary with the stamp that local circumstances and local organizers put on them. Most are in big cities where there are concentrations of hospitals, medical schools, and volunteers. Despite their medical intentions, many become multipurpose outposts. Generally open at night when much medical practice closes down, they are used variously not only as medical dispensaries but also as social and counseling agencies, "crisis centers," meeting places, and for telephone advice and referral. In daytime hours, they are often used as "pads," and sometimes like settlement houses.

To view the free clinics only as new volunteer community

services for special people, not unlike hospital and private clinics for patients with special diseases, would overlook their other intentions. Indeed, while their major users are special clienteles of either white youth, poor minorities, or neighborhood residents, the clinics are also political acts and organizational reforms. In the politics of education, medical students as organizers of clinics have argued for a community-based site of education as legitimate as that of the hospital.[37] In the politics of medical care, at least at the interinstitutional level, black and minority organizers of clinics for "their people" argue for socialized payment. They can also argue, if not bargain collectively from the clinic, for better access to and a bigger voice in the hospitals' outpatient departments. In the politics of treatment, the clinics for youth stand for social and medical care rather than legal control of drug users. The clinic's organizational reforms propose more peer, less rigid, hierarchial staff; more simplified, less elaborate treatment; easier access, fewer bureaucratic routines; professional yet more self-treatment; broader, less specialized definitions of the jobs of all health workers; and more personal encounters in getting care.

Looking back to their beginnings, the free clinics, as political acts, may have had an impact since public agencies are now funding them for both drug users and youth. Their patients are more readily accepted and treated in "established practices," and their self-help strategies are being widely adopted.[38] Yet, their original reforms seem less successful and slow to be adopted, if they ever are. A few reforms, such as the use of ex-patient street workers in outpatient clinics and on-the-spot dispensing in hospital walk-in services are only a trickle of change in the routines of large-scale medical organizations. This is not surprising, for their organizational features run counter to management values in health care. Large-scale efficiency, technological care and accounting are the values sought by the press for better management. Antitechnological and antibureaucratic in spirit, the clinics value open access, communication with patients, and treatment for stigmatized groups. The invention of free clinics outside the constraints of big institutions is, in part, a withdrawal, and in part a utopian attempt to invent the more perfect organization that it is hoped, will convert professionals into new ways of behaving and so change the depersonalization of the bigger organization. In part it is also a human concern of class or clan to "take care of one's own kind," whether they be white suburban kids, blacks, or one's own neighbors, all of whom may be left out—in particular, out of the health care system.

Since these expectations and energies are hard to sustain, especially with so little money, can the free clinics survive— or does it matter? Because of the uncertainties of resources, personnel, and motivation, some will argue that the clinics cannot last. Because their care is sporadic, limited, and often uneven in quality, some would argue that they should not. With both fragile support and uneven care, some would add that they are not a viable model for community-based services. But they are not in the bureaucratic tradition to be franchised standard outlets for community medical services. They are local self-help efforts, products of both a lingering voluntary tradition and a radical critique of the depersonalization of both patients and staff in large, modern treatment organizations. Their fate is uncertain.[39] Even if coopted by support from public funds and receipts from national health insurance they may become like the very public ones they stand against, bigger, technical, and impersonal.

Some of the free clinic reforms for both patients and staff may be adopted as good management by private and public practices, or the clinics themselves may be formally associated with a larger medical organization—in effect rationalizing the informal basis by which they now exist. Such a development acknowledges the need for local, miniature organizations for specialized access, communication, and immediate treatment that larger medical practices with different goals and orientation are unwilling to undertake. But even if the organizational reforms are not adopted and the short half-life of the clinics begins to run out, as it now seems, they will have served useful purposes by making new groups of patients visible and acceptable and by creating new conditions of clinical work. In the future, too, similar transient free clinic organizations may be invented again for still newer minorities at the bottom (homosexuals, women, former convicts) who, even as paying patients with national health insurance, might still not secure help in the established institutions, and for still other health workers seeking an opportunity to experiment and to change.

FOUNDATIONS FOR MEDICAL CARE, SOLO PRACTICE, SELF-REGULATED

While health centers, OPDs, and prepaid practice try to convert solo practices into groups, foundations for medical care are trying to preserve them as such.[40] Foundations are corporations organized by local county or state medical societies for the provision of medical services and for the control of their costs, use, and quality. Technically, "corporations" and foundations suggest a large collective group practice, but they are only auditing and collecting claims for solo practices, not organizing them. Care is provided by the solo practitioner of the insured subscriber's choice—a basic goal of foundations. Costs, use, and quality of the medical service given subscribers are controlled through audits done by committees of doctors. Such a peer review of fees that are excessive, services that are unnecessary and of a quality that is not optimal, can restrict or withhold the payment of the doctor's fee. As a result of such controls, large purchasers of medical services, like the government and insurance companies, are willing to have their clients and subscribers use solo practices. So far, costs are said to approach within 10 percent of the Kaiser Plan. In some instances, a prepayment insurance scheme of a foundation may help control costs while still paying physicians on a fee-for-service basis. Not all of the forty or more foundations are the same. Some deal only with peer review for insurance and governmental programs such as Medicaid, while others also are involved with setting standards for or operating prepaid comprehensive insurance as well as the provision of medical services.

Competition with solo practice from the Kaiser Plan of prepaid practice, with its closed panel of physicians, was the original impetus for the beginning of foundations in San Joaquin County, California, in 1954. The continued impetus for their growth has been the demand for cost control of governmental programs under Medicaid, and its enforcement mechanism—peer review of the doctor's work. At present some 25 percent of California physicians participate in foundations that cover 620,000 individuals. Compared to the twenty-five to fifty physicians in a closed panel of prepaid practice, the size of foundations is large, ranging from 120 to 1,000 physicians. While foundations have a numerical superiority, this is not likely to be an advantage to the poor in the decision to seek help.

As recipients of Medicaid, the poor have been included in several California foundations. Their care is financed by prepayment to a foundation. The results in costs and scope of services are not available for comparison with other programs, nor are patterns of care and patient experience known. One might expect such a mechanism to direct

Medicaid patients to private practice and away from health centers and clinics and to limit medical services.

PROBLEMS AND ACHIEVEMENTS

These out-of-hospital treatment organizations differ in their direction, size, costs, orientation, specialization-generalization, nonphysician health workers, location, financing, and community participation-factors that may determine whether the poor have access to, use, and receive quality services. In an age of universal entitlement to health care, these themes of access, use, and quality dominate our concerns about care and treatment for the poor and for everyone. What are the problems and achievements of these organizations?

Looking at their direction, all emphasize out-of-hospital practice, whether as a cost-saving device to reduce overall medical expenditures or to enlarge the scope and possibilities of practice in the community. Practices may handle these trade-offs in different ways. The Kaiser Plan and others like it have sometimes been praised for reducing hospitalization but criticized for not expanding services or access in order to maintain staff incomes. The absence of community-subscriber participation may account for such implicit decisions. Nonetheless, the emphasis of these organizations on ambulatory care is needed for the illness problems of the poor.

Because of increasing medical specialization the size of the group organization of practice in health centers, OPDs, and prepaid groups is also increasing. Only in foundations does practice remain a solo organization; in free clinics the size remains miniature, not usually over three physicians, with the practice unspecialized. Accompanying this trend toward the group organization of doctors, and in response to a rising demand for care as well, is an increase in the numbers of nonphysician health workers. They are involved not only in their traditional technical tasks of taking patient tests but in actual treatment, namely, in the traditional dyadic domain of the doctor-patient relation—giving examinations, advice, counsel, and prescriptions as nurses, aides, physician assistants.[41] Both the size of practice and the use of non-physician health workers increase the formal bureaucratic organization needed to coordinate services. So far, since the poor are viewed as having difficulty with impersonal bureaucratic services of any kind, whether in banks, stores, or clinics, the division of clinical work that these changes bring makes treatment less accessible to them. If so, small organizations like free clinics and patient advocates in the community are needed to provide easy entry and to remove these barriers to access.

If nonphysician health workers are also regarded as cutrate medicine, all right for the poor but no one else, they will be used far below their full potential. While such health workers care for the poor outside the hospital and for everyone inside the hospital, acceptance of such arrangements outside may be based more on generation than income. Older persons, irrespective of background, may prefer the single doctor. Younger persons, experiencing such arrangements in school, college, the army, and industry, may more readily accept teams of doctors and health workers. Indeed, the idea of the single doctor-patient relationship as the exclusive model for all treatment and communication in out-of-hospital practices may give way to acceptance of and preference for team treatment.

Not only do health centers, prepaid practices, and OPDs emphasize out-of-hospital care, but they provide for more primary care—for example, preventive services, health maintenance, and chronic illness management—services that are often viewed as mere "after care," leftovers in the emphasis on the hospital. Yet these services are most important in maintaining the health of the poor already handicapped by other disadvantages. While primary care is not an explicit goal of foundations for medical care and free clinics, these practices do provide some. The efforts are the greatest in prepaid group practices, where 60 percent of the medical staff are pysicians in primary care (internists, general practitioners, pediatricians) compared to 30 to 40 percent in solo practices. This difference is due to the organizational policies of prepaid practices and to the educational policies, or the lack of them, in medical schools. In the last four decades, the training programs of hospitals and medical schools have responded more to the technological needs of the hospital itself and to the interests of specialty societies than to the needs for practice in the community.[42] As a result specialists have been trained without regard to their need and, over-all, fewer physicians trained than needed. If primary care is to be expanded, it will depend not only on organization but on educational programs for primary care different from those for traditional medical specialization. Both health centers and prepaid groups bring this component to community practice to complement but not supplant the dysfunctional growth of specialization.[43] In addition, these group practices make an organization rather than a solo doctor the site of access for care, so that the patient may be confronted with health workers other than the doctor at his initial encounter. So far, the development of prepaid groups and centers is limited. So far, too, the medical schools with their heavy emphasis on specialization are ambivalent about the need for primary care, viewing education that responds to the service needs of the community with disdain, as compromising the intellectual basis of medicine. They fill a critical role in the development of primary care. As producers of medical services and personnel, the hospitals and medical schools, not the consumers, may determine what medical care the public should want by what, in fact, they are willing to offer. As a result, the development of more primary care for the poor (and non-poor alike) may well depend on what the leadership elite in this "industry" wants to offer. So far, the consensus is not complete, least of all in the schools.

While services are to be comprehensive in both the health center and group practices in which some poverty groups have been enrolled, such comprehensive care may not mean that the particular services that the poor need are available. Prepaid groups have successfully marketed a conventional package of in-and out-of-hospital medical services. Yet some treatment needs of the poor, for such problems as alcoholism, drug use, family planning, and mental health, are now often met in special subsidized public programs or in the voluntary efforts of free clinics. Unless there is a willingness to handle certain illness problems that the poor and others have, they will hardly feel that institutions are accessible, and few will use them.

To get care in any of these organizations, the poor have to pay for it. The various schemes of national health insurance will, of course, provide for this. But it would be unrealistic to expect that insurance schemes alone will pay all the bills. Other federal programs continue to support these treatment organizations, although indirectly. The Regional Medical Program (P.L. 89-239, 90-574, 91-515) for heart and kidney disease, cancer and stroke, the Hill-Burton Act for hospital construction, the Community Health and Mental Health Service Acts, the Children's Bureau, Vocational Rehabilitation, the Health Assistance Program, and the Manpower Development and Training Program all deal with particular problems of treatment organizations and with services available to everyone. By dealing separately with the financing of facilities, equipment, education, and health manpower training, these programs introduce tax moneys mostly into hospitals but some into community medical organizations. This approach is different from still another pattern of tax support, namely, special disease grants for tuberculosis, venereal diseases, mental illness hospitalization, and for the newer "special diseases" in the federal budget such as alcoholism and drug abuse, and for family planning, each of which receives a special subsidy. In effect, the tax moneys properly subsidize some of the work of treatment organizations that could not be realistically covered by insurance alone. In all likelihood these programs or some like them will be needed in the future as a form of indirect financing of health services for the poor and everyone.

If free clinics, health centers, and OPDs are indifferent to cost control, prepaid group practice, in its competition with solo practice, is obsessed with it. Because such plans have provided successful counter-incentives to expensive hospital use while providing expanded alternative ambulatory care use, they have become prominent in government proposals for the reorganization of practice and the control of costs. How physician behavior reduces hospitalization in prepaid group practices is not entirely clear. An economic study of internal medicine practice indicates that doctors in solo practice earn 35 percent of their income in hospital care while group practice doctors earn only 10 percent that way. [44] The solo doctor may be availing himself of hospital support services for efficiency and assured payment while group practice doctors derive proportionately more of their income from laboratory services done by others under their control. These economic variables may not be the whole explanation. Acceptance of queueing and waiting lists that can always insure a full hospital occupancy and an actual lower incidence of hospital need may be other factors that reduce hospital costs and use. Still another is a different handling of the patient-physician demand for hospitalization by "going through the clinic." Hospitalization as a social as well as medical experience not only provides technical care but meets the patient's dependency needs that accompany illness and is status-enhancing as well. Except for an office visit, the solo doctor has no such out-of-hospital experience to offer his patient; in group practice, the social experience of multiple ambulatory contacts may substitute, and for the doctor be a suitable way to obtain colleague consultation and maintain patient control.

The health maintenance legislation and the program for Family Medical Practice make it possible to refinance health centers and OPDs, changing them from tax-subsidized to insurance-supported prepaid practices. For example, the Family Medical Practice program of the Department of Health, Education, and Welfare permits per capita prepaid payments in place of Medicaid. To the extent that cost controls, as part of new financing mechanisms, permit these treatment organizations to remain viable, they help the poor; to the extent that controls limit services, as they may explicitly and implicitly do by fiscal indifference to whether services are optimally used or whether people come for treatment, they will not help the poor a bit.

Both the health center and free clinic have strategies of decentralized community-based locations which optimize local access, while more distant, centralized hospital-based group practice and outpatient departments with larger staffs and more technology can offer more complex treatment services. If transportation is improved, the difference in access may be removed and the need for decentralization questioned.

If the poor are looking for participation in the policies of health agencies, they are likely to experience it mostly in health centers and perhaps in free clinics. Proponents question the form, degree, and goals of community participation; skeptics, doubtful that it increases patients' utilization, improves patients' identification and satisfaction with the center, or contributes to management efficiency of services would reject it as an important organizational feature. Nonetheless, for the participants themselves, the rational search for instrumental effects of community participation on organization is irrelevant. To participate is a felt need of people now more dependent on large organizations for services; organizations cannot ignore it. Here and there even OPDs and prepaid practice plans are trying some version of participation, some including the poor. For example, the trustees of the Peter Bent Brigham Hospital in Boston and its outpatient department now have local community members. Similarly, HIP in New York is adding consumer representatives while the Group Health Cooperative of Puget Sound, Washington, has this feature built into its original organization.

Quality, a general concern in nearly all organizations, will be defined differently by public patients and professionals. Procedures for quality review are generally available. In centers, prepaid groups, and OPDs, where doctors are working together, professional behavior may respond to informal peer opinions on medical decisions that bear on quality; in foundations for medical care, formal peer review is an explicit function of the "corporation" but not of each solo practice itself. With new insurance and hospital regulations, formal peer review will also take place in OPDs and group practice. Free clinics have no peer review of quality. The nature of quality itself is often a matter of debate, not unexpectedly since the "criteria" are basically value judgments. Thus, so much of the evaluation literature on quality of medical care is one value versus another and a search to confirm its presence or absence.[45] For the most part, quality studies have had an entirely technical dimension, not only because technical aspects of care (e.g., the number of examinations, diagnostic tests, etc.) can be measured and compared, but also because this feature is more exclusively valued. [46] Yet other dimensions of quality might include (1) efficiency, (2) communication to patients (about diagnoses, illness, and prognosis), (3) continuity of treatment (through records, staff assignments, organization itself, referrals, and interprofessional communication), (4) comprehensiveness (full scope of services), (5) complexity (full scope of therapies), and (6) patient satisfaction.

OPDs and groups are likely to score high on technical performance, comprehensiveness, and complexity simply because they are organized for these aspects of services. OPDs, on the other hand, will rate less on continuity, other than through records, unless their part-time staff becomes more full-time, and they will remain less efficient, particularly if they are a site of training as well. Because of the limited scope of their dispensary medicine and their loose staff organization, free clinics are likely to be low in technical performance, but with their concern for communication of information to patients, they are likely to be high on this criterion. Similarly, health centers with close contacts in the community might also be expected to rate high on communication and patient satisfaction. Yet these deductive generalizations about organization should be taken with caution. Treatment can be shoddy, depersonalized, and technically less optimal in any structure. So much of quality depends on the dynamics of how organizations are supported and work, not just how they are structured.

OPTIMAL CARE AND EQUITABLE DISTRIBUTION

The poor are not only concerned about structural factors in treatment organizations—how to pay the doctor, organize treatment teams, find the right size, location, and appropriate mix of services, and then to manage it all for efficiency—but about their own encounters in access and treatment. They complain that they are received and treated indifferently in urban medical practices and health bureaucracies. These are unjustified complaints, some would say, if studies of the British system are a measure. These studies suggest that the poor use treatment organizations—and use reflects access—with the same frequency as those with higher incomes.[47] Nevertheless, their personal experience in reception and communication as patients, not structure, concerns the poor. Only the free clinics have an ideology that affirms acceptance of the poor and minorities with deviant lives and that asserts communication with patients and open access to be of major importance. Such reorientation of attitudes and relations of health workers with patients is as important as reorganization but because it cannot be measured by a cost-effectiveness estimate, it is difficult to express as public policy.

The increasing size and complexity of all the community medical organizations affects the poor and everyone else. Private groups, health maintenance organizations, outpatient departments, and health centers are essentially alike and represent group practice at the hospital and in the community, both of which are needed. These larger organizations invariably bring public or private bureaucratic arrangements for coordination and control that, historically, the poor have endured and those better off have avoided. It is to be hoped that more health workers (and resources) may produce arrangements that create a therapeutic milieu, not simply more barriers to medical help. In a traditional, pessimistic view, treatment differences between the poor and others, hence handicaps for the poor, persist when everyone uses similar organizations. The poor, for example, will more likely confront the formal administrative routines that others circumvent; they may also receive less communication, since they are perceived as having little need for information about health and illness. The more complex and expensive services of community medical organizations raise still other issues, like those of allocation. The allocation of limited, expensive treatment may depend less on random numbers than on one's social worth, a decision where the poor may not be so valued, even if they belong to health care plans and treatment organizations.

Whether the redefinition and reorganization of OPDs, health centers, and private practices as HMOs will distribute medical care more equitably depends on whether the care is viewed as a commodity or as a right. Although current rhetoric claims medical care to be a right, the HMO legislation views it as a commodity, a private good to be purchased by large groups of consumers in a free, competitive, but regulated market. Public and private insurance will subsidize some purchases. Competition among HMOs will control costs, as will their internal incentives to operate with some profit, even if without regard to services to be offered. Simply because costs may be reduced, better distribution of medical care is assumed to follow; distribution itself is being viewed as an attribute of the HMO. But the important distributive issue is who is left out of treatment organizations under schemes where medical care is purchased as a commodity. If people do not enroll in plans, and if organizations, in turn, do not seek out people in need, will they solve the problem of distribution? Certainly they may improve it but unless they can be required to enroll the disadvantaged poor whose treatment costs may be high, they will not solve distribution any more than solo practice has done in the past; and they may only be able to meet the tests of efficiency and cost control if they limit their services.

If health care is truly a right, then needed health services can be taken to those deprived regions and communities that are unlikely to meet the strictures of the competitive model. To do this will, in the long run, require a national health service. The idea of a health service was implicit in the earlier health center reform of the 1900s. The center was to be an institution like the school, open to everyone, its resources for health care allocated out of the taxes that financed other district services such as education. But so firmly rooted is the tradition of entrepreneurial practice and the public skepticism of large-scale medical practice that it seems unlikely that the organization of medical care in the community will immediately take the full direction of a national health service; neither will the traditional form of private solo practice altogether disappear. Indeed, the HMO as a practice at the hospital and in the community, along with schemes of national health insurance, is simply a strategy for subsidizing private practice as a group as opposed to an individual solo enterprise. Meanwhile, solo practice, although diminishing, is likely to persist, but may no longer be the major organization for care in the community. It may find itself limited to those with more money who are willing to pay more for treatment outside larger organizations. Looking ahead, the reforms are likely to be incremental. Future local public control of HMOs, health centers, OPDs, more public regulation of medical care practices and costs, more public subsidy of medical care, education, facilities, and research may transform the current HMO-health center idea into a national health service with appropriate central planning but local control, initiative, and management by public and professionals alike.

THE IMPACT OF TREATMENT AND CARE ON HEALTH STATUS AND POVERTY

The organization of health services in the community has been our major concern. Looking beyond this problem, two further questions arise. First, what care is most important for improving the health status of the poor? Second, what medical intervention might be important for reducing poverty? The first raises an issue of priorities, the second, an issue of strategy. Both are difficult to answer, for health care is not invariably linked to health status and much less to poverty as so commonly is assumed.

A common-sense view of health services is that they naturally must have effects on our health, in particular on our statistical measures of morbidity and mortality, and that all improvements in our health can be readily attributed to health services. We attribute so much disease control to health services because we are so accustomed to viewing health care as a specific treatment with specific outcomes, as, for example, the cure of bacterial pneumonia with penicillin, and to viewing such cures by medical treatment as the only means by which disease has been controlled. Those who hold this common-sense view are surprised to find that health care may have no demonstrable effect on those health indicators that we can most easily measure and objectify—morbidity and mortality—and to learn that these indicators have been improved by gains in public sanitation, nutrition, and living standards rather than by the use of health services. This note of caution, however, should not mean that the system of health care services is not without its effects, only that these may be more accurately seen in the disability that attends disease and the experience of patients with illness. The effects of health services are powerful and important for the poor and non-poor alike in reducing disability and the distress of illness. They are also much more difficult to measure.

Improved health programs in dental, psychiatric, and maternal-infant care are most needed. In dental care, fluoridation and restorative work must have the highest priorities, but both face great obstacles. Fluoridation, although endorsed by health authorities, still has limited application because of political and social resistance. Restorative work is hampered by a manpower shortage, although the profession and dental schools are now willing to train and employ dental aides. Furthermore, public resistance to reasonable dental treatment must also be considered. In clinical practice, it was observed that regular dental care given to children in a free municipal program did not carry over into later years when private sources were expected to be used.[48] While these findings indicate a need for continuing dental services, they also raise questions about the durability of types of medical practice.

For example, if the health centers—HMOs and other institutions are successful in remodeling people to fit the economy, they may, in poverty districts, become victims of their own success. Leaving a district to live in a better place may be a mark of successful change, but such people will no longer be around to use the health center-HMO practice. Supported by their improved economic status, they may seek the offices of private practitioners. Will health center-HMOs, then, be institutions of transition leading to something else? In the past, health planning for the poor often had expectations that any plan would be only temporary.

For example, the hospital outpatient department was viewed both as a "medical soup kitchen" for the poor and as an institution teaching good standards of practice and correct use of services for those who later would afford to see private doctors. The health center-HMO, however, will still be needed even after its patients are no longer poor because, as previous studies have observed, the patients will not "go private" as soon as they have more money. Accordingly, one can expect that the instant medical help and crisis medicine of health centers, free clinics, and hospital emergency rooms, so often disparaged, might still be with all of us for quite some time to come.

It is even more difficult to evaluate the long-range effect of these several organizations upon the care of psychiatric problems. The specific nature of clinical psychiatric disorders, including alcoholism, is so complicated that no simple prescription for preventive intervention can be written for them. Yet, appropriate and comprehensive services at general hospitals and in the community are certainly needed.[49] It is doubtful that they can be organized within group practices without employing a large and complex staff. A community health aide may be of some importance in this respect by recognizing treatable situations, surveying families at certain critical points, and generally making accommodations for the early symptoms of clinical disorders.

Probably the most important point of interaction of health services and poverty is the connection between educational methods and techniques of psychotherapy. If psychotherapy is viewed as a means of emotional re-education conducted either in a one-to-one relationship or in family and group therapy, then it may be important in dealing with some of the developmental problems of the dropouts, slow learners, and overactive children. It is rarely considered, however, whether therapeutic group work will be offered by the group practice staff or be built into the educational bureaucracy of the school health programs, student counseling or into education itself. The results of conventional school health programs are not impressive, and their historical bases are no longer tenable. An important function of any of the group practices could be to handle referrals from local schools. The other important task of psychiatric intervention, consultation with teachers on classroom problems, has been done by psychiatry but, in the future, may be done by educators with special skills.

The much publicized social class difference in perinatal mortality rates requires renewed efforts in the field of maternal and infant care. The clinical team of pediatrician, nurse, and health aide may be able to make this care available, although one cannot expect that the provision of more care and treatment alone would continue to reduce these rates. Part of the increased perinatal mortality rate seems related to prematurity which, in turn, is related to the early age of the mother's conception and antecedent periods of nutritional imbalance in her earlier life, factors not altogether related to health services.

Community medical practices have always been viewed more as organizations for maintenance and support compared to the medical-surgical cures expected in hospitals. In this tradition, John B. Grant, like many others, viewed one of these out-of-hospital organizations, the early health centers, as a means for the social rehabilitation of the community.[50] Indeed, to some extent they were, for through improved environmental sanitation and the control of infectious disease, more people had longer lives to live in the community; through improved nutrition they had greater physical vitality for living. While our expectations of community medical practice today may be the same, the modern problems and the solutions are not. Treatment organizations in the community now have complex problems of chronic medical and psychological disorders as well as dental and maternal-infant health. The major means of medical care in the community are still comprehensive personal health services, but their scope is changing. Much of this is caused by the blurring of distinctions between health and illness. Thus, what constitutes "medical treatment" is also undergoing change. Just as the halfway house, now the first step in leaving treatment institutions, has become a necessary variety of living and so a preventive first step for containing illness in the community, out-of-hospital organizations may do the same. They can offer relief and rehabilitation to many handicapped so that such persons can be their best even with their disorders—provided, of course, that the services are sufficiently complex to deal with complicated illness. An expectation that the medical care at centers, HMOs, or group practices can offer more, that treatment will result in a cure, is true in only a few instances. Yet, the limited outcomes are no less important. While medical therapies and the use of personal health services at community practices do not promise cures, they do provide some control and relief. By making such services more available and accessible, much can be achieved to provide patient satisfaction, relief from health problems, and maintenance of the ill. Such an achievement will make life better for the poor and the non-poor alike.

Notes
Index

Notes

Chapter 1: The Nature of Poverty

1. William Graham Sumner, *What Social Classes Owe to Each Other* (Harper & Bros. 1883), pp. 19-20.
2. Suzanne Keller, *The American Lower Class Family* (Albany, N.Y.: State Division of Youth, 1966); Arthur B. Shostak and William Gomberg, eds., *Blue-Collar World* (Englewood Cliffs, N.J.: Prentice-Hall, 1964).
3. Henry E. Sigerist, *Medicine and Human Welfare* (New Haven: Yale University Press, 1941); Raymond S. Duff and August B. Hollingshead, *Sickness and Society* (New York: Harper & Row, 1968); John Kosa, "Entrepreneurship and Charisma in the Medical Profession," *Social Science and Medicine*, 4 (July 1970), 25-40.
4. Gunnar Myrdal, *The Challenge of World Poverty* (New York: Pantheon, 1970); Peter Townsend, ed., *The Concept of Poverty* (London: Heinemann, 1970); Louis A. Ferman, Joyce L. Kornbluh and Alan Haber, eds., *Poverty in America* (Ann Arbor: University of Michigan Press, 1968); Frances Fox Piven and Richard A. Cloward, *Regulating the Poor* (New York: Pantheon, 1971).
5. John Hope Franklin, *From Slavery to Freedom* (New York: Alfred A. Knopf, 1948), p. 70.
6. Milton I. Roemer, *Medical Care in Latin America* (Washington, D.C.: Pan American Union, 1963); Alfred Yankauer, "National Planning and the Construction of Maternal and Child Hygiene Norms in Latin America," *American Journal of Public Health,* 57 (May 1967), 751-761.
7. Marion D. de B. Kilson, "Towards Freedom: An Analysis of Slave Revolts in the United States," *Phylon*, 25 (Summer 1964), 175-187.
8. Walter B. Miller, "Lower Class Culture as a Generating Milieu of Gang Delinquency," *Journal of Social Issues,* 14 (1958), 5-19; Oscar Lewis, *La Vida* (New York: Random House, 1965), pp. 1-1i.
9. Charles Nordhoff, *The Communistic Societies of the United States* (New York: Hillary House, 1960).
10. Michael Harrington, *The Other America* (New York: Macmillan Company, 1962).
11. Dwight MacDonald, "Our Invisible Poor," *The New Yorker,* January 19, 1963, p. 84.
12. Concerning the theory of the paradox see Hubert H. Humphrey, *War on Poverty* (New York: McGraw-Hill, 1964); Burton A. Weisbrod, *The Economics of Poverty: An American Paradox* (Englewood Cliffs, N.J.: Prentice-Hall, 1965); Robert E. Will and Harold G.

Vatter, eds., *Poverty in Affluence* (New York: Harcourt, Brace & World, 1965).

13. Max Weber, *The Protestant Ethic and the Spirit of Capitalism* (New York: Charles Scribner's Sons, 1948).

14. Robert S. Lynd and Helen M. Lynd, *Middletown* (New York: Harcourt, Brace, 1929); David Riesman, *The Lonely Crowd* (New Haven: Yale University Press, 1950); William H. Whyte, Jr., *The Organization Man* (New York: Simon and Schuster, 1956); Mark Lefton, "The Blue Collar Worker and the Middle Class Ethic," *Sociology and Social Research,* 51 (January 1967), 158-170.

15. Robert H. Bremmer, *From the Depths* (New York: New York University Press, 1965).

16. Jacob A. Riis, *How the Other Half Lives* (New York: Charles Scribner, 1890); W. I. Thomas and Florian Znaniecki, *The Polish Peasant in Europe and America* (5 vols.; Chicago: University of Chicago Press, 1918-1920); John Kosa, *Land of Choice* (Toronto: University of Toronto Press, 1957); and Kosa, "The Emergence of a Catholic Middle Class" in William T. Liu and Nathaniel Pallone, eds., *Catholics U.S.A.* (New York: John Wiley & Sons, 1970), pp. 15-24.

17. John Kosa, Aaron Antonovsky, and Irving K. Zola, eds., *Poverty and Health* (1st ed.; Cambridge, Mass: Harvard University Press, 1969), pp. 15-18.

18. Harry Caudill, *Night Comes to the Cumberlands* (Boston: Atlantic-Little, Brown, 1963); Mary Jean Bownian and W. Warren Haynes, *Resources and People in East Kentucky* (Baltimore: John Hopkins Press, 1963).

19. Carolyn Jackson and Terri Velten, "Residence, Race and Age of Poor Families," *Social Security Bulletin,* 32 (June 1969), 3-11.

20. Also see Oscar Ornati, *Poverty Amid Affluence* (New York: Twentieth Century Fund, 1966); Herman P. Miller, *Rich Man, Poor Man* (New York: Thomas Y. Crowell, 1964); Alan B. Batchelder, *The Economics of Poverty* (New York: John Wiley & Sons, 1966); Thomas I. Ribich, *Education and Poverty* (Washington, D.C.: Brookings Institution, 1968); Charles A. Valentine, *Culture and Poverty* (Chicago: University of Chicago Press, 1968).

21. Patricia Cayo Sexton, *Spanish Harlem* (New York: Harper & Row, 1965); Arthur J. Rubel, *Across the Tracks: Mexican-Americans in a Texas City* (Austin: University of Texas Press, 1966); Alphonso Pinkney and Roger R. Woock, *Poverty and Politics in Harlem* (New Haven: College and University Press, 1970); Benjamim Schlesinger, *Poverty in Canada and the United States* (Toronto: University of Toronto Press, 1966); Arthur M. Ross and Herbert Hill, *Employment, Race and Poverty* (New York: Harcourt, Brace & World, 1967); Lester

C. Thurow, *Poverty and Discrimination* (Washington, D.C.: Brookings Institution, 1970).

22. Kenneth B. Clark and Jeannette Hopkins, *A Relevant War Against Poverty* (New York: Harper & Row, 1969); Warner Bloomberg, Jr. and Henry J. Schmandt, eds., *Urban Poverty* (Beverly Hills, Calif.: Sage Publications, 1970).

23. Albert K. Cohen and Harold M. Hodges, Jr., "Characteristics of the Lower-Blue-Collar Class," *Social Problems,* 10 (Spring 1963), 303-334; and W. B. Miller, "Lower Class Culture."

24. Bernard C. Rosen, Harry J. Crockett and Clyde Z. Nunn, *Achievement in American Society* (Cambridge, Mass.: Schenkman, 1969(; Andrew Billingsley, *Black Families in White America* (Englewood Cliffs, N.J.: Prentice-Hall, 1968); Stephen Richter, "The Economics of Child Rearing," *Journal of Marriage and the Family,* 30 (August 1968), 462-466.

25. Louis Schneider and Sverre Lysgaard, "Deferred Gratification Pattern," *American Sociological Review,* 18 (April 1953), 142-149; Lee Rainwater, "Crucible Identity: The Negro Lower-Class Family," *Daedalus,* 95 (Winter 1966), 172-216.

26. W. Lloyd Warner, *American Life, Dream and Reality* (Chicago: University of Chicago Press, 1953), p. 87.

27. August B. Hollingshead, *Elmtown's Youth* (New York: John Wiley & Sons, 1949); Seymour M. Lipset and Reinhard Bendix, *Social Mobility in Industrial Society* (Berkeley: University of California Press, 1962).

28. Alfred C. Kinsey, Wardell B. Pomeroy, and Clyde E. Martin, *Sexual Behavior in the Human Male* (Philadelphia: W. B. Saunders Company, 1948), chap. 10.

29. Bernard Rosenberg and Joseph Bensman, "Sexual Patterns in Three Ethnic Subcultures," *Annals of the American Academy of Political and Social Science,* 376 (March 1968), 61-75; Carlfred B. Broderick, "Social Heterosexual Development Among Urban Negroes and Whites," *Journal of Marriage and the Family,* 27 (May 1965), 200-203.

30. Lewis, *La Vida.*

31. Mirra Komarovsky, *Blue Collar Marriage* (New York: Random House, 1964); Kingsley Davis, "Statistical Perspective on Divorce," *Annals of the American Academy of Political and Social Science,* 272 (November 1950), 9-21; William M. Kephart, "Occupational Level and Marital Disruption," *American Sociological Review,* 20 (August 1955), 456-465.

32. Edmund W. Vaz, ed., *Middle-Class Juvenile Delinquency* (New York: Harper & Row, 1967).

33. Lenore E. Bixby and Eleanor Ring, "Work Experience of Men Claiming Retirement Benefits," *Social Security Bulletin*, 32 (August 1969), 3-14; Lawrence D. Haber, *The Disabled Worker Under OASDI* (Washington, D.C.: U.S. Department of Health, Education, and Welfare, Social Security Administration, Division of Research and Statistics, Research Report No. 6, October 1964).

34. John Kenneth Galbraith, *The Affluent Society* (Boston: Houghton Mifflin Company, 1958); Mollie Orshansky, "The Shape of Poverty in 1966," *Social Security Bulletin*, 31 (March, 1968), 3-32.

35. Leon H. Keyserling, *Progress or Poverty* (Washington, D.C.: Conference on Economic Progress, December 1964); Milton Friedman, *Capitalism and Freedom (Chicago: University of Chicago Press, 1962)*.

36. Saul D. Alinsky, *Rules for Radicals* (New York: Random House, 1971); Michael Harrington, *The Accidental Century* (New York: Macmillan Company 1965), chap. 4.

37. George A. Brager and Francis P. Purcell, *Community Action Against Poverty* (New Haven: College and University Press, 1967); Mayer N. Zald, ed., *Organizing for Community Welfare* (Chicago: Quadrangle Books, 1967); Clark and Hopkins, *A Relevant War Against Poverty*.

38. Wilbur J. Cohen, "A Ten-point Program to Abolish Poverty," *Social Security Bulletin*, 31 (December 1968), 3-13.

39. Daniel P. Moynihan, *Maximum Feasible Understanding* (New York: Free Press, 1969); S.M. Miller and Pamela A. Roby, *The Future of Inequality* (New York: Basic Books, 1970).

40. Martin K. White, Joel J. Alpert, and John Kosa, "The Hard-to-Reach Families in a Comprehensive Care Program," *Journal of the American Medical Association*, 201 (September 11, 1967), 123-128; Charles H. Goodrich, Margaret C. Olendzki, and George S. Reader, *Welfare Medical Care* (Cambridge, Mass.: Harvard University Press, 1970).

Chapter II: The Social Aspects of Health and Illness

1. Galen, *De sanitate tuenda*, 1.5.20, ed. K. Koch et al., *Corpus Medicorum Graecorum* (Leipsig: Teubner, 1923).

2. World Health Organization, *Official Records*, no. 2 (June 1948), p. 100.

3. Robert P. Hudson, "The Concept of Disease," *Annals of Internal Medicine*, 65 (1966), 600.

4. Edward Zigler and Leslie Phillips, "Psychiatric Diagnosis and Symptomatology," *Journal of Abnormal and Social Psychology*, 63 (July 1961), 69-75.

5. Hudson, "The Concept of Disease," p. 599.

6. George L. Engel, "Is Grief a Disease?" *Psychosomatic Medicine,* 23 (January-February 1961), 18-22.

7. Owsei Temkin, "The Scientific Approach to Disease," in Alistair Crombie, ed., *Scientific Change* (New York: Basic Books, 1963); Rene J. Dubos, *The Mirage of Health* (New York: Harper & Row, 1959); and George L. Engle, *Psychological Development in Health and Disease* (Philadelphia: W. B. Saunders Company, 1962).

8. Saxon Graham and Leo Reeder, "Social Factors in the Chronic Diseases," in Howard E. Freeman, Sol Levine and Leo G. Reader, eds., *Handbook of Medical Sociology* 2d ed.; (Englewood Cliffs, N. J.: Prentice-Hall, 1972).

9. Stanley H. King, "Social Psychological Factors in Illness," in Freeman, Levine and Reader, eds., *Handbook of Medical Sociology.*

10. Allan Mazur and Leon S. Robertson, *Biology and Social Behavior* (New York: Free Press, 1972).

11. Hans Selye, *The Stress of Life* (New York: McGraw-Hill, 1956).

12. Harold E. Simmons, *The Psychogenic Theory of Disease* (Sacramento, Calif.: Citadel Press, 1966).

13. Hans J. Eysenck, *Smoking, Health and Personality* (New York: Basic Books, 1965).

14. Stanley H. King, "Psychosocial Factors Associated with Rheumatoid Arthritis," *Journal of Chronic Diseases,* 2 (September 1955), 287-302.

15. Roger J. Meyer and Robert J. Haggerty, "Streptococcal Infections in Families: Factors Altering Individual Suseptibility," *Pediatrics,* 29 (April 1962), 539-549.

16. Richard H. Rake et al., "Social Stress and Illness Onset," *Journal of Psychosomatic Research,* 8 (July 1964), 35-44.

17. Thomas H. Holmes and Minoru Masuda, "Life Changes and Illness Susceptibility," paper presented at the American Association for the Advancement of Science, Chicago, Illinois, December 1970.

18. Daniel H. Funkenstein, Stanley H. King, and Margaretta E. Drolette, *Mastery of Stress* (Cambridge, Mass.: Harvard University Press, 1957).

19. Kurt W. Back and Morton D. Bogdonoff, "Plasma Lipid Responses to Leadership, Conformity and Deviation," in P. Herbert Leiderman and David Shapiro, eds., *Psychobiological Approaches to Social Behavior* (Stanford: Stanford University Press, 1964).

20. Roy Coleman, Milton Greenblatt, and Harry C. Solomon, "Physiological Evidence of Rapport During Psychotherapeutic Interviews," *Diseases of the Nervous System,* 17 (March 1956), 71-77; Alberto Di Mascio, Richard W. Boyd, and Milton Greenblatt, "Physio-

logical Correlates of Tension and Antagonism During Psychotherapy," *Psychosomatic Medicine,* 19 (March-April 1957), 99-104.

21. Howard B. Kaplan, Neil R. Burch, and Samuel W. Bloom, "Physiological Covariation and Sociometric Relationships in Small Peer Groups," in Leiderman and Shapiro, eds., *Psychobiological Approaches to Social Behavior.*

22. Seymour S. Kety, "Biochemical Theories of Schizophrenia," *Science,* 129 (June 1959), 1528-1532.

23. Stanley Schachter, *The Psychology of Affiliation* (Stanford: Stanford University Press, 1959).

24. Robert R. Sears, Eleanor E. Maccoby, and Harry Levin, *Patterns of Child Rearing* (Evanston, Ill.: Row, Peterson, 1957).

25. Leon S. Robertson and Louis E. Dotson, "Perceived Parental Expressivity, Reaction to Stress, and Affiliation," *Journal of Personality and Social Psychology,* 12 (July,1969), 229-234.

26. Barbara S. Dohrenwend and Bruce P. Dohrenwend, "Stress Situations, Birth Order, and Psychological Symptoms," *Journal of Abnormal Psychology,* 71 (June 1966), 215-223.

27. A. P. MacDonald, Jr., "Anxiety, Affiliation, and Social Isolation," *Developmental Psychology,* 3 (September 1970), 242-254.

28. U. S. National Health Survey, *Family Income in Relation to Selected Health Characteristics,* Vital and Health Statistics, Public Health Service Publication No. 1000, series 10, no. 2 (Washington, D. C.: Public Health Service, 1963).

29. Warner Wilson, "Correlates of Avowed Happiness," *Psychological Bulletin,* 67 (April 1967), 294-306.

30. "The Special Position of the Sick," originally published in 1929, and reprinted in Henry E. Sigerist, *On the Sociology of Medicine,* ed. Milton I. Roemer (New York: M. D. Publications, 1960), pp. 9-22; see further Henry E. Sigerist, *Medicine and Human Welfare* (New Haven: Yale University Press, 1941).

31. Talcott Parsons and Rene Fox, "Illness, Therapy, and the Modern Urban American Family," *Journal of Social Issues,* 8 (1952), 31-44; Talcott Parsons, "Definitions of Health and Illness in the Light of American Values and Social Structure," in E. Gartly Jaco, ed., *Patients, Physicians and Illness* (Glencoe, Ill.: Free Press, 1958), pp. 165-187.

32. John Kosa et al., "The Place of Morbid Episodes in the Social Interaction Pattern," paper presented at the Sixth Congress of the International Sociological Association, 1966.

33. Stanley H. King, *Perceptions of Illness and Medical Practice* (New York: Russell Sage Foundation, 1962).

34. David Mechanic, "The Concept of Illness Behavior," *Journal of Chronic Diseases,* 15 (February 1962), 189-194; and "Some Impli-

cations of Illness Behavior for Medical Sampling," *New England Journal of Medicine,* 269 (August 1963), 244-247.

35. Edward A. Suchman, "Stages of Illness and Medical Care," *Journal of Health and Human Behavior,* 6 (Fall 1965), 114-128.

36. Stanislav V. Kasl and Sidney Cobb, "Health Behavior, Illness Behavior and Sick Role Behavior," *Archives of Environmental Health,* 12 (February 1966), 246-266.

37. Monroe Lerner and Odin W. Anderson, *Health Progress in the United States* (Chicago: University of Chicago Press, 1963); John Fry, *Profiles of Disease* (Edinburgh: Livingstone, 1966); Ronald Anderson and Odin W. Anderson, *A Decade of Health Services* (Chicago: University of Chicago Press, 1967); J. Whitney Brown et al., "A Study of General Practice in Massachusetts," *Journal of the American Medical Association,* 216 (April 1971), 301-306.

38. Thomas S. Szasz, *The Myth of Mental Illness* (New York: Harper & Row, 1962).

39. John Kosa et al., "Crises and Stress in Family Life," *Wisconsin Sociologist,* 4 (Summer 1965), 11-19; Joel J. Alpert, John Kosa, and Robert J. Haggerty, "A Month of Illness and Health Care Among Low-income Families," *Public Health Reports,* 82 (August 1967), 705-713; John Kosa, Joel J. Alpert, and Robert J. Haggerty, "On the Reliability of Family Health Information," *Social Science and Medicine,* 1 (July 1967), 265-181.

40. Paul R. Robbins, "Some Explorations into the Nature of Anxieties Relating to Illness," *Genetic Psychology Monographs,* 66 (August 1962), 91-141; Gene N. Levine, "Anxiety About Illness," *Journal of Health and Human Behavior,* 3 (Spring 1962), 30-34.

41. Kosa et al., "The Place of Morbid Episodes in the Social Interaction Pattern."

42. Norman B. Gordon and Bernard Kutner, "Long Term and Fatal Illness and the Family," *Journal of Health and Human Behavior,* 6 (Winter 1965), 190-197; Theodor J. Litman, "The Family and Physical Rehabilitation," *Journal of Chronic Diseases,* 19 (February 1966), 211-217.

43. Clyde Z. Nunn, John Kosa, and Joel J. Alpert, "Causal Locus of Illness and Adaptation to Family Disruptions," *Journal for the Scientific Study of Religion,* 7 (Fall 1968), 210-218.

44. Benjamin D. Paul, ed., *Health, Culture and Community* (New York: Russell Sage Foundation, 1955).

45. Joel J. Alpert, John Kosa, and Robert J. Haggerty, "Medical Help and Maternal Nursing Care in the Life of Low-income Families," *Pediatrics,* 39 (May 1967), 749-755; Milton S. Davis and Robert L. Eichhorn, "Compliance with Medical Regimens," *Journal of Health and Human Behavior,* 4 (Winter 1963), 240-249.

46. Walter I. Wardwell, "Christian Science Healing," *Journal for the Scientific Study of Religion,* 4 (Spring 1965), 175-181.

47. Eliot Freidson, *Profession of Medicine* (New York: Dodd, Mead, 1971); John D. Stoeckle, Irving K. Zola, and Gerald E. Davidson, "On Going to See the Doctor," *Journal of Chronic Diseases,* 16 September 1963), 975-989.

48. M. W. Susser and W. Watson, *Sociology in Medicine* (New York: Oxford University Press, 1971), chap. 8.

49. Leon S. Robertson et al., "Family Size and the Use of Medical Resources," in William T. Liu, ed., *Family and Fertility* (Notre Dame, Ind.: University of Notre Dame Press, 1967), pp. 131-144.

50. Theodor J. Litman, "Health Care and the Family," *Medical Care,* 9 (January 1971), 67-81.

51. Edith Chen and Sidney Cobb, "Family Structure in Relation to Health and Disease," *Journal of Chronic Diseases,* 12 (November 1960), 544-567; Joseph H. Meyerowitz and Howard B. Kaplan, "Familial Responses to Stress," *Social Science and Medicine,* 1 (September 1967), 249-264.

52. Leon S. Robertson et al., *Changing the Medical Care System* (New York: Praeger, 1974); M. W. Susser and W. Watson, *Sociology in Medicine,* chap 7; Jerome L. Schwartz, *Medical Plans and Health Care* (Springfield, Ill.: Charles C. Thomas, 1968); Irwin M. Rosenstock, "Why People Use Health Services," *Millbank Memorial Fund Quarterly,* 44 (July 1966), 94-124.

53. John Kosa, "Entrepreneurship and Charisma in the Medical Profession," *Social Science and Medicine,* 4 (July 1970), 25-40.

54. John A. Ryle, *The Natural History of Disease* (London: Cumberlege 1948); see further Max B. Clyne, *Night Calls: A Study in General Practice* (London: Tavistock Publications, 1961).

55. Joel J. Alpert et al., "The Types of Families That Use an Emergency Clinic," *Medical Care,* 7 (January 1969), 55-61; Margaret C. Heagarty et al., "Some Comparative Costs in Comprehensive versus Fragmented Pediatric Care," *Pediatrics,* 46 (October 1970), 596-603; John Kosa et al., "Social Distance and Medical Care," paper presented at the meeting of the American Sociological Association, 1970.

56. Abraham B. Bergman and Richard J. Werner, "Failure of Children to Receive Penicillin by Mouth," *New England Journal of Medicine,* 268 (June 1963), 1334-1338; Evan Charney et al., "How Well Do Patients Take Oral Penicillin?" *Pediatrics,* 40 (August 1967), 188-195.

57. William R. Rosengren and Mark Lefton, *Hospitals and Patients* (New York: Atherton Press, 1969); Frederick H. Lovejoy et al., "Unnecessary and Preventable Hospitalizations," *Journal of Pediatrics,* 79 (November 1971), 868-872.

58. See the "radical" literature on health politics, particularly the periodicals *Health-PAC Bulletin* and *Health Rights News*. From the professional side see Rosemary Stevens and Robert Stevens, "Medicaid: Anatomy of a Dilemma," *Law and Contemporary Problems,* 35 (Spring 1970), 348-425; Loring Conant, Jr., et al., "Anticipated Patient Acceptance of New Nursing Roles and Physicians' Assistants," *American Journal of Diseases of Children,* 122 (September 1971), 202-205; Marcel A. Fredericks et al., "Physicians and Poverty Programs," *Hospital Progress,* 52 (March 1971), 57-61.

Chapter III: Social Differences in Physical Health

1. Daniel F. Sullivan, "Conceptual Problems in Developing an Index of Health," in *Vital and Health Statistics: Data Evaluation and Methods Research,* National Center for Health Statistics, ser. 2, no. 17 (Washington, D. C.: U. S. Government Printing Office, May 1966); Theodore D. Woolsey, *Measurements of the Nation's Health,* address at the meeting of the Washington Chapters of the American Statistical Association and the American Marketing Association, 1967; and Monroe Lerner, discussion of the paper by Theodore D. Woolsey.

2. Alvin L. Schorr, *Slums and Social Insecurity: An Appraisal of the Effectiveness of Housing Policies in Helping to Eliminate Poverty in the United States,* U. S. Social Security Administration; Division of Research and Statistics, Research Report No. 1 (Washington, D. C.: U. S. Government Printing Office, 1963); and Daniel M. Wilner, et al., "How does the quality of housing affect health and family adjustment?" *American Journal of Public Health,* 46 (April 1956), 736-744.

3. Anselm L. Strauss, "Medical ghettos: Medical care must be reorganized to accept the life-styles of the poor," *Trans-action,* 4 (January 1967), 7.

4. Lola M. Irelan, ed., *Low Income Life Styles,* Welfare Administration Publication No. 14 (Washington, D. C.: U. S. Government Printing Office, 1966).

5. William P. Shepard, "Does the modern pace really kill?" *Journal of the American Geriatric Society,* 3 (January 1955), 139-145.

6. M. Allen Pond, "Interrelationship of Poverty and Disease," *Public Health Reports,* 76 (November 1961), 967-968.

7. Odin W. Anderson and George Rosen, "An Examination of the Concept of Preventive Medicine," Health Information Foundation, *Research Series,* no. 12 (New York: The Foundation, 1960).

8. Robert M. Woodbury, *Causal Factors in Infant Mortality,* U. S. Children's Bureau Publication No. 142 (Washington, D. C.: U. S. Government Printing Office, 1925), p. 148.

9. Monroe Lerner and Odin W. Anderson, *Health Progress in the*

United States, 1900-1960 (Chicago: University of Chicago Press, 1963), pp. 143-150.

10. Various articles by William M. Gafafer cited in Selwyn D. Collins, "Long-Time Trends in Illness and Medical Care," *Public Health Monographs* no. 48 (Washington, D. C.: U. S. Public Health Service, 1957).

11. This situation may not be restricted to the United States. See Timothy D. Baker, "Problems in measuring the influence of economic levels on morbidity," *American Journal of Public Health*, 56 (April 1966), 499-507.

12. U. S. National Center for Health Statistics,*Monthly Vital Statistics Report: Provisional Statistics*, 20 (February 1972), 1-8.

13. For a detailed discussion of this and the subsequent paragraphs see Lerner and Anderson, *Health Progress in the United States.*

14. Chicago Board of Health, Planning Staff of the Health Planning Project, *A Report on Health and Medical Care in Poverty Areas of Chicago and Proposals for Improvement* (Chicago: Board of Health, 1965); and Mark H. Lepper et al., "Approaches to Meeting Health Needs of Large Poverty Populations," *American Journal of Public Health*, 57 (July 1967), 1153-1157.

15. Evelyn M. Kitagawa and Karl E. Taeuber, eds., *Local Community Fact Book, 1960* (Chicago: Community Inventory, University of Chicago, 1963), 324-325.

16. Samuel M. Andelman, "Tuberculosis in Large Urban Centers," address at the meeting of the American Public Health Association, 1965.

17. Lerner and Anderson, *Health Progress in the United States*, pp. 105-113, 122-130.

18. Irelan, *Low Income Life Styles.*

19. Eleanor P. Hunt and Earl E. Huyck, "Mortality of White and Nonwhite Infants in Major U. S. Cities," *Health, Education, and Welfare Indicators*, January 1966, pp. 1-19.

20. National Center for Health Statistics, "Medical Care, Health Status, and Family Income, United States," *Vital Statistics: Data from the National-Health Survey*, ser. 10, no. 9 (Washington, D. C.: U. S. Government Printing Office, 1964), pp. 66,67.

21. Z. M. Stadt et al., "Socio-economic Status and Dental Caries Experience of 3,911 Five-Year-Old Natives of Contra Costa County, California," *Journal of Public Health Dentistry*, 27 (Winter 1967), 2-6.

22. L. F. Szwejda, "Observed Differences of Total Caries Experience Among White Children of Various Socio-Economic Groups," *Journal of Public Health Dentistry*, 20 (Fall 1960), 59-66.

23. L. F. Szwejda, "Dental Caries Experience by Race and Socio-

Economic Level After Eleven Years of Water Fluoridation in Charlotte, North Carolina," *Journal of Public Health Dentistry,* 22 (Summer 1962), 91-98.

24. National Center for Health Statistics, "Dental Visits, Volume and Interval Since Last Visit, United States, 1969," *Vital Statistics,* ser. 10, no. 76 (Washington, D. C.: U. S. Government Printing Office, 1972), table 5, p. 14.

25. National Center for Health Statistics, "Volume of Dental Visits, United States, July 1963- June 1964," *Vital Statistics,* ser. 10, no. 23 (Washington, D.C.: 1965), table 17, p. 32.

Chapter IV: Social Differences in Mental Health

1. The problem of formulating a useful and highly general definition of mental health for empirical analysis is, of course, no different from the problem of defining physical health, although the use of specific and widely accepted indicators in the field of physical health obscures the underlying normative issue.

2. Erik H. Erikson, "Growth and Crises of the Health Personality," *Psychological Issues,* 1 (1959), 50-100; Marie Jahoda, *Current Concepts of Positive Mental Health* (New York: Basic Books, 1958); M. Brewster Smith, "Optima of Mental Health," *Psychiatry,* 13 (November 1950), 503-510.

3. Michel Foucault, *Madness and Civilization* (New York: Pantheon Books, 1965).

4. Sigmund Freud, *Civilization and Its Discontents* (1930), in vol. 21 of *Complete Psychological Works* (standard ed., London: Hogarth Press, 1961).

5. Ornulv Odegaard, "Current Studies of Incidence and Prevalence of Hospitalized Mental Patients in Scandinavia," in Paul H. Hoch and Joseph Zubin, eds., *Comparative Epidemiology of the Mental Disorders* (New York: Grune and Stratton, 1961), pp. 45-56.

6. Bernard J. Bergen and Claudewell S. Thomas, eds., *Issues and Problems in Social Psychiatry* (Springfield, Ill.: Charles C Thomas, 1966); John Cumming and Elaine Cumming, *Ego and Milieu* (New York: Atherton Press, 1962); Alfred Stanton and Morris Schwartz, *The Mental Hospital* (New York: Basic Books, 1954).

7. Howard E. Freeman and Ozzie G. Simmons, "Feeling of Stigma Among Relatives of Former Mental Patients," *Social Problems,* 8 (Spring 1961), 312-321; Freeman and Simmons, "Mental Patients in the Community," *American Sociological Review,* 23 (April 1958); 147-153; and Simmons and Freeman, "Familial Ex-Patients," *Human Relations,* 12 (1959), 233-242.

8. Emile Durkheim, *Suicide,* trans., John A. Spaulding and George Simpson (Glencoe, Ill.: Free Press, 1951).

9. See Robert E. Clark, "Psychoses, Income and Occupational Prestige," *American Journal of Sociology,* 54 (March 1949), 433-440; Robert E. Clark, "The Relationship of Schizophrenia to Occupational Income and Occupational Prestige," *American Sociological Review,* 13 (June 1948), 325-330; John A. Clausen and Melvin L. Kohn, "Relation of Schizophrenia to the Social Structure of a Small City," in Benjamin Pasamanick, ed., *Epidemiology of Mental Disorder* (Washington, D. C.: American Association for Advancement of Science, 1959), pp. 69-95; B. B. Cohen, Ruth Fairbank, and Elizabeth Greene, "Personality Disorder in the Eastern Health District in 1933," *Human Biology,* 11 (February 1939), 112-129; Bruce P. Dohrewend, "Social Status and Psychological Disorder," *American Sociological Review,* 31 (February 1966), 14-34; J. Warren Dunham, *Community and Schizophrenia* (Detroit: Wayne State University Press, 1965); Robert E. Faris and J. Warren Dunham, *Mental Disorders in Urban Areas* (Chicago: University of Chicago Press, 1939); Robert M. Frumkin, "Occupation and Major Mental Disorders," in Arnold M. Rose, *Mental Health and Mental Disorder* (New York: W. W. Norton, 1955); Robert M. Frumkin, "Occupation and Mental Illness," *Ohio Public Welfare Statistics* (September 1952), 4-13; Edith M. Furbush, "Social Facts Relative to Patients With Mental Disease," *Mental Hygiene,* 5 (July 1921), 587-611; W. M. Fuson, "Occupation of Functional Psychotics," *American Journal of Sociology,* 48 (March 1943), 612-613; Donald L. Gerard and Lester G. Houston, "Family Setting and the Social Ecology of Schizophrenia," *Psychiatric Quarterly,* 27 (January 1953), 19-37; E. M. Goldberg and S. L. Morrison, "Schizophrenia and Social Class," *British Journal of Psychiatry,* 109 (November 1963), 785-802; August B. Hollingshead and Frederick C. Redlich, *Social Class and Mental Illness* (New York: John Wiley & Sons, 1958); Robert W. Hyde and Lowell V. Kingsley, "Relation of Mental Disorders to Community Socio-Economic Level," *New England Journal of Medicine,* 231 (October 1944), 543-548; E. Gartly Jaco, *The Social Epidemiology of Mental Disorders* (New York: Russell Sage Foundation, 1960); A. J. Jaffe and E. Shanas, "Economic Differentials in the Probability of Insanity," *American Journal of Sociology,* 44 (January 1935), 534-539; Eva Johnson, "A Study of Schizophrenia in the Male," *Acta Psychiatrica et Neurologica Scandinavia,* 33 (1958), supplement 125; Bert Kaplan, Robert B. Reed, and Wyman Richardson, "A Comparison of the Incidence of Hospitalized and Non-Hospitalized Cases of Psychosis in Two Communities," *American Sociological Review,* 21 (August 1956), 472-479; Thomas S. Langner, "Environmental Stress and Mental Health," in Paul H. Hoch and Joseph Zubin,

eds., *Comparative Epidemiology of Mental Disorders* (New York: Grune and Stratton, 1961), pp. 32-45; R. Lapouse, M. S. Monk, and M. Terris, "The Drift Hypothesis and Socio-Economic Differentials in Schizophrenia," *American Journal of Public Health,* 46 (August 1956), 978-986; Everett S. Lee, "Socio-Economic and Migration Differentials in Mental Disease," *Milbank Memorial Fund Quarterly,* 41 (July 1963), 249-268; Dorothea Leighton et al., *The Character of Danger* (New York: Basic Books, 1963); P. Lemkau, C. Tietze, and M. Cooper, "Mental Hygiene Problems in an Urban District," *Mental Hygiene,* 26 (January 1941), 100-119; Ben Z. Locke et al., "Problems in Interpretation of Patterns of First Admissions to Ohio State Public Mental Hospitals," *Psychiatric Research Reports,* no. 10 (1958); Benjamin Malzberg, *Social and Biological Aspects of Mental Disease* (New York: State Hospitals Press, 1940); Norbert L. Mintz and David T. Schwartz, "Urban Ecology and Psychosis," *International Journal of Social Psychiatry,* 10 (1964), 101-118; W. J. Nolan, "Occupation and Dementia Praecox," *New York State Hospital Quarterly,* 3 (1917), 127-154; Ornulv Odegaard, "Emigration and Insanity," *Acta Psychiatrica et Neurologica Scandinavia* (1932), supplement 4; Benjamin Pasamanick, "A Survey of Mental Disease in an Urban Population," *American Journal of Psychiatry,* 119 (October 1962), 299-305; Benjamin Pasamanick, ed., *Epidemiology of Mental Disorder* (Washington, D. C.: American Association for Advancement of Science, 1959), pp. 183-203; A. J. Rosanoff, "Survey of Mental Disorders in Nassau County, New York," *Psychiatric Bulletin,* 2 (1917), 109-231; Leonard G. Rowntree, Kenneth H. McGill, and Louis P. Hellman, "Mental and Personality Disorders in Selective Service Registrants," *Journal of the American Medical Association,* 128 (1945), 1084-1087; C. W. Schroeder, "Mental Disorders in Cities," *American Journal of Sociology,* 48 (July 1942), 40-47; Ama Sreenivasan and J. Hoenig, "Caste and Mental Hospital Admissions in Mysore State, India," *American Journal of Psychiatry,* 117 (July 1960), 37-43; Lilli Stein, "Social Class Gradient in Schizophrenia," *British Journal of Preventive Social Psychiatry,* 11 (1957), 181-195; Dorothy Thomas and Ben Z. Locke, "Marital Status, Education and Occupational Differentials in Mental Disease," *Milbank Memorial Fund Quarterly,* 41 (April 1963), 145-160; Christopher Tietze, Paul Lemkau and Marcia Cooper, "Schizophrenia, Manic-Depressive Psychosis and Docial-Economic Status," *American Journal of Sociology,* 47 (September 1941), 167-175.

10. The two earliest studies we have located are Rosanoff's "Survey of Mental Disorders," and Nolan's "Occupation and Dementia Praecox," both published in 1917. Since the original publication of the present review, relatively few additional studies have reported new data on social class and mental disorder. A recent study, (William A.

Rushing, "Two Patterns in the Relationship Between Social Class and Mental Hospitalization," *American Sociological Review,* 34 (1969) 533-541 on data from three state hospitals reports a continuous inverse relationship between psychiatric hospitalization and occupational status. An analytic review of the implicit causal hypotheses about social class and psychiatric disorder has also appeared which cites a number of additional studies mainly in foreign journals (Bruce P. Dohrenwend and Barbara Snell Dohrenwend, *Social Status and Psychological Disorder* [New York: Wiley-Interscience, 1969]). None of these data have been incorporated in the summary of findings given in the text.

11. Nolan, Occupation and Dementia Praecox."

12. Jaco, *The Social Epidemiology;* Locke et al., "Problems in Interpretation of First Admissions."

13. Furbish, "Social Facts Relative to Patients"; Kaplan et al., "A Comparison of the Incidence."

14. Clark, "Psychosis, Income and Occupational Prestige"; Faris and Dunham, *Mental Disorder in Urban Areas;* Frumkin, "Occupation and Mental Illness"; Fuson, "Occupation of Functional Psychotics"; Hollingshead and Redlich, *Social Class and Mental Illnesss;* Jaco, *The Social Epidemiology;* Odegaard, "Emigration and Insanity"; and Tietze et al., "Schizophrenia, Manic-Depressive Psychosis."

15. The four studies based on data beyond psychiatric hospitalization that provide ambiguous or negative evidence are Dunham, *Community and Schizophrenia;* Jaco, *Social Epidemiology;* Dohrenwend, "Social Status and Psychological Disorder"; and Kaplan et al., "A Comparison of Incidence."

16. For recent evidence on the biasing effects of state psychiatric hospital data, see R. Jay Turner et al., "Field Survey Methods in Psychiatry," *Journal of Health and Social Behavior,* 10 (December 1969), 289-297.

17. Hollingshead and Redlich, *Social Class and Mental Illness;* O. Eugene Baum, Stanton G. Felzer, and Elaine Shumaker, "Psychotherapy, Dropouts and Lower Socio-Economic Patients," *American Journal of Orthopsychiatry,* 36 (July 1966), 629-635; Nyla J. Cole, E. H. Hardin Branch, and Roger B. Allison, "Some Relationships Between Social Class and the Practice of Dynamic Psychotherapy," *American Journal of Psychiatry,* 118 (August 1961), 1004-1012; John A. Clausen, "Ecology of Mental Disorders," in *Symposium on Preventive Social Psychiatry* (Washington, D.C.: Walter Reed Army Institute of Research, 1957), 97-109; David Fanshel, "A Study of Caseworkers," *Social Casework,* 39 (December 1958), 543-551; R. More, E. Benedek, and J. Wallace, "Social Class, Schizophrenia and the Psychiatrist," *American Journal of Psychiatry,* 120 (August 1963), 149-154;

J. Myers, L. Bean, and Max P. Pepper, "Social Class and Psychiatric Disorders," *Journal of Health and Human Behavior,* 6 (Summer 1965), 74-79; David W. Rowden et al., "Judgments About Candidates for Psychotherapy," *Journal of Health and Social Behavior,* 11 (March 1970), 51-58.

18. Durkheim, *Suicide,* p. 243.
19. Louis I. Dublin and Bessie Bunzel, *To Be or Not To Be* (New York: Smith and Haas, 1933).
20. Louis I. Dublin, *Suicide* (New York: Ronald Press, 1963), p. 61.
21. Jack P. Gibbs and Walter Martin, *Status Integration and Suicide* (Eugene: University of Oregon Press, 1964).
22. Peter Sainsbury, *Suicide in London* (London: Chapman and Hall, 1955).
23. Warren Breed, "Occupational Mobility and Suicide Among White Males," *American Sociological Review,* 28 (April 1963), 179-188; Andrew F. Henry and James F. Short, Jr., *Suicide and Homicide* (Glencoe, Ill.: Free Press, 1954); Sainsbury, *Suicide in London.*
24. Dublin, *Suicide;* Breed, "Occupational Mobility"; Breed, "Suicide, Migration and Role," *Journal of Social Issues,* 22 (January 1966), 30-43; Henry and Short, *Suicide and Homicide;* Sainsbury, *Suicide in London;* Elwin H. Powell, "Occupation, Status and Suicide," *American Sociological Review,* 23 (April 1958), 131-139.
25. Stuart Perry, "The Middle-Class and Mental Retardation in America," *Psychiatry,* 28 (May 1965), 107-118.
26. J. Wortis, "Prevention of Mental Retardation," *American Journal of Orthopsychiatry,* 35 (October 1965), 886-895.
27. Hollingshead and Redlich, *Social Class and Mental Illness;* R. Moses and J. Shanan, "Psychiatric Out-Patient Clinic," *Archives of General Psychiatry,* 4 (January 1961), 60-73; Leo Srole et al., *Mental Health in the Metropolis* (New York: McGraw-Hill, 1962); Cohen et al., "Personality Disorder"; Hyde and Kingsley, "Relation of Mental Disorders"; Kaplan et al., "A Comparison of Incidence"; Leighton et al., *The Character of Danger;* Lemkau et al., "Mental Hygiene"; Rowntree et al, "Mental and Personality Disorders."
28. Cohen et al., "Personality Disorder"; Dohrenwend, "Social Status and Psychological Disorder"; Dunham, *Community and Schizophrenia;* Elmer A. Gardner and Haroutun M. Babigian, "A Longitudinal Comparison of Psychiatric Services," *American Journal of Orthopsychiatry,* 36 (October 1966), 818-828; R. W. Hyde and R. M. Chisholm, "The Relation of Mental Disorders to Race and Nationality," *New England Journal of Medicine,* 231 (1944), 612-618; Jaco, *Social Epidemiology of Mental Disorder;* Robert J. Kleiner, Jacob Tuckman, and Martha Lavell, "Mental Disorder and Status Based on

Race," *Psychiatry,* 23 (August 1960), 271-274; Judith Lazarus, Ben Z. Locke and Dorothy Thomas, "Migration Differentials in Mental Disease," *Milbank Memorial Fund Quarterly,* 41 (January 1963), 25-42; Lee, "Socio-Economic and Migration Differentials"; Leighton et al., *The Character of Danger;* Lemkau et al., "Mental Hygiene Problems"; Locke et al., "Problems in Interpretation"; Malzberg, *Social and Biological Aspects;* Pasamanick, "Survey of Mental Disease"; E. S. Pollack et al., "Socio-Economic and Family Characteristics of Patients Admitted to Psychiatric Services," *American Journal of Public Health,* 54 (1964), 506-518; Thomas F. Pugh and Brien MacMahon, *Epidemiologic Findings in United States Mental Hospital Data* (Boston: Little, Brown, 1962); W. F. Roth and F. B. Luton, "The Mental Hygiene Program in Tennessee," *American Journal of Psychiatry,* 99 (March 1943), 662-675; Rowntree et al., "Mental and Personality Disorders"; Rosanoff, "Survey of Mental Disorders"; Thomas and Locke, "Marital Status and Education"; D. G. Wilson and E. M. Lantz, "The Effect of Culture Change on the Negro Race in Virginia," *American Journal of Psychiatry,* 114 (July 1957), 25-32.

29. Dohrenwend, "Social Status and Psychological Disorder."

30. Malzberg, *Social and Psychological Aspects;* Pugh and MacMahon, *Epidemiologic Findings.*

31. Malzberg, *Social and Psychological Aspects,* p. 226.

32. Wilson and Lantz, "The Effect of Culture Change."

33. Pollack et al., "Socio-Economic and Family Characteristics."

34. Lee, "Socio-Economic and Migration Differentials"; Lazarus et al., "Migration Differentials"; Thomas and Locke, "Marital Status and Education."

35. Faris and Dunham, *Mental Disorders in Urban Areas;* Donald L. Gerard and Joseph Siegal, "The Family Background of Schizophrenia," *Psychiatric Quarterly,* 24 (January 1950), 47-73; Gerard and Houston, "Family Setting and Social Ecology"; E. H. Hare, "Family Setting and the Urban Distribution of Schizophrenia," *Journal of Mental Science,* 102 (1956), 753-759; E. H. Hare, "Mental Illness and Social Conditions in Bristol," *Journal of Mental Science,* 102 (1956), 349-357.

36. Dohrenwend, "Social Status and Psychological Disorder"; Mintz and Schwartz, "Urban Ecology and Psychosis"; Joan L. Burke, Hugh Lafave, and Grace Kurtz, "Minority Group Membership as a Factor in Chronicity," *Psychiatry,* 28 (August 1965), 235-238; Henry Wechsler and Thomas F. Pugh, "Fit of Individual and Community Characteristics and Rates of Psychiatric Hospitalization," *American Journal of Sociology,* 73 (November 1967), 331-338.

37. Clausen and Kohn, "Relation of Schizophrenia"; Lapouse et al., "The Drift Hypothesis"; Lee, "Socio-Economic and Migration

Differentials"; Odegaard, "Emigration and Insanity"; Lazarus et al., "Migration Differentials"; Locke et al., "Immigration and Insanity"; Benjamin Malzberg and Everett Lee, *Migration and Mental Disease* (New York: Social Science Research Council, 1956); F. M. Martin, J. H. F. Brotherston, and S. P. W. Chave, "Incidence of Neurosis in a New Housing Estate," *British Journal of Preventive and Social Medicine*, 11 (1957), 196-202; H. B. M. Murphy, "Social Change and Mental Health," in *Causes of Mental Disorders* (New York: Milbank Memorial Fund, 1961), pp. 280-329; H. B. M. Murphy, "Migration and the Major Mental Disorders," in Mildred Kantor, ed., *Mobility and Mental Health* (Springfield, Ill.: Charles C Thomas, 1965), pp. 5-24; Marc Fried, "Effects of Social Change on Mental Health," *American Journal of Orthopsychiatry*, 34 (January 1964), 3-28.

38. Jaco, *Social Epidemiology of Mental Disorders.*

39. The data indicating disproportionately high rates of psychiatric hospitalization among migrants is given in Lazarus et al., "Migration Differentials"; Lee, "Socio-Economic and Migration Differentials"; and Thomas and Locke, "Marital Status and Education." The study of psychiatric hospitalization in Philadelphia that reveals a reversal of these trends among blacks is Seymour Parker and Robert J. Kleiner, *Mental Illness in the Urban Negro Community* (New York: Free Press, 1966).

40. Henry S. Shryock, Jr., *Population Mobility Within the United States* (Chicago: Community and Family Study Center, 1964).

41. Basil G. Zimmer, "Participation of Migrants in Urban Structures," *American Sociological Review*, 20 (April 1955), 218-224.

42. Faris and Dunham, *Mental Disorders.*

43. Gerard and Siegel, "Family Background of Schizophrenia."

44. Mintz and Schwartz, "Urban Ecology and Psychosis."

45. Wechsler and Pugh, "Fit of Individual."

46. Murphy, "Migration and the Major Mental Disorders."

47. Arnold Rose, *Mental Health and Mental Disorder;* Neil A. Dayton, *New Facts on Mental Disorders* (Springfield, Ill.: Charles C Thomas, 1940); Jaco, *Social Epidemiology;* Locke et al., "Problems in Interpretation"; Malzberg, *Social and Biological Aspects;* Thomas and Locke, "Marital Status, Education."

48. Marc Fried, "Social Problems and Psychopathology," in Leonard J. Duhl, ed., *Urban America and the Planning of Mental Health Services* (New York: Group for the Advancement of Psychiatry, 1964), pp. 403-446.

49. Marc Fried, "Deprivation and Migration," in Daniel P. Moynihan, ed., *On Understanding Poverty* (New York: Basic Books, 1969).

50. Rowntree et al., "Mental and Personality Disorders."

51. Jaco, *Social Epidemiology.*

52. Fried, "Social Problems and Psychopathology."

53. Dayton, *New Facts on Mental Disorders;* Harvey Brenner, *Mental Illness and the Economy.* To be published by Harvard University Press.

54. Dublin, *Suicide;* Breed, "Occupational Mobility"; Breed, "Suicide, Migration and Role"; Henry and Short, *Suicide and Homicide;* Sainsbury, *Suicide in London;* and Powell, "Occupation, Status and Suicide."

55. Nyla J. Cole et al., "Socio-Economic Adjustment of a Sample of Schizophrenic Patients," *American Journal of Psychiatry,* 120 (November 1963), 465-471.

56. Marc Fried, "The Role of Work in a Mobile Society," in Sam B. Warner, Jr., ed., *Planning for a Nation of Cities* (Cambridge, Mass.: MIT Press, 1966), pp. 81-105; Eugene A. Friedmann et al., *The Meaning of Work and Retirement* (Chicago: University of Chicago Press, 1954); Alex Inkeles, "Industrial Man," *American Journal of Sociology,* 66 (July 1960), 1-31; Arthur Kornhauser, *Mental Health of the Industrial Worker* (New York: John Wiley 1965); Nancy C. Morse and Robert S. Weiss, "The Function and Meaning of Work and the Job," *American Sociological Review,* 20 (April 1955), 191-198.

57. Kornhauser, *Mental Health of the Industrial Worker.*

58. Clausen and Kohn, "Relationship of Schizophrenia"; Dunham, *Community and Schizophrenia;* Gerard and Houston, "Family Background of Schizophrenia"; Goldberg and Morrison, "Schizophrenia and Social Class"; Hare, "Mental Illness and Social Conditions"; Hollingshead and Redlich, *Social Class and Mental Illness;* Jaco, *Social Epidemiology;* Lapouse et al., "The Drift Hypothesis"; Thomas S. Langner and Stanley T. Michaels, *Life Stress and Mental Health* (New York: Free Press, 1963); M. H. Lystad, "Social Mobility Among Selected Groups of Schizophrenic Patients," *American Sociological Review,* 22 (June 1957), 288-292. We have not included in this summary one recent study which reveals lower rates of upward intergenerational mobility and higher rates of downward intergenerational mobility than in a random sample of the population. On the other hand, these data show a high degree of intragenerational occupational stability among schizophrenic patients, indicating selective factors that are quite different from the simple notion of downward drift due to schizophrenic pathology. See R. Jay Turner, "Class and Mobility in Schizophrenic Outcome," *Psychiatric Quarterly,* 42 (October 1968), 712-725; and R. Jay Turner and Morton O. Wegenfeld, "Occupational Mobility and Schizophrenia," *American Sociological Review,* 32 (February 1967), 104-113.

59. Clausen and Kohn, "Relationship and Schizophrenia"; Jaco, *Social Epidemiology;* Lapouse et al., "The Drift Hypothesis.."

60. Lapouse et al., "The Drift Hypothesis."

61. Gerard and Houston, "Family Setting and Social Ecology."

62. Dunham, *Community and Schizophrenia;* Clausen and Kohn, "Relationship of Schizophrenia."

63. Eli M. Bower, Thomas A. Shallhamer, and John M. Daily, "School Characteristics of Male Adolescents Who Later Became Schizophrenic," *American Journal of Orthopsychiatry,* 30 (October 1960), 712-729.

64. Goldberg and Morrison, "Schizophrenia and Social Class," p. 786; Dunham, *Community and Schizophrenia.*

65. Cole et al., "Socio-Economic Adjustment."

66. Joseph Kahl and James Davis, "A Comparison of Indexes of Socio-Economic Status," *American Sociological Review,* 20 (June 1955), 317-325.

67. Warren C. Haggstrom, "The Power of the Poor," in Frank Riessman, Jerome Cohen, and Arthur Pearl, eds., *Mental Health of the Poor* (New York: Free Press, 1964), pp. 205-223.

68. Langner and Michaels, *Life Stress and Mental Health;* Jerome Myers and Bertram Roberts, *Family and Class Dynamics in Mental Illness* (New York: John Wiley & Sons, 1959).

69. Moore et al., "Social Class, Schizophrenia"; Norman Q. Brill and Hugh A. Storrow, "Social Class and Psychiatric Treatment," *Archives of General Psychiatry,* 3 (October 1960), 340-344; Dewitt L. Crandell and Bruce P. Dohrenwend, "Some Relations Among Psychiatric Symptoms, Organic Illness, and Social Class," *American Journal of Psychiatry,* 123 (June 1967), 1527-1538.

70. Lloyd H. Rogler and August B. Hollingshead, *Trapped: Families and Schizophrenia* (New York: John Wiley & Sons, 1965).

71. Charles Kadushin, "Social Class and the Experience of Ill Health," in Reinhard Bendix and Seymour M. Lipset, eds., *Class, Status and Power* (New York: Free Press, 1966), pp. 406-412.

72. Howard Freeman and Ozzie G. Simmons, *The Mental Patient Comes Home* (New York: John Wiley & Sons, 1963); Dunham, *Community and Schizophrenia;* Hollingshead and Redlich, *Social Class and Mental Illness.*

73. William Haase, "The Role of Socio-Economic Class in Examiner Bias," in Riessman, Cohen, and Pearl, eds., *Mental Health of the Poor,* pp. 241-247.

74. Fanshel, "A Study of Caseworkers"; Rowden et al., "Judgments About Candidates for Psychotherapy." Kandel's data lend themselves to a similar interpretation; Denise B. Kandel, "Status Homophily, Social Context, and Participation in Psychotherapy," *American Journal of Sociology,* 71 (May 1966), 640-650.

75. Howard T. Blane, Willis F. Overton, and Morris E. Chafetz,

"Social Factors in the Diagnosis of Alcoholism," *Quarterly Journal of Studies on Alcoholism,* 24 (December 1963), 640-663.

76. Hollingshead and Redlich, *Social Class and Mental Illness;* Fanshel, "A Study of Caseworkers"; Moore et al., "Social Class, Schizophrenia"; Brill and Storrow, "Social Class and Psychiatric Treatment."

77. Kadushin, "Social Class."

78. U.S. Department of Health, Education, and Welfare, *Family Income in Relation to Selected Health Characteristics,* National Center for Health Statistics Series 10, no. 2, July, 1963; U. S. Department of Health Education, and Welfare, *Medical Care, Health Status, and Family Income,* National Center for Health Statistics Series 10, no. 9, May, 1964; U. S. Department of Health, Education, and Welfare, *Selected Health Characteristics by Occupation,* National Center for Health Statistics Series 10, August, 1965, p. 21.

79. Langner and Michaels, *Life Stress and Mental Health.*

80. Dohrenwend, "Social Status and Psychological Disorder"; Edward Zigler and Leslie Phillips, "Psychiatric Diagnosis," *Journal of Abnormal and Social Psychology,* 63 (November 1961), 607-618.

81. Fried, "Social Problems and Psychopathology."

Chapter V: Prevention of Illness and Maintenance of Health

1. Stanislav V. Kasl and Sidney Cobb, "Health Behavior, Illness Behavior, and Sick-Role Behavior," *Archives of Environmental Health,* 12 (February 1966), 246-266; and (April 1966), 531-541.

2. Monroe Lerner and Odin W. Anderson, *Health Progress in the United Statees, 1900-1960: A Report of the Health Information Foundation* (Chicago: University of Chicago Press, 1963); Herman M. Somers and Anne R. Somers, *Doctors, Patients, and Health Insurance: The Organization and Financing of Medical Care* (Washington, D. C.: Brookings Institution, 1961); U. S. Department of Health, Education, and Welfare, *Health, Education, and Welfare Trends, 1963 Edition* (Washington, D. C.; U. S. Government Printing Office, 1963); U. S. Department of Health, Education, and Welfare, Public Health Service, *Health Statistics From the U.S. National Health Survey: Dental Care, Interval and Frequency of Visits, United States, July 1957-June 1959,* Public Health Service Publication No. 584-B14 (Washington, D.C.: U.S. Government Printing Office, 1960); Stephen S. Kegeles, Stanley Lotzkar, and Lewis W. Andrews, "Predicting the Acceptance of Dental Care by Residents of Nursing Homes," *Journal of Public Health Dentistry,* 26 (Summer 1966), 290-302; U.S. Department of Health, Education, and Welfare, Public Health Service, *Health Statistics From*

the U.S. National Health Survey: Volume of Physician Visits, United States, July 1957-June 1959, Public Health Service Publication No. 584-B19 (Washington, D.C.: U.S. Government Printing Office, 1960); U.S. Department of Health, Education, and Welfare, Public Health Service, *Health Statistics From the U.S. National Health Survey, Hospital Discharges and Length of Stay: Short-Stay Hospitals, United States*, 1958-1960, Public Health Service Publication No. 584-B32 (Washington, D.C.: U.S. Government Printing Office, 1962); John D. Stoeckle, Irving K. Zola, and Gerald E. Davidson, "On Going to See the Doctor," *Journal of Chronic Diseases*, 16 (1963), 975-989; Irving K. Zola, "Illness Behavior of the Working Class," in ed. Arthur B. Shostak and William Gomberg, eds., *Blue-Collar World*, (Englewood Cliffs, N.J.: Prentice-Hall, 1964), pp. 351-361; Eliot Freidson, *Patients' Views of Medical Practice* (New York: Russell Sage Foundation, 1961); Edward A. Suchman, "Social Patterns of Illness and Medical Care," *Journal of Health and Human Behavior* 6 (Spring 1965), 2-16.

3. Paul N. Borsky and Oswald K. Sagen, "Motivations Toward Health Examinations," *American Journal of Public Health*, 49 (April 1959), 514-527; S. Stephen Kegeles et al., "Survey of Beliefs About Cancer Detection and Taking Papanicolaou Tests," *Public Health Reports*, 80 (September 1965), 815-824; Irwin M. Rosenstock, Mayhew Derryberry, and Barbara K. Carriger, "Why People Fail to Seek Poliomyelitis Vaccination," *Public Health Reports*, 74 (February 1959), 98-103; Godfrey M. Hochbaum, *Public Participation in Medical Screening Programs*, U.S. Public Health Service Publication No. 572 (Washington, D.C.: U.S. Government Printing Office, 1958); S. Stephen Kegeles, "Some Motives for Seeking Preventive Dental Care," *Journal of the American Dental Association*, 67 (July 1963), 90-98; Fred Heinzelmann, "Determinants of Prophylaxis Behavior with Respect to Rheumatic Fever," *Journal of Health and Human Behavior*, 3 (1962), 73-81; Elizabeth Flack, "Participation in Case Finding Program for Cervical Cancer," administrative report, Cancer Control Program, U.S. Public Health Service (Washington, D.C.: U.S. Government Printing Office, 1960); Howard Leventhal et al., "Epidemic Impact on the General Population in Two Cities," in *The Impact of Asian Influenza on Community Life*, U.S. Public Health Service Publication No. 766 (Washington, D.C.: U.S. Government Printing Office, 1960); S. Stephen Kegeles, "Why People Seek Dental Care," *Journal of Health and Human Behavior*, 4 (Fall 1963), 166-173; Don P. Haefner et al., "Preventive Actions in Dental Disease, Tuberculosis and Cancer," *Public Health Reports*, 82 (May 1967), 451-460; Irwin M. Rosenstock, "Why People Use Health Services," *Milbank Memorial Fund Quarterly*, 44 (July 1966), 94-127.

4. Haefner, "Preventive Actions in Dental Disease, Tuberculosis and Cancer."

5. Charles Kadushin, "Social Class and the Experience of Ill Health," *Sociological Inquiry,* 34 (Winter 1964), 67-80.

6. Kegeles, "Survey of Beliefs about Cancer Detection."

7. Ibid.

8. Haefner, "Preventive Actions in Dental Disease, Tuberculosis and Cancer."

9. Kurt Lewin, *A Dynamic Theory of Personality* (New York: McGraw-Hill, 1935).

10. Jerome Bruner and Cecile C. Goodman, "Value and Need as Organizing Factors in Perception," *Journal of Abnormal and Social Psychology,* 42 (1947), 37-39; and Irwin M. Rosenstock and Jean Hendry, "Epidemic Impact on Community Agencies," in *The Impact of Asian Influenza on Community Life,* Public Health Service Publication No. 766 (Washington, D.C.: U.S. Government Printing Office, 1960).

11. Paul Robbins, "Some Explorations Into the Nature of Anxieties Relating to Illness," *Genetic Psychology Monographs,* No. 66, (U.S. Department of Health, Education, and Welfare, Public Health Service, 1962), 91-141.

12. Freidson, *Patients' Views of Medical Practice,* p. 144.

13. Hochbaum, *Public Participation in Medical Screening Programs.*

14. Kegeles, "Some Motives for Seeking Preventive Dental Care."

15. Leon Festinger, *A Theory of Cognitive Dissonance* (Evanston, Ill.: Row Peterson, 1957).

16. Howard Leventhal et al., "Epidemic Impact on the General Population in Two Cities."

17. Kegeles, "Some Motives for Seeking Preventive Dental Care."

18. Irwin M. Rosenstock, "Why People Use Health Services."

19. Don P. Haefner and John P. Kirscht, "Motivational and Behavioral Effects of Modifying Health Beliefs," *Public Health Reports,* 85 (June 1970), 478-484.

20. Marshall H. Becker, Robert H. Drachman, and John P. Kirscht, "Predicting Mothers' Compliance with Pediatric Medical Regimens," *Journal of Pediatrics* (in press, July 1972).

21. Irving K. Zola, "Illness Behavior of the Working Class."

22. Kegeles, "Survey of Beliefs about Cancer Detection."

23. Daniel Rosenblatt and Edward A. Suchman, "Blue-Collar Attitudes and Information Toward Health and Illness," in Shostak and Gomberg, eds., *Blue-Collar World,* pp. 324-333.

24. Irwin M. Rosenstock et al., "Public Knowledge, Opinion and Action Concerning Three Public Health Issues," *Journal of Health and Human Behavior,* 7 (Summer 1966), 91-98.

25. Paul F. Lazarsfeld and Patricia Kendall, "The Communication Behavior of the Average American," in Wilbur L. Schramm, ed., *Mass Communications,* (Urbana: University of Illinois Press, 1960), pp. 425-437; Elihu Katz and Paul F. Lazarsfeld, *Personal Influence* (Glencoe, Ill.: Free Press, 1955).

26. Leo Bogart, "The Mass Media and the Blue-Collar Worker," in Shostak and Gomberg, eds., *Blue-Collar World,* pp. 416-428; James W. Swinehart, "Voluntary Exposure to Health Communications," *American Journal of Public Health,* 58 (July 1968), 1265-1275.

27. Earl L. Koos, *The Health of Regionville* (New York: Columbia University Press, 1954).

28. Kadushin, "Social Class and the Experience of Ill Health"; and Gene N. Levine, "Anxiety About Illness: Psychological and Social Bases," *Journal of Health and Human Behavior,* 3 (Spring 1962), 30-34.

29. Ozzie G. Simmons, *Social Status and Public Health,* Social Science Research Council, Pamphlet No. 13 (New York, 1958).

30. U.S. Department of Health, Education, and Welfare, Public Health Service, *Medical Care, Health Status, and Family Income: United States,* Public Health Service Publication No. 1000, series 10, no. 9 (Washington, D.C.: U.S. Government Printing Office, 1965).

31. Elizabeth Herzog, "Some Assumptions About the Poor," *Social Service Review,* 37 (December 1963), 389-402; Albert K. Cohen and Harold M. Hodges, Jr., "Characteristics of the Lower-Blue-Collar-Class," *Social Problems,* 10 (Spring 1963), 303-334.

32. Freidson, *Patients' Views of Medical Practice.*

33. J. Whitney Brown et al., "A Study of General Practice in Massachusetts," *Journal of the American Medical Association,* 216 (April 12, 1971), 301-306.

34. Mary W. Herman, "The Poor: Their Medical Needs and the Health Services Available to Them," *Annals of the American Academy of Political and Social Science,* 399 (January 1972), 12-21.

35. Lawrence Bergner and Alonzo S. Yerby, "Low Income and Barriers to Use of Health Services," *New England Journal of Medicine,* 278 (March 7, 1968), 541-546.

36. Herman, "The Poor: Their Medical Needs and the Health Services."

37. U.S. Department of Health, Education, and Welfare, Public Health Service, "Cooperation in Health Examination Surveys," National Center for Health Statistics, Public Health Service Publication No. 1000, series 10, no. 9 (Washington, D.C.: U.S. Government Printing Office, July 1965).

38. U.S. Department of Health, Education and Welfare, Public Health Service, "Visits for Medical and Dental Care During the Year Preceding Childbirth, United States—1963 Births," National Center

for Health Statistics, Public Health Service Publication No. 1000, series 22, no. 4 (Washington, D.C.: U.S. Government Printing Office, 1968).

39. Joel J. Alpert et al., "Attitudes and Satisfactions of Low-Income Families Receiving Comprehensive Pediatric Care," *American Journal of Public Health*, 60 (March 1970), 499-506.

40. Theodore J. Colombo, Ernest W. Saward, and Merwyn R. Greenlick, "The Integration of an OEO Health Program Into a Prepaid Comprehensive Group Practice Plan," *American Journal of Public Health*, 59 (April 1 69), 641-650.

41. U.S. Department of Health, Education, and Welfare, Public Health Service, "Volume of Physician Visits, United States—July 1966-June 1967," National Center for Health Statistics, Public Health Service Publication No. 1000, series 10, no. 49 (Washington, D.C.: U.S. Government Printing Office, 1968).

Chapter VI: The Help-Seeking Behavior of the Poor

1. The results of many useful studies are reviewed and discussed in J. N. Morris, *Uses of Epidemiology* (London: E. and S. Livingston, 1967).

2. C. H. Goodrich, M. C. Olendzki, and G. G. Reader, *Welfare Medical Care: An Experiment* (Cambridge, Mass.: Harvard University Press, 1970).

3. W. H. McBroom, "Illness, Illness Behavior and Socio-Economic Status," *Journal of Health and Social Behavior*, 11 (December 1970), 319-326.

4. L. Pratt, "The Relationship of Socioeconomic Status to Health," *American Journal of Public Health*, 61 (February 1971), 281-291. See also N. Q. Brill, R. Weinstein, and J. Garratt, "Poverty and Mental Illness: Patients' Perceptions of Poverty as an Etiological Factor in Their Illness," *American Journal of Psychiatry*, 125 (March 1969), 1172-1179.

5. O. Brim, D. Blass, D. Lavin, and N. Goodman, *Personality and Decision Processes: Studies in the Social Psychology of Thinking* (Stanford, Calif.: Stanford University Press, 1962); G. Fulcher, *Common Sense Decision Making* (Evanston, Ill.: Northwestern University Press, 1965); A. Shostak and W. Gomberg, eds., *Blue-Collar World* (Englewood Cliffs, N.J.: Prentice-Hall, 1964); D. Wolfe, "Power and Authority in the Family," in D. Cartwright, ed., *Studies in Social Power* (Ann Arbor: University of Michigan), pp. 99-117.

6. I. K. Zola and M. Spivak, "Psychological and Cultural Factors in Seeing a Doctor," unpublished manuscript, Brandeis University, 1963. See also, J. D. Stoeckle, I. '. Zola, and G. E. Davidson, "On Going to

see the Doctor, the Contributions of the Patient to the Decision to Seek Medical Aid," *Journal of Chronic Diseases*, 16 (September 1963), 975-989.

7. J. B. McKinlay, "The Concept 'Patient Career' as a Heuristic Device for Making Medical Sociology Relevant to Medical Students," *Social Science and Medicine*, 5 (October 1971), 441-460; E. Goffman, "The Moral Career of the Mental Patient," *Psychiatry*, 22 (May 1959), 123-142; R. M. Swanson and S. P. Spitzer, "Stigma and the Psychiatric Patient Career," *Journal of Health and Social Behavior*, 11 (March 1970), 44-51.

8. D. Mechanic, *Medical Sociology* (New York: Free Press, 1968), p. 141 (italics added); and "Illness and Cure" in the first edition of this book (Cambridge, Mass.: Harvard University Press, 1969), p. 199.

9. E. A. Suchman, "Stages of Illness and Medical Care," *Journal of Health and Human Behavior*, 6 (Fall 1965), 114-128.

10. Mechanic, "Illness and Cure," p. 202 (my emphasis).

11. I. H. Pearse and L. H. Crocker, *The Peckham Experiment* (London: George Allen and Unwin, 1944).

12. E. L. Koos, *The Health of Regionville* (New York: Columbia University Press, 1954). For more recent data with respect to another culture see M. E. J. Wadsworth, W. J. H. Butterfield, and R. Blaney, *Health and Sickness: The Choice of Treatment* (London: Tavistock Publications, 1971); J. R. Butler, "Illness and the Sick Role: An Evaluation in Three Communities," *British Journal of Sociology*, 21 (September 1970), 241-261.

13. I. K. Zola, "Culture and Symptoms: An Analysis of Patients Presenting Complaints"; M. Zborowski, "Cultural Components in Response to Pain," *Journal of Social Issues*, 8 (1952), 16-30; R. N. Anderson, O. W. Anderson, B. Smedby, "Perception of and Response to Symptoms of Illness in Sweden and the United States," paper presented at American Sociological Association, 1967.

14. I. K. Zola, "Illness Behavior of the Working Class," in Shostak and Gomberg, eds., *Blue-Collar World*, pp. 350-361.

15. J. W. Eaton and R. J. Weil, *Culture and Mental Disorders* (Glencoe, Ill.: Free Press, 1955).

16. S. Dinitz et al., "Psychiatric and Social Attributes as Predictors of Case Outcome in Mental Hospitalization," *Social Problems*, 8 (Spring 1961), 322-328; S. Dinitz et al., "Instrumental Role Expectations and Post-hospital Performance of Female Mental Patients," *Social Forces*, 40 (1962), 248-254; M. Lefton et al., "Social Class, Expectations, and Performance of Mental Patients," *American Journal of Sociology*, 68 (July 1962), 79-87; "Former Mental Patients and the Neighbors: A Comparison of Performance Levels," *Journal of Health and Human Behavior*, 7 (Summer 1966), 106-113; M. R. Yarrow et

al., "The Psychological Meaning of Mental Illness in the Family," *Journal of Social Issues*, 11 (1955), 12-24; H. Sampson, S. L. Messinger, and R. D. Towne, "Family Processes and Becoming a Mental Patient," *American Journal of Sociology*, 68 (July 1962) 88-96; A. K. Daniels, "Normal Mental Illness and Understandable Excuses," *American Behavioral Scientist*, 14 (December 1970), 167-184.

17. E. Ludwig and G. Gibson, "Self-Perception of Sickness and the Seeking of Medical Care," *Journal of Health and Social Behavior*, 10 (June 1969), 125-133.

18. Ibid., p. 133.

19. J. B. McKinlay, "Some Aspects of Lower Working Class Utilization Behavior," unpub. Ph.D. diss., Aberdeen University, Aberdeen, Scotland, 1970; E. M. Biles, "The Use of Child Welfare Clinics by Primigravidal in Alberdeen," unpublished report, Aberdeen University, 1954.

20. L. Rainwater, "Fear and the House-as-Haven in the Lower Class" in I. Deutscher and E. J. Thompson, eds., *Among the People* (New York: Basic Books, 1968), pp. 84-95; A. K. Cohen and H. M. Hodges, "Characteristics of the Lower-Blue-Collar-Class," *Social Problems*, 10 (Spring 1962), 303-335.

21. Koos, *Health of Regionville*, p. 37.

22. D. Apple, "How Laymen Define Illness," *Journal of Health and Human Behavior*, 1 (Fall 1960), 219-225.

23. L. H. Garland, "Studies of the Accuracy of Diagnostic Procedures," *American Journal of Roentgenology, Radium Therapy, Nuclear Medicine*, 82 (July-December 1959), 25-38; H. Bakwin, "Pseudoxia Pediatricia," *New England Journal of Medicine*, 232 (June 1945), 691-97.

24. Koos, *Health of Regionville*.

25. D. Mechanic, "Correlates of Frustration Among British General Practitioners," *Journal of Health and Social Behavior*, 11 (June 1970), 87-104; D. Mechanic and R. Faich, "Doctors in Revolt: The Crisis in the English National Health Service," *Medical Care*, 8 (November-December 1970); See also A. Cartwright, *Patients and Their Doctors: A Study of General Practice* (London: Routledge and Kegan Paul, 1967); G. W. Horobin and M. Bloor, "Role Taking and Illness," paper to Social Science and Medicine International Conference, Aberdeen Scotland, September 1970.

26. This kind of process is described by T. J. Scheff in both "Decision Rules, Types of Error, and the Consequences in Medical Diagnosis," *Behavioral Science*, 8 (April 1963), 97-107 and "Preferred Errors in Diagnosis," *Medical Care*, 2 (July-September 1964), 166-172.

27. Extracted from material gathered during field work for a study

of lower-class use of services. See J. B. McKinlay, "Some Aspects of Lower Working Class Utilization Behavior."

28. H. S. Becker, "Notes on the Concept of Commitment," *American Journal of Sociology,* 66 (July 1960), 32-40.

29. E. Freidson, "Client Control and Medical Practice," *American Journal of Sociology,* 65 (January 1960), 3374-382; Mechanic, *Medical Sociology;* R. M. Coe, *Sociology of Medicine* (New York: McGraw-Hill, 1970).

30. This is rather vividly described in S. R. Kauner, "Taking the Medical System's Pulse," and L. K. Altman, "The High Cost of Medicine," *New York Times,* January 9, 1972.

31. E. Freidson, *Profession of Medicine* (New York: Dodd, Mead and Co., 1970). How the poor are exploited in various ways is discussed by D. Caplovitz, *The Poor Pay More* (New York: Free Press, 1963).

32. D. Rosenblatt and E. A. Suchman, "The Underutilization of Medical-Care Services by Blue-Collarites," in Shostak and Gomberg, eds., *Blue-Collar World,* p. 344.

33. M. Jefferys, J. H. F. Brotherstone, and A. Cartwright, "The Consumption of Medicines on a Working Class Estate," *British Journal of Preventive and Social Medicine,* 14 (1960), 64-76.

34. Yarrow et al., "The Psychological Meaning of Mental Illness in the Family"; Sampson et al., "Family Processes and Becoming a Mental Patient."

35. Suchman, "Stages of Illness and Medical Care"; and Zola, "Illness Behavior of the Working Class."

36. Freidson, *Profession of Medicine,* pp. 290-291; M. Young and P. Willmott, *Family and Kinship in East London* (London: Routledge and Kegan Paul, 1957).

37. Z. D. Blum and P. H. Rossi, "Social Class Research and Images of the Poor: A Bibliographic Review" in D. P. Moynihan, ed., *On Understanding Poverty,* (New York: Basic Books, 969), pp. 343-397; Shostak and Gomberg, eds., *Blue-Collar World;* Rainwater, "Fear and the House-as-Haven in the Lower Class," pp. 84-95.

38. Freidson, *The Profession of Medicine,* p. 291.

39. A. Davis, "The Motivation of the Underprivileged Worker," in W. F. Whyte, ed., *Industry and Society* (New York: McGraw-Hill, 1946), pp. 84-106; H. A. Halbertsma, "Working-Class Systems of Mutual Assistance in Case of Childbirth, Illness and Death," *Social Science and Medicine,* 3 (1970), 321-328. A number of pertinent papers appear in Shostak and Gomberg's *Blue-Collar World.*

40. E. Freidson, "Client Control and Medical Practice," *American Journal of Sociology,* 65 (January 1960), 377.

41. Freidson, "Client Control and Medical Practice"; see also his *Profession of Medicine*, pp. 290-295, and *Patients' Views of Medical Practice* (New York: Russell Sage Foundation, 1961).

42. J. B. McKinlay, "Some Aspects of Lower-Working Class Utilization Behavior"; J. B. McKinlay, "Social Networks and Utilization Behavior," paper to Social Science and Medicine International Conference, Aberdeen, Scotland, September, 1970; E. Freidson, "The Organization of Medical Practice and Patient Behavior," *American Journal of Public Health*, 51 (January 1961), 43-52.

43. E. Bott, *Family and Social Network: Roles, Norms and External Relationships in Ordinary Urban Families* (London: Tavistock Publications, 1957).

44. For a discussion of the type of process involved see W. Goode, "A Theory of Role Strain," *American Sociological Review*, 25 (April 1960), 483-496; T. J. Scheff, "Negotiating Reality: Notes on Power in the Assessment of Responsibility," *Social Problems*, 16 (Summer 1968), 3-17; M. Balint, *The Doctor, His Patient and the Illness* (London: Pitman Paperbacks, 1968).

45. J. B. McKinlay and S. M. McKinlay, "Some Social Characteristics of Lower Working Class Utilizers and Underutilizers of Maternity Care Services," *Journal of Health and Social Behavior*, 14 (March 1973), 00-000.

46. A. W. Gouldner, "The Norm of Reciprocity: A Preliminary Statement," *American Sociological Review*, 25 (April 1960), 161-179; D. E. Muir and E. A. Weinstein, "The Social Debt: An Investigation of Lower-Class and Middle-Class Norms of Social Obligation," *American Sociological Review*, 27 (August 1962), 532-539.

47. J. B. McKinlay, "The Sick Role—Illness and Pregnancy," *Social Science and Medicine*, 6 (1972), 561-572; F. A. Petroni, "Social Class, Family Size, and the Sick Role," *Journal of Marriage and the Family*, 31 (November 1969), 728-735.

48. L. Rainwater, *And the Poor Get Children* (Chicago: Quadrangle Books, 1960); and *Family Design: Marital Sexuality, Family Size and Family Planning* (Chicago: Aldine Publishing Co., 1964).

49. Scheff, "Preferred Errors in Diagnosis."

50. Freidson, "Client Control and Medical Practice," p. 378.

51. C. H. Goodrich, M. C. Ólendzki, and G. G. Reader, *Welfare Medical Care: An Experiment* (Cambridge, Mass: Harvard University Press, 1970).

52. R. Fink, "The Measurement of Medical Care Utilization," in M. R; Greenlick, ed., *Conceptual Issues in the Analysis of Medical Care Utilization Behavior* (Washington, D.C.: Department of Health, Education and Welfare, Public Health Service, 1969), pp. 5-32.

53. C. R. Pope, S. S. Yoshioka, and M. R. Greenlick, "Determi-

nants of Medical Care Utilization: The Use of the Telephone for Reporting Symptoms," paper to American Sociological Association, San Francisco, 1969; M. C. Heagarty, C. Robertson, J. Kosa, and J. J. Alpert, "Use of the Telephone by Low-Income Families," *Journal of Pediatrics*, 73 (November 1968), 740-744.

54. J. Kitsuse and A. Cicourel, "A Note on the Uses of Official Statistics," *Social Problems*, 11 (Fall 1963), 131-139.

55. M. Rein, "Social Class and the Health Service," *New Society*, November 20, 1969, pp. 807-810; M. Rein, "Social Class and the Utilization of Medical Care Services," *Hospitals*, 43 (July 1969), 43-54. See also G. Forsyth, "Is the Health Service Doing Its Job?" *New Society*, October 19, 1967, pp. 545-550; R. M. Titmuss, *Commitment to Welfare* (London: George Allen and Unwin, 1968); R. M. Titmuss, *The Gift Relationship* (New York: Pantheon Books, 1971).

56. L. A. Coser, "Unanticipated Conservative Consequences of Liberal Theorizing," *Social Problems*, 16 (Winter 1969(, 263-272.

57. F. Tannenbaum, *Crime and the Community* (Boston: Ginn, 1938); D. R. Cressey, "Theoretical Foundations for Using Criminals in the Rehabilitation of Criminals," in H. W. Mattick, ed., *The Future of Imprisonment in a Free Society, Key Issues* 2 (1965), 96-97; J. I. Kitsuse, "Societal Reactions to Deviant Behavior: Problems of Theory and Method," in H. Becker, ed., *The Other Side* (New York: Free Press, 1964), pp. 87-102; H. Becker, *Outsiders: Studies in the Sociology of Deviance* (New York: Free Press, 1963).

58. See R. K. Merton, *Social Theory and Social Structure* (Glencoe, Ill.: Free Press, 1957), pp. 421-436; E. M. Lemert, *Social Psychology* (New York: McGraw-Hill, 1951); and for additional readings see E. Rubington and M. S. Weinberg, *Deviance: The Interactionist Perspective* (New York: Macmillan Company, 1968); E. Schur and J. P. Gibbs, "Conceptions of Deviant Behavior: The Old and the New," *Pacific Sociological Review*, 9 (Spring 1966), 9-14.

59. J. B. McKinlay, "Some Observations on the Concept of a Subculture," unpublished paper, 1970; W. Yancey, "The Culture of Poverty—Not So Much Parsimony," unpublished paper, Washington University; C. A. Valentine, *Culture and Poverty* (Chicago: University of Chicago Press, 1968); J. L. Roach and O. R. Gursslin, "An Evaluation of the Concept 'Culture of Poverty,' " *Social Forces*, 45 (1967), 383-392; M. M. Gordon, "The Concept of the Subculture and Its Application," *Social Forces*, 26 (October 1947), 40-43; W. B. Miller, "Implications of Urban Lower-Class Culture for Social Work," *Social Service Review*, 33 (September 1959), 219-236; A. L. Schorr, "The Nonculture of Poverty," *American Journal of Orthopsychiatry*, 34 (October 1964), 907-912; J. Cohen, "Social Work and the Culture of Poverty," *Social Work*, 9 (January 1964), 3-11; S. M. Miller and F.

Riessman, "The Working Class Subculture: A New View," *Social Problems,* 9 (Summer 1961), 86-97.

60. C. A. Valentine, "Culture and Poverty: Critique and Counter-Proposals," *Current Anthropology,* 10 (April-June 1969), 181-201.

61. F. S. Jaffe and S. Polgar, "Family Planning and Public Policy: Is he 'Culture of Poverty' the New Cop-Out?" *Journal of Marriage and the Family,* 30 (May 1968), 228-235.

62. H. S. Becker, "Whose Side Are You On?" *Social Problems,* 14 (Winter 1967), 239-247. See also A. W. Gouldner, "Anti-Minotaur: The Myth of a Value-Free Sociology," *Social Problems,* 9 (Winter 1962), 199-213.

63. S. G. Lubeck and L. T. Empey, "Mediatory vs. Total Institution: The Case of the Runaway," *Social Problems,* 16 (1966), 242-260; A. C. Higgins, "Two Thirds of a Medical Equation—Pathology and Patients," in I Deutscher and E. J. Thompson, eds., *Among the People* (New York: Basic Books, 1968), pp. 279-293; E. Freidson, "Disability as Social Deviance," in M. B. Sussman, ed., *Sociology and Rehabilitation* (American Sociological Association, 1965), pp. 71-99.

64. McKinlay, "Some Approaches and Problems in the Use of Service—An Overview"; J. L. Roach, "A Theory of Lower Class Behavior" in L. Gross, ed., *Sociological Theory: Inquiries and Paradigms* (New York: Harper International, 1967), pp. 294-314.

65. L. Schneiderman, "Social Class, Diagnosis and Treatment," *American Journal of Orthopsychiatry,* 35 (January 1965), 99-105.

66. G. Sjoberg, R. A. Brymer, and B. Farris, "Bureaucracy and the Lower Class," *Sociology and Social Research,* 50 (April 1963), 325-337; F. Reissman, J. Cohen, and A. Pearl, eds., *Mental Health of the Poor* (New York: Free Press, 1964); J. B. McKinlay, "Clients and Organizations," in J. B. McKinlay, ed., *Processing People: Studies of Organizational Behavior* (London: Holt, Rinehart and Winston, forthcoming); J. B. McKinlay, "Better Maternity Care For Women?" *Medical Officer,* 120 (November 1968), 275-276.

67. H. J. Gans, "The Subcultures of the Working Class, Lower Class, and Middle Class," in *The Urban Villagers* (New York: Free Press, 1962), pp. 229-254; H. Rodman, "On Understanding Lower-Class Behavior," *Social and Economic Studies,* 8 (1959), 441-450; L. Rainwater, "The Lower Class: Health, Illness and Medical Institutions," *Pruitt Igoe Occasional Paper No. 15,* March, 1965; C. K. Riessman, "Birth Control, Culture, and the Poor," *American Journal of Orthopsychiatry,* 40 (July 1968), 693-699.

68. A. L. Strauss, "Medical Organization, Medical Care and Lower Income Groups," *Social Science and Medicine,* 3 (1969), 143-177; A. L. Strauss, "Medical Ghettos," *Trans-action,* (May 1968), 7-15, 62.

69. M. Jefferys, "Social Class and Health Promotion," *Health*

Education Journal, 15 (May 1967), 109-117; L. Pratt, A. Seligman, and G. Reader, "Physicians' Views on the Level of Medical Information Among Patients," *American Journal of Public Health,* 47 (October 1957), 1277-1283; A. Segal, "Workers' Perceptions of Mentally Disabled Clients: Effect on Service Delivery," *Social Work,* 15 (July 1970), 39-46.

70. H. J. Osofsky, "The Walls Are Within—An Exploration of Barriers Between Middle-Class Physicians and Poor Patients," in Deutscher and Thompson, eds., *Among the People,* pp. 239-258.

71. L. Schatzman and A. Strauss, "Social Class and Modes of Communication," *American Journal of Sociology,* 60 (January 1955), 329-338; B. Bernstein, "Social Class and Linguistic Development: A Theory of Social Learning," in A. H. Halsey, J. Floud, and C. A. Anderson, eds., *Education, Economy and Society* (New York: Free Press, 1971), pp. 288-314.

72. K. Davis, "Mental Hygiene and the Class Structure," *Psychiatry,* 1 (February 1938), 55-56; O. G. Simmons, "Implications of Social Class for Public Health," *Human Organization,* 16 (Fall 1957), 7-10.

73. E. Freidson, *Professional Dominance* (Chicago: Atherton, 1970); J. L. Walsh and R. H. Elling, "Professionalism and the Poor—Structural Effects and Professional Behavior," *Journal of Health and Social Behavior,* 9 (March 1968), 16-28; J. B. McKinlay, "Clients and Organizations," and A. K. Daniels, "Professionalism and Organizations," in J. B. McKinlay, ed., *Processing People;* Editors of the Yale Law Journal, "The American Medical Association: Power, Purpose, and Politics in Organized Medicine," *Yale Law Journal,* 63 (May 1954).

74. R. M. Sade, "Medical Care as a Right: A Refutation," *New England Journal of Medicine,* 285 (December 1971), 1288-1292.

75. M. R. Haug and M. B. Sussman, "Professional Autonomy and the Revolt of the Client," *Social Problems,* 17 (Fall 1969), 153-161; M. R. Haug and M. B. Sussman, "Professionalism and the Public," *Social Inquiry,* 39 (1969), 57-64.

76. McKinlay and McKinlay, "Some Social Characteristics of Lower Working Class Utilizers and Underutilizers of Maternity Care Services."

77. Kornhauser, *The Politics of Mass Society* (Glencoe, Ill.: Free Press, 1959), pp. 93-110.

78. D. Bell, "America as a Mass Society: A Critique," in *The End of Ideology* (Glencoe, Ill.: Free Press, 1960), pp. 21-36; J. R. Gusfield, "Mass Society and Extremist Politics," *American Sociological Review,* 27 (February 1962), 19-30.

79. C. W. Mills, *The Power Elite* (New York: Oxford University

Press, 1956). See also K. Boulding, *The Organizational Revolution* (New York: Harper & Bros., 1953).

80. A. G. Neal and M. Seeman, "Organizations and Powerlessness: A Test of the Mediation Hypothesis," *American Sociological Review,* 29 (April 1964), 216-226; C. M. Bonjean and M. D. Grimes, "Bureaucracy and Alienation: A Dimensional Approach," *Social Forces,* 48 (March 1970), 365-373; E. Josephson and M. Josephson, *Man Alone: Alienation in Modern Society* (New York: Dell, 1962).

Chapter VII: The Treatment of the Sick

1. Robert E. Coker, Jr., John Kosa, and Bernard G. Greenberg, "Medical Careers in Public Health," *Milbank Memorial Fund Quarterly,* 44 (April 1966), part 1,147-258; Frances S. McConnell, John Kosa, and Robert E. Coker, Jr., "The Selection of the Field of Public Health," *American Journal of Public Health,* 56 (May 1966), 764-775; John D. Stoeckle and Irving K. Zola, "After Everyone Can Pay for Medical Care," *Medical Care,* 2 (January 1964), 36-41.

2. John Kosa, "Entrepreneurship and Charisma in the Medical Profession," *Social Science and Medicine,* 4 (July 1970), 25-40.

3. Leon S. Robertson et al., "Race, Status, and Medical Care," *Phylon,* 28 (Winter 1967), 353-360.

4. Richard I. Feinbloom et al., "The Physician's Knowledge of Low-income Families," paper presented at the meeting of the American Public Health Association, 1967.

5. Barbara Ehrenreich and John Ehrenreich, *The American Health Empire* (New York: Randon House, Vintage Books, 1971).

6. U.S. Department of Health, Education, and Welfare, *Health Manpower Source Book* (Washington, D.C.: U.S. Government Printing Office, 1969).

7. Robert R. Cadmus and John H. Ketner, *Organizing Ambulance Services in the Public Interest,* (Chapel Hill, N.C., January 1965).

8. Bert Ellenbogen, Charles E. Ramsey, and Robert A. Danley, "Health Need, Status, and Subscription to Health Insurance," *Journal of Health and Human Behavior,* 7 (Spring 1966), 63.

9. Jerry Solon, "Patterns of Medical Care," *American Journal of Public Health,* 50 (December 1960), 1905-1913.

10. Joel J. Alpert et al., "Types of Families That Use An Emergency Clinic," *Medical Care,* 7 (January 1969), 55-61; Joel J. Alpert, John Kosa, and Robert J. Haggerty, "A Month of Illness and Health Care Among Low-income Families," *Public Health Reports,* 82 (August 1967), 705-713.

11. Robert J. Haggerty, "Community Pediatrics," *New England Journal* of Medicine, 278 (January 1968), 15-21; George A. Silver,

Family Medical Care, (Cambridge, Mass.: Harvard University Press, 1963).

12. "Comprehensive Health Planning," a symposium of articles in the *American Journal of Public Health,* 58 (June 1968), 1015-1089.

13. Joel J. Alpert et al., "Effective Use of Comprehensive Pediatric Care," *American Journal of Diseases of Children,* 116 (November 1968), 529-533.

14. J. Whitney Brown et al., "Study of General Practice in Massachusetts," Journal of the American Medical Association, 216 (April 1971), 301-306.

15. Marcel A. Fredericks, John Kosa, and Leon S. Robertson, "The Doctor and the Poor," a paper presented at the meeting of the Eastern Sociological Soc., 1969.

16. Julius A. Roth et al., "Who Will Treat The Poor?", paper presented at the meeting of the American Sociological Association, 1967.

17. See Marvin B. Sussman et al., *The Walking Patient* (Cleveland: Western Reserve University Press, 1967); Malcolm W. Klein et al., "Problems of Measuring Patient Care in the Out-Patient Department," *Journal of Health and Human Behavior,* 2 (Summer 1961), 138-144; Norman Berkowitz, Mary F. Malone, and Malcolm W. Klein, "Patient Care as a Criterion Problem," *Journal of Health and Human Behavior,* 3 (Fall 1962), 171-176.

18. Howard S. Becker et al., *Boys in White* (Chicago: University of Chicago Press, 1961), esp. chap. 16.

19. Julius A. Roth et al., "Who Will Treat The Poor?"; and Marcel A. Fredericks et al., "Physicians and Poverty Programs," *Hospital Progress,* March 1971.

20. Earl L. Koos, *The Health of Regionville* (New York: Columbia University Press, 1954) pp. 88-94; Lyle Saunders, *Cultural Difference and Medical Care* (New York: Russell Sage Foundation, 1954), pp. 79-87; David Elesh, "Pharmacists and Physicians: The Issue of Access," University of Wisconsin Institute for Research on Poverty (mimeographed, 1971).

21. For further details on the study of the hospital emergency department, see the following; Julius A. Roth, "Utilization of the Hospital Emergency Department," *Journal of Health and Social Behavior,* 12, (December 1971), 312-320; Julius A. Roth, "Some Contingencies of the Moral Evaluation and Control of Clientele: The Case of the Hospital Emergency Service," *American Journal of Sociology* 77 (March 1972), 00-000; Julius A. Roth, "Staff and Client Control Strategies in Urban Hospital Emergency Services," *Urban Life and Culture* 1 (April 1972), pp. 39-60.

22. Raymond S. Duff and August B. Hollingshead, *Sickness and Society* (New York: Harper and Row, 1968), p. 115.

23. Ibid., especially pp. 61, 68, 129-133, 140, 155, 224, 232, 381.

24. Herbert E. Klarman, "Characteristics of Patients in Short-Term Hospitals in New York City," *Journal of Health and Human Behavior*, 3 (Spring 1962), 46-52.

25. Duff and Hollingshead, *Sickness and Society*, p. 111.

26. Personal communication from Walter Klink.

27. *The TB Clinic Attitudes, Management and Standards*, (New York: National Tuberculosis Association, 1967), p. 10.

28. The information is taken from the author's studies of tuberculosis hospitals. See his "Behavior Control in Tuberculosis," *T: International Union Against Tuberculosis*, July 1963, pp. 17-23.

29. Dorothy Miller and Michael Schwartz, "County Lunacy Commission Hearings," *Social Problems*, 14 (Summer 1966), 26-35; Thomas J. Scheff, "The Societal Reaction to Deviance," *Social Problems*, 11 (Spring 1964), 401-413.

30. August B. Hollingshead and Frederick G. Redlich, *Social Class and Mental Illness* (New York: John Wiley & Sons, 1958); Jerome K. Myers, Lee L. Bean and Max P. Pepper, "Social Class and Psychiatric Disorders," *Journal of Health and Human Behavior*, 6 (Summer 1965), 74-79; Raymond G. Hunt, Orville Gurrslin, and Jack L. Roach "Social Status and Psychiatric Service in a Child Guidance Clinic," *American Sociological Review*, 23 (February 1958), 81-83; Georges Sabagh et al., "Social Class and Ethnic Status of Patients Admitted to a State Hospital for the Retarded," *Pacific Sociological Review*, 2 (Fall 1959), 75-80.

31. Hollingshead and Redlich, *Social Class and Mental Illness*, p. 295; Sabagh et al., "Social Class and Ethnic Status"; Robert Hardt and Sherwin Feinhandler, "Social Class in Mental Hospitalization Prognosis," *American Sociological Review*, 24 (December 1959) 815-821.

32. Julius A. Roth and Elizabeth M. Eddy, *Rehabilitation for the Unwanted* (New York: Atherton Press, 1967).

33. See note 23, and Ehrenreich and Ehrenreich, *The American Health Empire*, chaps. 4,5,6, and 15.

34. Ibid., chap. 17.

Chapter VIII: Readjustment and Rehabilitation of Patients

1. Marvin B. Sussman, "Use of the Longitudinal Design in Studies of Long-Term Illness: Some Advantages and Limitations," *Gerontologist*, 2, Part II (June 1964), 25-29.

2. Robert A. Scott, *The Making of Blind Men* (New York: Russell Sage Foundation, 1969); Thomas J. Scheff, "Typification in the Diagnostic Practices of Rehabilitation Agencies," Robert A. Scott,

"Comments About Interpersonal Processes of Rehabilitation," and Albert F. Wessen, "The Rehabilitation Apparatus and Organization Theory," in Marvin B. Sussman, ed., *Sociology and Rehabilitation* (Washington, D.C.: American Sociological Association, 1966), pp. 132-178; Elliott A. Krause, "After the Rehabilitation Center," *Social Problems,* 14 (Fall 1966), 197-206.

3. Robert A. Scott, "The Selection of Clients by Social Welfare Agencies: The Case of the Blind," *Social Problems,* 14 (Winter 1967), 248-257; Peter H. Rossi, "Boobytraps and Pitfalls in the Evaluation of Social Action Programs," paper presented at the meeting of the American Statistical Association, 1967.

4. Marie R. Haug and Marvin B. Sussman, "Professional Autonomy and the Revolt of the Client," *Social Problems,* 17 (Fall 1969), 153-161.

5. Organized opposition to the medical establishment has taken various forms, one being a people's movement to improve the delivery of heatlh care services. The Medical Committee for Human Rights is an activist health movement with an ideology of "Health Care is a Human Right" and a program to develop a new system of health care in the United States. See *Health Rights News,* a monthly publication of MCHR for their description of activities in such areas as community, occupational, prison, women's rights, rural, and mental health and with such problems as sickle cell anemia projects, patients' rights and advocacy.

6. A fuller explanation of this "client rebellion" is offered in Marvin B. Sussman, "A Policy Perspective on the United States Rehabilitation System," *Journal of Health and Social Behavior,* 13 (June 1972), 152-161.

7. Charles Kadushin, "Social Class and the Experience of Ill Health," *Sociological Inquiry,* 34 (Winter 1964), 67-80; and Aaron Antonovsky, "Social Class and Illness: A Reconsideration," *Sociological Inquiry,* 37 (Spring 1967), 311-322. See further Charles Kadushin, "Social Class and Ill Health: The Need for Further Research. A Reply to Antonovsky," *Sociological Inquiry,* 37 (Spring 1967), 323-332.

8. Frank Reissman and Sylvia Scribner, "The Under-Utilization of Mental Health Services by Workers and Low Income Groups," *American Journal of Psychiatry,* 121 (February 1965), 798-801.

9. Ibid.

10. Elliott A. Krause, *Factors Related to Length of Mental Hospital Stay* (Boston: Massachusetts Department of Mental Health, 1967).

11. Ibid.

12. Benjamin Pasamanick, Frank R. Scarpitti, and Simon Dinitz, *Schizophrenics in the Community* (New York: Appleton-Century-Crofts, 1967).

13. Simon Dinitz, Mark Lefton, Shirley Angrist, and Benjamin Pasamanick, "Psychiatric and Social Attributes as Predictors of Case Outcome in Mental Hospitalization," *Social Problems*, 8 (Spring 1961), 322-328.

14. H. Warren Dunham and Bernard N. Meltzer, "Predicting Length of Hospitalization of Mental Patients," *American Journal of Sociology*, 52 (September 1946), 123-131.

15. August B. Hollingshead and Frederick C. Redlich, *Social Class and Mental Illness* (New York: John Wiley & Sons, 1958).

16. Robert H. Hardt and Sherwin J. Feinhandler, "Social Class and Mental Hospitalization Prognosis," *American Sociological Review*, 24 (December 1959), 815-821.

17. Ibid., 821. Some analyses of variables affecting discharge from the hospital are found in Benjamin Pasamanick, et al., *Schizophrenics in the Community: An Experimental Study in the Prevention of Hospitalization* (New York: Appleton-Century-Crofts, 1967), and in Howard E. Freeman and Ozzie G. Simmons, *The Mental Patient Comes Home* (New York: John Wiley & Sons, 1963).

18. Julius A. Roth and Elizabeth M. Eddy, *Rehabilitation For the Unwanted* (New York: Atherton Press, 1967), p. 58.

19. Elliott A. Krause, *Factors Related to Length of Mental Hospital Stay* (Boston: Massachusetts Department of Mental Health, Division of Mental Hygiene: Community Mental Health Monograph Series, n.d.).

20. Ibid., p. 60

21. See Arthur Pearl and Frank Riessman, *New Careers for the Poor* (New York: Free Press, 1965) and William E. Henry and James G. Kelley, eds., *Nonprofessionals in the Human Services* (San Francisco: Jossey-Bass, 1969).

22. Gerald S. Berman, Marie R. Haug, and Marvin B. Sussman, "Bridges and Ladders: A Descriptive Study in New Careers," Institute on the Family and Bureaucratic Society, Case Western Reserve University, November 1971.

23. Theodore R. Sarbin, "Schizophrenia is a Myth, Born of Metaphor, Meaningless," *Psychology Today*, (June 1972), 18-27.

24. Scott, *Making of Blind Men*, p. 74.

25. F. T. Kolouch, "Computer Shows How Patient Stays Vary," *Modern Hospital*, 105 (November 1965), 130-134.

26. Morris W. Stroud, III, Marvin B. Sussman, and Sherwood B. Slater, "Rehabilitation of the Disabled and the Hospital: A Look at the Past and a Glimpse of the Future" (unpublished manuscript).

27. Marvin B. Sussman et al., *Rehabilitation and Tuberculosis: Predicting the Vocational and Economic Status of Tuberculosis Patients* (Cleveland: Western Reserve University, 1964).

28. D. M. Kissen, "Relapse in Pulmonary Tuberculosis Due to Special Psychological Causes," *Health Bulletin* (Department of Health for Scotland) 15, no. 1 (1957); and D. M. Kissen, "Some Psychological Aspects of Pulmonary Tuberculosis," *International Journal of Social Psychiatry*, 3, no. 4 (1958).

29. Charles M. Wylie, "Delay in Seeking Rehabilitation After Cerebrovascular Accidents," *Journal of Chronic Disease*, 14 (October 1961), 442-451.

30. Stroud et al., "Rehabilitation of the Disabled and the Hospital" (unpublished manuscript).

31. C. W. Tempel et al., "An Analysis of Hospital Records of Patients Discharged from a Large Tuberculosis Service," *U.S. Armed Forces Medical Journal*, 4 (December 1953), 1719-1733; W. B. Tollen, "Irregular Discharge: The Problem of Hospitalization of the Tuberculous," *Public Health Reports*, 63 (November 1948), 1441-1473.

32. Louis J. Moran et al., "The Use of Demographic Characteristics in Predicting Response to Hospitalization for Tuberculosis," *Journal of Counseling Psychology*, 19, 1 (1955), 65-70.

33. Sussman et al., *Rehabilitation and Tuberculosis*.

34. Sidney Katz and Austin Chinn, "Multidisciplinary Studies of Illness in Aged Persons," *Journal of Chronic Disease*, 13 (1961), 453-464.

35. Daniel Rosenblatt and Edward A. Suchman, "The Underutilization of Medical-Care Services by Blue-Collarites," and "Blue-Collar Attitudes and Information Toward Health and Illness," in Arthur B. Shostak and William Gomberg, eds., *Blue-Collar World: Studies of the American Worker* (Englewood Cliffs, N.J.: Prentice-Hall, 1964), pp. 324-349.

36. L. Schneiderman, "Social Class, Diagnosis, and Treatment," *American Journal of Orthopsychiatry*, 35 (January 1965), 99-105.

37. Sussman, *Sociology and Rehabilitation*, pp. 179-222.

38. Marvin B. Sussman et al., *The Walking Patient: A Study in Outpatient Care* (Cleveland: Western Reserve University Press, 1967).

39. See Eliot Freidson, "Disability as Social Deviance," in Sussman, *Sociology and Rehabilitation*, pp. 71-99; and A. S. Yerby, "The Disadvantaged and Health Care," *American Journal of Public Health*, 56 (January 1966), 5-9.

40. George James, "Poverty as an Obstacle to Health Progress in Our Cities," *American Journal of Public Health*, 55 (November 1965), 1757-1771.

41. Jack T. Conway, "The Beneficiary, The Consumer," *American Journal of Public Health*, 55 (November 1965), 1784.

42. Erving Goffman, *Stigma* (Englewood Cliffs, N. J.: Prentice-Hall, 1963).

43. George A. Streeter, "Phantasies of Tuberculosis Patients," *Psychosomatic Medicine,* 19 (July-August 1957), 287-292.

44. Scheff, "Typification in the Diagnostic Practices," p. 141.

45. Michael Balint, *The Doctor, His Patient, and the Illness* (New York: International Universities Press, 1957), p. 216.

46. Stroud et al., "Rehabilitation of the Disabled and the Hospital."

47. Howard E. Freeman and Ozzie G. Simmons, "Social Class and Posthospital Performance Levels," *American Sociological Review,* 24 (June 1959), 345-351.

48. Marvin B. Sussman, William B. Weil, and Alan J. Crain, "Family Interaction, Diabetes, and Sibling Relationships," *International Journal of Social Psychiatry,* 12 (Winter 1966), 35-43; and "Effects of .a Diabetic Child on Marital Integration and Related Measures of Family Functioning," *Journal of Health and Human Behavior,* 7 (Summer 1966), 122-127; Stroud et al., "Rehabilitation of the Disabled and the Hospital" (unpublished manuscript); Reuben Hill, "Social Stresses on the Family," *Social Casework,* 39 (1958), 139-150.

49. Robert Maisel, "The Ex-Mental Patient and Rehospitalization," *Social Problems,* 15 (Summer 1967) 18-24.

50. Edward A. Suchman, "Medical 'Deprivation,'" *American Journal of Orthopsychiatry,* 36, (July 1966), 665-672; and "Social Patterns of Illness and Medical Care," *Journal of Health and Human Behavior,* 6 (1965), 2-16; Rodney M. Coe and Albert F. Wessen, "Social-Psychological Factors Influencing the Use of Community Health Resources," *American Journal of Public Health,* 55 (July 1965), 1024-1031.

Chapter IX: Patient Care, the Poor, and Medical Education

1. R. S. Duff and A. B. Hollingshead, *Sickness and Society* (New York: Harper & Row, 1968).

2. Leonard Tushnet, *The Medicine Men. The Myth of Quality Medical Care in America Today* (New York: St. Martin's Press, 1971).

3. Dickinson W. Richards, "The Hospital and the City," *Pharos of Alpha Omega Alpha,* 22 (April 1965), 35.

4. Eliot Freidson, *The Profession of Medicine* (New York: Dodd, Mead, 1970).

5. Elizabeth B. Drew, "The Health Syndicate: Washington's Noble Conspirators," *Atlantic Monthly,* December 1967, pp. 75-83.

6. Cecil G. Sheps and Conrad Seipp, "The Medical School: Its Products and Its Problems," *Annals of the American Academy of Political and Social Science,* 399 (January 1972), 38-50.

7. Gerald E. Thompson and Seymour M. Glick, "Municipal Hospital Care," *Archives of Internal Medicine,* 126 (October 1970), 673-678.

8. Gilbert Y. Steiner, *The State of Welfare* (Washington, D.C.: Brookings Institute, 1971).

9. Stephen J. Miller, *Prescription for Leadership: Training for the Medical Elite* (Chicago: Aldine Publishing Company, 1970).

10. Michael L. Glenn, "Challenge to the City Hospitals," *New England Journal of Medicine,* 274 (June 1966) 1476-1480.

11. House Staff Organization: "What Future Lies Ahead?" *Hospital Practice,* 7 (May 1972), 29-41.

12. Harris Chaiklin, "The House Staff of a University Teaching Hospital: A Study of Conflicting Norms," unpub. doctoral diss., Yale University, Department of Sociology, 1960.

13. R. S. Duff, D. S. Rowe, and F. P. Anderson, "Patient Care and Student Learning in a Pediatric Clinic," *Pediatrics* (in press), 1972.

14. David Mechanic, "Health Problems and the Organization of Health Care," *Annals of the American Academy of Political and Social Sciences,* 399 (January 1972), 1-11.

15. Elmer A. Gardner, "Emotional Disorders in Medical Practice," *Annals of Internal Medicine,* 73 (October 1970), 651-652.

16. Z. J. Lipowski, "Psychosocial Aspects of Disease," *Annals of Internal Medicine,* 71 (December 1969), 1197-1206.

17. G. Forsyth and R. F. Logan, *The Demand for Medical Care* (London: Oxford University Press, 1960)

18. Michael Balint et al., *Treatment or Diagnosis: A Study of Repeat Prescriptions in General Practice* (Philadelphia: J. B. Lippincott Company, 1970)

19. Raymond A. Gosselin, "Prescription Writing, 1970 and Beyond," *Medical Marketing and Media,* April 1970.

20. D. J. Wilson, "Domiciliary Prescribing," *Journal of the Royal College of General Practitioners,* 21 (August 1971), 509-510.

21. Charlotte Muller, "The Overmedicated Society: Forces in the Marketplace for Medical Care," *Science,* 176 (May 5, 1972), 488-492.

22. Charles E. Lewis, "Variations in the Incidence of Surgery," *New England Journal of Medicine,* 281 (October 1969), 880-884; John P. Bunker, "Surgical Manpower, A Comparison of Operations and Surgeons in the United States and in England and Wales," *New England Journal of Medicine,* 282 (January 15, 1970), 135-144.

23. R. S. Duff et al., "Use of Utilization Review to Assess the Quality of Pediatric Inpatient Care," *Pediatrics,* 72 (February 1972), 169-176.

24. Duff and Hollingshead, *Sickness and Society.*

25. R. M. Magraw, "Psychosomatic Medicine and the Diagnostic Process," *Postgraduate Medicine*, 25 (June 1959), 639-645.

26. Milton Davis, "Variations in Patients' Compliance with Doctors' Orders: Analysis of Congruence Between Survey Responses and Results of Empirical Investigations," *Journal of Medical Education*, 41 (November 1966), 1037-1048; Vida Francis, Barbara Korsch, and Marie Morris, "Gaps in Doctor-Patient Communication," *New England Journal of Medicine*, 280 (March 1969), 535-540; Ray Elling, Ruth Whitemore, and Morris Green, "Patient Participation in a Pediatric Program," *Journal of Health and Human Behavior*, 1 (Fall 1960), 183-191.

27. Paul Wilkes, "When Do We Have the Right to Die?" *Life*, January 14, 1972.

28. Anthony Shaw, "Doctor, Do We Have a Choice?" *New York Times Magazine*, January 30, 1972; "The Agonizing Decision of Joanne and Roger Pell," *Readers Digest*, February 1972. Raymond S. Duff and A.G.M. Campbell, "Moral and Ethical Dilemmas in a Special Care Nursery," *New England Journal of Medicine*, 289 (Oct. 25, 1973).

29. Jules V. Coleman, "Mental Health, Patient Care, and Medical Practice," *Proceedings of a Lecture Series Sponsored by Bank Street College of Education as a Memorial to Ruth Kotinsky*, 1962.

30. J. Thomas May, "The History of Medicine and the 'Crisis' in Medicine," *Inquiry*, 8 (July 1971), 62-66.

31. Martin L. Gross, *The Doctors* (New York: Random House, 1966).

32. Kenneth F. Clute, *The General Practitioner: A Study of Medical Education and Practice in Ontario and Nova Scotia* (Toronto: University of Toronto Press, 1963), pp. 160-163.

33. L. J. Henderson, "Physician and Patient as a Social System," *New England Journal of Medicine*, 212 (May 1935), 819-823.

34. Paul E. Lembcke, "Evolution of the Medical Audit," *Journal of the American Medical Association*, 199 (February 1967), 543-550.

35. E. A. Codman, "The Product of a Hospital," *Surgery, Gynecology and Obstetrics*, 18 (April 1914), 491-496.

Chapter X: The Reorganization of Practice in the Community

1. Michael M. Davis, Jr., *Clinics, Hospitals and Health Centers* (New York: Harper & Bros., 1927); Irwin M. Rosenstock, "Why People Use Health Services," *Milbank Memorial Fund Quarterly*, 44 (July 1966), 94-127; Rene Sand, *The Advance to Social Medicine* (London: Staples, 1952); George A. Rosen, *A History of Public Health* (New York: MD Publications, 1958); Anselm L. Strauss, "Med-

ical Ghettos," *Trans-Action,* 4 (May 1967), 7-16; John D. Stoeckle, "The O.P.D. as Ambulatory Care at the Hospital," in A. Lillienfeld and A. Gifford, eds., *Chronic Diseases and Public Health* (Baltimore: John Hopkins University Press, 1966), pp. 221-228.

2. "Physician Visits, Volume and Interval Since Last Visit, U.S. 1969," *National Center for Health Statistics,* ser. 10, no. 75 (Washington D.C. U.S. Department of Health, Education and Welfare); "Volume of Physician Visits, July, 1966- June 1967," *National Center for Health Statistics,* ser. 10, no. 49 (Washington, D.C.: U.S. Department of Health, Education and Welfare, 1968); "Current Estimates from Health Interview Survey, June 1963-July, 1964," *National Center for Health Statistics,* ser. 10, no. 13 (Washington, D.C.: U.S. Department of Health, Education and Welfare, 1964); Maurice E. Odoroll and Leslie Morgan Abbee, "Use of General Hospitals: Factors in Outpatient Visits," *Public Health Reports,* 72 (June 1957), 478-483; "Health Characteristics of Low-Income Persons," *National Center for Health Statistics,* ser. 10, no. 74 (Washington, D.C.: U.S. Department of Health, Education and Welfare 1972).

3. *Preliminary Report on Patterns of Medical and Health Care in Poverty Areas in Chicago* (Chicago: Chicago Board of Health Medical Care Report, 1966).

4. Jerry A. Solon, Cecil G. Sheps, and Sidney S. Lee, "Patterns of Medical Care: A Hospital's Outpatients," *American Journal of Public Health,* 50 (December 1960), 1905-1913.

5. Raymond C. Lerner and Corinne Kirchner, *Municipal General Hospital Outpatient Population Study in New York City Outpatients Departments, VII Utilization of Clinics and Other Sources of Medical Care* (New York: School of Public Health and Administrative Medicine, Columbia University, 1967).

6. *National Health Survey,* series 10, no. 18, (Washington, D.C.: National Center for Health Statistics, 1964); and series 10, no. 74 (1972).

7. Massachusetts Department of Public Welfare, Bureau of Research and Statistics, *Report on Vendor Payments for Medical Care Classified by Vendor* (Boston, 1966).

8. J. Romm, *Initial Analyses of Baseline Surveys for Neighborhood Health Centers* (Bethesda, Md.: System Sciences, 1971).

9. Barbara Blackwell, "The Literature on Delay in Seeking Medical Care for Chronic Illness," *Health Education Monographs,* 16 (1963), 3-32; George Forsyth and Richard Logan, *Gateway or Dividing Line: A Study of Hospital Outpatients in the 1960's* (London: Oxford University Press, 1968).

10. *Preliminary Report on Medical Care in Chicago;* Leon Robertson, John Kosa, Joel J. Alpert, "Race, Status, and Medical Care,"

Phylon, 28 (Winter 1967), 353-360; Joseph Dorsey, "Physician Distribution in Boston and Brookline, 1940-1961," *Medical Care,* 7 (November 1969), 429-440; personal communications, membership, Massachusetts Medical Society; local directories, Massachusetts Medical Society, 1925, 1930, 1940, 1950, 1965; and Leon Robertson, "On the Intraurban Ecology of Primary Care Physicians," *Social Science and Medicine,* 4 (August 1970), 227-237.

11. Richard Cabot, "Suggestions for the Reorganization of Hospital Outpatient Departments with Special Reference to the Improvement of Treatment," *Maryland Medical Journal,* 50 (March 1907), 1-10; Stoeckle, "The O.P.D. as Ambulatory Care at the Hospital"; and also see John D. Stoeckle and Irving K. Zola, "Views, Problems and Potentialities of the Clinic," *Medicine,* 43 (May 1964), 413-422.

12. Nora Piore, Deborah Lewis, and Jeanne Seeliger, *A Statistical Profile of Hospital Outpatient Services in the U.S.: Present Scope and Potential Role* (New York: Association for Aid to Crippled Children, 1971).

13. H. Waitzkin and J. Stoeckle, "Communication of Information about Illnesss," in *Advances in Psychosomatic Medicine,* 8 (Basel: Karger, 1972), 180-215.

14. C. Rufus Rorem, *Private Group Clinics* (Chicago: University of Chicago Press, 1931); Jerome L. Schwartz, "Early History of Prepaid Medical Care Plans," *Bulletin of the History of Medicine,* 39 (October 1965), 450-475; William A. MacColl, *Group Practice and the Prepayment of Medical Care* (Washington, D.C.: Public Affairs Press, 1966); Jerome L. Schwartz, "Prepayment Medical Clinics in the Mesabi Iron Range: 1904-1964," *Journal of History of Medicine and Allied Sciences,* 22 (April 1967), 139-151; and C. Todd, M. E. McNamara, and B. C. Martin, *Medical Groups in the U.S., 1969* (Chicago: American Medical Association, Center for Health Services Research and Development, 1971).

15. *Selected Notated Bibliography on Health Maintenance Organizations with Special Reference to Prepaid Group Practice* (Washington, D.C.: U.S. Department of Health, Education, and Welfare, May 1971); "The Role of Prepaid Group Practice in Relieving the Medical Care Crisis," *Harvard Law Review,* 84 (February 1971), 887-1001; *Group Practice, Guidelines to Joining or Forming a Medical Group* (Chicago: American Association of Medical Clinics, American Medical Association, Medical Group Management Association, 1970); Greer Williams, "Kaiser," *Modern Hospital,* February 1971, pp. 67-97; and Anne R. Somers, ed., *The Kaiser-Permanente Medical Care Program: A Symposium* (New York: Commonwealth Fund, 1971).

16. Ernest W. Saward, *The Relevance of Prepaid Group Practice in*

the Effective Delivery of Health Services (Washington, D.C.: U.S. Department of Health, Education, and Welfare, 1971).

17. George S. Perrot, *The Federal Employees Health Benefit Program* (Washington, D.C.: U.S. Department of Health, Education, and Welfare, 1971).

18. Martin K. White, Joel J. Alpert, and John Kosa, "Hard-to-Reach Families in a Comprehensive Care Program," *Journal of the American Medical Association*, 201 (September 1967), 123-128.

19. Alana S. Cohen and Howard Waitzkin, "A Critical Appraisal of the Harvard Community Health Plan," *Harvard Medical Alumni Bulletin*, 47 (September-October 1972), 12-18.

20. Merwyn R. Greenlick, "Medical Service to Poverty Groups, in Somers, ed., *Kaiser- Permanente*, pp. 138-148; and Merwyn R. Greenlick et al., "Determinants of Medical Care Utilization," *Health Services Research*, 3 (Winter 1968), 296.

21. H. Jack Geiger, "The Neighborhood Health Center," *Archives of Environmental Health*, 14 (June 1967), 912-916; Count D. Gibson, "The Neighborhood Health Center: The Primary Unit of Health Care," *American Journal of Public Health*, 58 (July 1968), 1188-1191; Luther J. Carter, "Rural Health," *Science*, June 16, 1967, pp. 1466-1468; Elinor Langer, "Medicine for the Poor: A New Deal in Denver," *Science*, July 29, 1966, 508-512; John D. Stoeckle, "Health Centers, Organization Goals, Results and Alternatives," *Chicago Medicine*, 74 (September 1971), 695-697; and John D. Stoeckle and Lucy Candib, "The Neighborhood Health Center—Reform Ideas of Yesterday and Today," *New England Journal of Medicine*, 280 (June 1969), 1385-1391. The historical origins and growth of the health center idea have been extensively covered in the essay, "The Future of Health Care," in the first edition of this book.

22. *Directory of Boston Neighborhood Health Centers* (Boston: Action for Boston Community Development, 1971).

23. Jack H. Medalie and Kalman J. Mann, "Evaluation of Medical Care: Methodological Problems in a 6-Year Follow-up of a Family and Community Health Center," *Journal of Chronic Disease*, 19 (January 1969), 17-33.

24. J. Zackler, S. L. Andelman, and F. Bauer, "The Young Adolescent as an Obstetric Risk," *American Journal of Obstetrics and Gynecology*, 103 (February 1969), 305-312.

25. Seymour S. Bellin, H. Jack Geiger, and Count D. Gibson, "Impact of Ambulatory-Health Care Services on the Demand for Hospital Beds," *New England Journal of Medicine*, 280 (April 1969), 808-812; and Seymour S. Bellin and H. Jack Geiger, "Actual Public Acceptance of the Neighborhood Health Center by the Urban Poor,"

Journal of the American Medical Association, 214 (December 1970), 2147-2151.

26. Louis I. Hochheiser, Kenneth Woodward, and Evan Charney, "Effect of the Neighborhood Health Center on the Use of Pediatric Emergency Departments in Rochester, New York, *New England Journal of Medicine,* 285 (July 1971), 148-152; and Gordon T. Moore, Roberta Bernstein, and Rosemary A. Bonanno, "The Effect of Neighborhood Health Centers on Hospital Emergency Room Use," *Medical Care,* 10 (May-June 1972), 240-247.

27. Leslie A. Falk, "Community Participation in the Neighborhood Health Center," *Journal of the National Medical Association,* 61 (November 1969), 493-497; and Milton S. Davis and Robert E. Tranquada, "A Sociological Evaluation of the Watts Neighborhood Health Center," *Medical Care,* 7 (March-April 1969), 105-117.

28. J. L. Falkson, "An Evaluation of Alternative Models of Citizen Participation in Urban Bureaucracy," unpub. Ph.D diss., University of Michigan, Department of Political Science, 1971.

29. Robert M. Hollister, "From Consumer Participation to Consumer Control," unpub. Ph.D diss., Massachusetts Institute of Technology, Department of Urban Studies and Planning, 1971.

30. Gerald Sparer and Joyce Johnson, "Cost Evaluation of OEO Neighborhood Health Centers," American Journal of Public Health, 61 (May 1971), 931-942; and Gerald Sparer and Arne Anderson, "Cost of Services at Neighborhood Health Centers, *New England Journal of Medicine,* 286 (June 1972), 1241-1245.

31. This description is derived from a previous essay by John D. Stoeckle, William H. Anderson, John Page, and Joseph Brenner, "Free Medical Clinics, *Journal of the American Medical Association,* 219 (January 1972), 603-605.

32. Jerome L. Schwartz, "Free Health Clinics: What Are They?" *Health Rights News,* 4 (1971), 5.

33. David Smith, "Runaways and Their Health Problems in Haight-Asbury During the Summer of 1967," *American Journal of Public Health,* 59 (November 1969), 2046-2050; and John D. Stoeckle, William H. Anderson, John Page, and Joseph Brenner, "The Free Clinic Movement: Present and Future," in D. Smith, D. J. Bentel, and J. L. Schwartz, eds., *Free Clinic: A Community Approach* to Health Care and Drug Abuse (Beloit, Wis.: STASH Press, 1971), pp. 127-142.

34; R. W. Revans, *Standards for Morale, Cause and Effect in the Hospital* (London: Oxford University Press, 1966), p. 134.

35. F. Cooper, "The Lady's Not for Burning: Women as Health Workers," and P. Montner, "One, Two, Three More People's Health

Centers," in *Street Medicine, A Newspaper for Health Politics,* 1 (Fall 1970), 10-12, and (Spring 1970), 4-5.

36. Mayor Daley Loses to YPO in Court," *The Firing Line,* newsletter of the Young Patriots Community Health Service, Chicago, 1970.

37. William R. Straughn, III, "Student Health Committee, Student Activists, the UNC School of Medicine," *University of North Carolina School of Medicine and Medical Alumni Association Bulletin,* 16 (1969), 32-36.

38. W. L. Minkowski, R. C. Weiss, and G. A. Heidbreder, "The County of Los Angeles Health Department Youth Clinics," *American Journal of Public Health,* 61 (April 1971), 757-762.

39. Michael J. Halberstam, "Liberal Thought, Radical Theory, and Medical Practice," *New England Journal of Medicine,* 284 (May 1971), 1180-1185; Jerome L. Schwartz, "First National Survey of Free Medical Clinics, 1967-1969," *Health Services Mental Health Administration Health Report,* 86 (September 1971), 775-787; *Free Clinics, Health PAC Bulletin,* no. 34 (New York: Health Policy Advisory Center, 1971).

40. Carollyn Steinwald, *Foundations for Medical Care* (Chicago: Blue Cross Reports, Research Series 7, August 1971).

41. John D. Stoeckle and Andrew C. Twaddle, "Introducing Non-Physician Health Workers: Some Problems and Prospects," *Social Science and Medicine,* 8 (February 1974), 71-77.

42. Julius B. Richmond, *Currents in American Medicine: A Developmental View of Medical Care and Medical Education* (Cambridge, Mass.: Harvard University Press, 1969).

43. Mark Field, "The Medical System and Industrial Society," in A. Sheldon, F. Baker, and C. P. McLaughlin, eds., *Systems and Medical Care* (Cambridge, Mass.: MIT Press, 1970), pp. 143-181.

44. Richard M. Bailey, "A Comparison of Internists in Solo and Fee-for-Service Group Practice in the San Francisco Bay Area," *Bulletin of the New York Academy of Medicine,* 44 (November 1968), 1293-1303.

45. A. Donabedian, "An Evaluation of Prepaid Group Practice," *Inquiry,* 6 (September 1969), 3-27.

46. M.A. Morehead, R. S. Donaldson, and M. R. Seravalli, "Comparisons Between OEO Neighborhood Health Centers and Other Health Care Providers of Ratings of the Quality of Health Care," *American Journal of Public Health,* 61 (July 1971), 1294-1306.

47. Martin Rein, "Social Class and Utilization of Health Services," *Hospitals,* 43 (July 1969), 43-52.

48. Howard E. Freeman and Camille Lambert, Jr., "Preventive

Dental Behavior of Urban Mothers," *Journal of Health and Human Behavior,* 6 (Fall 1965), 166-173; Camille Lambert, Jr., et al., "Public Clinic Care and Eligibility," *American Journal of Public Health,* 53 (August 1963), 1196-1204.

49. Jules V. Coleman and Paul Errara, "The General Hospital Room and Its Psychiatric Problems," *American Journal of Public Health,* 53 (August 1963), 1294-1301; Maurice E. Chafetz, Howard T. Blaine, and James J. Muller, "Acute Psychiatric Services in the General Hospitals," *American Journal of Psychiatry,* 123 (December 1966), 664-669.

50. Conrad Seipp, ed., *Selected Papers of John B. Grant* (Baltimore: Johns Hopkins University Press, 1963).

Index

Aberdeen, Scotland: health and welfare services in, 244-247, 267-269

Access to health services, 89; importance of, 382; of health centers and free clinics, 386

Accidents, 102, 115

Activities of daily living (ADL), and economic dependence, 319-321

Acute poverty: defined, 30-32; war on, 34

Affiliation, 50, 51

Affluence, and mortality, 96-97

Age: and poverty, 19-20, 31, 37; and nurturance, 67; and degenerative diseases, 96; and morbidity, impairment, and disability, 99; and mortality, 112-115; and lay-referral system, 249

Aged, the: in poverty stratum, 86; and Medicare, 299-300; length of hospital stay by, 306

Alcoholism, 183, 185; and emergency clinics, 289; and tuberculosis, 296; need for inclusion of in medical services, 384; federal grants for, 385

Alienation, and the mass society, 270-271

Alinsky, Saul, 33

Alpert, Joel J., 217-218

America. See United States

Andelman, Samuel M., 111

Anderson, F. P., 342

Anderson, Odin W., 100

Anomie, 214-215; and suicide, 152; and rehabilitation, 314-315

Antonovsky, Aaron, 305

Anxiety: arousal of by morbid episode, 57, 58-59; responses to, 59-63; and professional health care, 73

Appalachia, 17, 37, 86, 95

Apple, D., 234

Attitudes of communities toward poverty, 5-10; taken for granted and not perceived, 9-10; and perceived, 10; not taken for granted but perceived, 10-12; and not perceived, 12-15

Balint, Michael, 345

Becker, Marshall H., 210, 238, 255, 256

Bergner, Lawrence, 216

Berkeley Free Clinic, 374

Birth-order: and stress, 50-52; and nurturance, 67

Blacks, in poverty class, 86. See also Negroes

Blindness, treatment of, 312

Blue-collar working class, 85; life styles of, 87, 88-90; mortality in, 98-99; types of illness among, 103-104

Blue Cross-Blue Shield, 284, 294

Boston: schizophrenia among Italians in, 162; solo practice in, 359; health centers in, 368-369; Columbia Point Health Center, 371; Bunker Hill Health Center, 371

Boston Children's Hospital Emergency Clinic, 279, 281

Boston City Hospital, Harvard Medical Unit at, 340-341

Bott, E., 245-246

Brenner, Harvey, 166

British National Health Service, 240, 253. See also Great Britain

Bunker, John P., 345

Bunker Hill Health Center (Boston), 371
Bureaucratization, 332; threat to war on poverty, 37-38; barrier to the poor, 322, 389-390; and importance of access, 382

California: dental survey in, 130; medical foundations in, 380
Calvinism, and the Protestant ethic, 13
Cambridgeport Medical Clinic (Cambridge), 374
Cancer, 109-110; rise in, 96
Carmichael, Stokeley, 33
Chaiklin, Harris, 342
Charcot, Jean Martin, 138
Chicago Committee on Urban Opportunity, 106
Chicago Local Community Fact Book, 107
Chicago Poverty Study, 106-111; infant mortality in, 115-119
Children's Bureau, 384
Chiropractors, 287, 349
Christianity, and attitudes toward poverty, 10
Chronic disease vs. acute illness, in hospitalization, 317
Chronic patients, 294-300
Chronic poverty, defined, 30-32
Cigarette smoking, 97
Cities, private physicians in, 277-278
Clausen, John A., 169
Client revolt, 261
Cobb, Sidney, 55, 194
Codman, E. A., 350
Coe, R. M., 239
Cohen, Alana S., 367
Cohen, Wilbur J., 36
Cole, Nyla J., 167
Coleman, Jules V., 348
Collins, Selwyn D., 101
Colombo, Theodore J., 218
Columbia Point Health Center (Boston), 371
Communicable diseases: and the poor, 93-94, 95; decline in, 96, 100
Communication: as feature of quality

control, 388; important to patient, 389
Community action programs, 35
Compensatory education, 38-39
Complementarity, psychosocial, 189-190
Comprehensive care program, 282-283
Congenital malformations, and infant mortality, 118-119, 121
Coser, L. A., 254
Cressey, D. R., 255
Crime, and social class, 185
Curative (treatment) service, 262; class utilization of, 264-265; studied in Aberdeen, 268
Cure, attitudes toward, 74-75
Cybernetics, 31

Dayton, Neil A., 166
Deep South: poverty in, 17, 86; mortality rates in, 95, 98
Degenerative diseases, rise in, 96
Delayed gratification, class differences in, 25-26
Delinquency, 183, 185
Dementia praecox (schizophrenia), 144
Dental care: of the poor, 95; need for, 128-131; and income, 217; in Aberdeen study, 268-269; priorities for, 393
Dental morbidity, 128-131
Deviance: labeling of, 255; and posthospital follow-up, 324
Diagnosis: function of in professional health care, 70; differences in, due to social class, 180-181; stereotypes of, 325
Diphtheria, 103
Disability: and SES, 99-104; and age, 99; differentials in, 121; date on length of, 123-124; and income, 123-128
Discrimination, 23
Disease, crusade against, 338
Disordered functioning: and patterns of health services, 182-186; cumulative impact of determinants of,

186-192. *See also* Mental illness; Schizophrenia

Divorce, and mental illness, 163, 177, 306

Dix, Dorothea, 137

Dohrenwend, Barbara S., 51

Dohrenwend, Bruce P., 51, 158

Drew, Elizabeth B., 338

Drug addiction, 183, 185; treatment of in health programs, 384; federal grants for, 385

Druggists, 349; advice from, 287

Dublin, Louis L., 152; on suicide, 153

Duff, Raymond S., 292, 293, 335-350

Dunham, H. Warren, 143, 162, 169, 307

Durkheim, Emile, 142, 152

East South Central states, mortality rates in, 113-114

Eaton, J. W., 231

Economic factors: and length of hospitalization, 313-314; and rehabilitation, 332. *See also* Socioeconomic strata

Eddy, Elizabeth M., 308

Education, level of: and preventive health care, 198, 222; and use of private physicians, 276

Elizabethan Poor Laws, 137

Elling, Ray, 347

Emergency clinics, social atmosphere of, 287-291

Emergency service. *See* Survival service

Emergency wards, of HMOs, 367-368

Employment status: and mental illness, 164-168; and suicide, 166

Epinephrine, 48, 50

Erikson, Erik, 255

Eysenck, Hans J., 46

Family: structure of, and poverty, 20-22; interaction pattern of, 67-72; and lay referral, 240-243, 248-249; rehabilitation of isolates from, 314-315; tolerance of deviant behavior by, 330

Family doctor: use of, and income, 275-276, 283-284; vs. team treatment, 382. *See also* Private physicians; Solo practice

Family planning: inclusion of in health services, 384; federal grants for, 385

Faris, Robert E., 162

Federal programs, for health services, 384-385

Feedback, 50, 51. *See also* Communication

Feinhandler, Sherwin J., 307

Females, and degenerative diseases, 97

Feudalism: and freedom of competition, 8; attitude toward poverty, 8, 10

Financing; federal, 299-300, 368-369, 384-385; of hospitalization, 326-330; in medical centers, 339; of physicians, 348; of outpatient departments, 362; of health maintenance organizations, 365-366; of health centers, 368-370; of free clinics, 373-374; of foundations, 379-380, 385

Fink, R., 252

Flexner Report, 338, 349

Fluoridation, 129-130, 393

Follow-up studies, difficulties of, 303-305

Forsyth, G., 344

Foundations for medical care, 379-381; primary care by, 383

Francis, Barbara Forsch, 347

Franklin, Benjamin, 13

Free clinics, 353, 373-379; characteristics of, 373-374; non-bureaucratic nature of, 374-375; de-emphasis of professional status in, 375; self-help and group help in, 375-376; diversity of, 376; political implications of, 377-378; future of, 378-379; access to, 382, 386; primary care by, 383; participation of poor in policies of, 387

Freidson, Eliot, 205, 239; on lay referral systems, 241-243, 245; on crusade against disease, 338
French Canadians, and minority status, 22-24
Freud, Sigmund, 138-139
Fried, Marc, 135-192
Funkenstein, Daniel H., 48, 50

Galbraith, John Kenneth, 30
Galen, 41, 53
Gardner, Elmer A., 344
Geographic divisions (U.S.), mortality rates in, 111-115
Geographic factors of poverty, 16-18; removal of, 36-37
George, Henry, 14
Gibson, G., 232
Glick, Seymour M., 339
Goffman, Erving, 325
Graham, Saxon, 44
Grant, John B., 395
Great Britain: patient-physician relationship in, 236-237; self-medication in, 240; accessibility of health services in, 389
Group Health Association of Washington, D. C., 365
Group Health Cooperative of Puget Sound, 365, 387

Haase, William, 181
Haefner, Don P., 209
Haggstrom, Warren C., 174-175
Halfway house, 396
Hardt, Robert H., 307
Harrington, Michael, 12, 33
Hartley, Robert M., 14
Harvard Community Health Plan, 367
Haug, M. R., 261
Health: medical view of, 41-44; determinants of illness, 44-48; and SES, 90-104; maintenance of, 193. *See also* Mental health; Physical health
Health Assistance Program, 384
Health behavior: defined, 194; study

of, 195-197; consistency of, 196-197; effect of health beliefs on, 200-205; health supervision visits, 216-221; general considerations, 221-223
Health beliefs: perceived susceptibility, 201, 206; perceived seriousness, 201-202; perceived benefits of action, 202, 206; perceived barriers to action, 202-203; cues to action, 204-205; empirical evidence on, 205-211; and income, 211-216, 222
Health, Education and Welfare, Department of, 368; Family Medical Practice program of, 386
Health insurance: lack of in rural population, 278; national, 384. *See also* Blue Cross-Blue Shield; Medicaid; Medicare
Health Insurance Plan of Greater New York, 365, 368, 387
Health maintenance organizations (HMO), 353, 364-368; background of, 364; examples of, 365; aims of, 365; elements of, 365-366; reservations concerning, 367; accessibility of, 386; participation policies of, 387
Health services: as privileges of life, 3-4; use of by the poor, 250-273; utilization studies of, 251-253; bureaucratization of, 257-262; types of, 262-270; reorganization of, 351-396; equitable distribution of, 389-392; and the reduction of poverty, 392-396
Health supervision visits, 216-221
Heart disease, 109-110; rise in, 96
Help-seeking behavior: "career" approach to study of, 227; role of symptoms in, 228-233; mediatory factors, 233-238; lay referrals and self-medication, 238-250; use of services by the poor, 250-273
Henderson, L. J., 92, 349
Herman, Mary W., 216
Hill-Burton Act, 384

Hochbaum, Godfrey M., 205, 206, 212
Hollingshead, August B., 181, 292, 293, 307-308, 336, 344, 346
Hollister, Robert M., 372
Hormones: and health, 45-47; in situations of stress, 48-50
Hospitalization: and psychiatric disorder, 179-182; by social class, 216; duration of, 307-314; paying for, 326-330; reduction of, 381
Hospitals: long-stay vs. short-stay, 352-353; reorganization of practice outside, 353. *See also* Hospitals, private; Hospitals, public
Hospitals, private: emergency service in, 290-291; inpatient care, 291-292
Hospitals, public: treatment of the poor in, 293-294; and chronic patients, 294; tuberculars in, 295-297; mental cases in, 297-298. *See also* Inpatient service; Outpatient department
Housing, and SES, 85
Hutterites, tolerance of deviation by, 231

Illness: medical views of, 41-44; determinants of, 44-48; and stress, 44-47, 48-52; role of hormones in, 45-47; social situations as factor in, 47; sociological view of, 52-56; concept of morbid episode, 57-59; professional control of, 73-78; increase in minor, 100; and interference with routine, 234-235. *See also* Health; Mental illness; Professional health care
Illness behavior, defined, 194
Immigrants, and poverty, 15
Impairment: and SES, 99-104; and age, 99; differentials in, 121
Income: and disruption by morbid episodes, 69; and choice of network of health care, 72; mortality rates by geographic location and, 111-115; and disability, 123-128;

and dental care, 130-131; and seeking of preventive medical care, 193-199, 222; and health beliefs, 211-216; and prenatal care, 217; and use of family doctor, 275-277; and public clinics, 279-280. *See also* Socioeconomic strata
Indians on reservations, 86, 95
Infant mortality: and SES, 97-98; differentials in, 115-121; Chicago Study, 115-119; causes of, 118-119, 121; in ten largest cities, 119-121
Influenza, and infant mortality, 118, 121
Inhibitory system: class differences in, 27-28; in professional health care, 73-74
Inpatient service, 291-294; in private hospitals, 291-293; in public hospitals, 293; and Medicare, 293-294
Insurance, medical, and health maintenance organizations, 364. *See also* Health insurance; Medicaid; Medicare
Insurance status, and income, 214
Interns, in outpatient clinics, 286
Irelan, Lola M., 88
Isolation: and progression of disease, 316; of tuberculosis patient, 324-325

Jaco, E. Gartly, 161, 165
Jaffe, F. S., 256
Janet, Pierre, 138
Johnson Administration, war on poverty by, 36

Kadushin, Charles, 185, 197, 214, 254, 305
Kaiser Foundation Health Plan, 365, 367, 368, 380, 381
Kaiser Foundation Hospitals, 365
Kaiser Medical Care Program, 365-366
Kasl, Stanislav V., 55, 194
Kegeles, S. Stephen, 198
Kentucky, poverty in, 17

King, Martin Luther, 33
King, Stanley H., 45, 54-55
Kirscht, John P., 209
Kissen, D. M., 316
Kitsuse, J. I., 255
Kohn, Melvin L., 169
Koos, E. L., 230, 236
Kornhauser, 270
Kosa, John, 1-79, 367
Kraepelin, 138
Krause, Elliott A., 309

Langner, Thomas N., 189
Lay referral, 238-250; importance of, 241; systems of, 242; and social networks, 245-247; consequences of, 247-248
Lembke, Paul E., 350
Lemert, E. M., 255
Leprosy, 94
Lerner, Monroe, 80-134, 100
Levine, Gene N., 214
Lewin, Kurt, 200
Lewis, Charles E., 345
Life styles: and socioeconomic strata, 86-90; level of living, 86-88; access to private medical care, 87, 88-89; occupation of family head, 87, 89; nature of social milieu, 87, 90
Lipowski, Z. J., 344
Logan, R. F., 344
Lower respiratory conditions, 102
Ludwig, E., 232
Lunatics, imprisonment of, 137

MacDonald, A. P., Jr., 51
Magraw, R. M., 347
Malaria, 103
Males: degenerative diseases of, 97; psychiatric disorder of, after divorce, 177
Malzberg, Benjamin, 158
Manipulative actions, 62-67; therapeutic, 64; gratificatory, 65
Manpower Development and Training Program, 384
Marginality, social, and length of hospitalization, 309
Marital status, and mental illness, 163-164. See also Divorce

Marx, Karl, 12
Mass society, theory of, 270-272
Massachusetts, welfare benefits in, 18
May, J. Thomas, 349
Mayo Clinic, 365
McBroom, W. H., 225-226
McKinlay, John B., 224-273
Means of subsistence: deficiency in, 2-3; availability of, 7
Mechanic, David, 55, 228-229, 233, 236, 239, 253, 344
Mediatory factors in help-seeking behavior, 233-238; hierarchy of needs, 233-234; interference with routine, 234-235; accessibility of medical care, 235-237; changing pattern of health problems, 237-238
Medicaid: effect of, 292; and medical foundations, 380
Medical care system, and rehabilitation, 321-326
Medical centers: interests of, 337-344; and crusade against disease, 338-339; care of the poor in, 339-341; physicians-in-training at, 341-344
Medical education: technology vs. healing, 335; sources of clinical material for, 336-337; broadening of, 350; lack of emphasis on primary care, 383. See also Physicians-in-training
Medical school care facilities, treatment of the poor in, 301
Medicare: Title XVIII, 88; and treatment of the aged, 292; hospital attitude toward, 293-294; and nursing homes, 299-300
Medicare-Medicaid, 71, 274, 284; effect of on Outpatient Departments, 362
Meltzer, Bernard N., 307
Mental health: social differences in, 135-192; emergence of contemporary conceptions of, 137-139; definitions of, 139-142; inclusion of in health programs, 384
Mental hospitals, 297-299; length of stay in, 306-307

Mental illness: 19th-century reconceptualization of, 138; and social
class, 142-155; dynamic relation
between poverty and, 155-172; and
powerlessness, 175-179; and hospitalization, 179-182; interrelationship between forms of, 182-
186; diverse causes of, 186-192;
treatment of, and SES, 297-298,
305; grants for, 385
Mental retardation, and social class,
154-155, 185
Merton, R. K., 255
Mexican-Americans, in poverty
stratum, 86
Michaels, Stanley T., 189
Middle Atlantic states, mortality
rates in, 113-115
Middle class: advantaged position of,
259-261; utilization of health
services by, 264-265
Middle and upper classes: highest
socioeconomic stratum, 84; life
styles of, 87-90; increase of minor
illnesses in, 103. *See also* Blue-
collar working class
Midtown study, 187
Midwestern states, mortality rates in,
114
Migration and social disruption: and
mental illness, 160-161; and social
class, 164
Migratory laborers, 86
Mills, C. Wright, 271
Minority status, and mental illness,
162-163
Mississippi, welfare benefits in, 18
Mobility, social: rate of, 8; and
American immigrants, 15-16;
limitations on in rural America, 18
Morbid episode: concept of, 57-59;
assessment of threat, 57-58; arousal
of anxiety, 57, 58-59; application
of general knowledge, 57, 61-62;
performance of manipulative
actions, 57, 62-67; and family
interaction, 67-69; and professional
health care, 69-72
Morbidity, impairment, and disability: by Socioeconomic status,

99-104; and age, 99; differentials
in, 121-131; dental, 128-131;
impact of health care on, 392-393
Morris, Marie, 347
Mortality: in poverty class, 90-95; in
white-collar middle class, 96-98; in
blue-collar working class, 98-99;
differentials in, 104-115; impact of
health care on, 392-393. *See also*
Infant mortality; Morbidity
Mortality rates: as indicators of
health level, 82; trends in, 131-134;
perinatal, 395
Motivation, in perception, 200
Muller, Charlotte, 345

National Center for Health Statistics,
122
National health insurance, as network
of professional health care, 71-72
National health service, 353, 391-392
National Health Survey, 122-123,
186, 217, 219, 357
National Institutes of Health, 339
Naturopaths, 287
Needs, hierarchy of, 233-234
Negroes: and minority status, 22-24;
mental illness among, 155-160;
unemployment of, 167; use of
private physicians by, 276-277; use
of public clinics by, 281; tubercu-
losis among, 296
Neighborhood health centers, 353,
368-373; characteristics of, 369-
370; performance of, 370-371;
effect of transportation on, 371;
cost of, 372
Neonatal mortality rate, 117-118
Neuroses, 152, 154-155
"New careerists," effect of on health
care, 309-310
New York Association for Improving
the Condition of the Poor, 14
New Yorker, 12
New Zealand, 240
Nolan, W. J., 143, 144
Nonpsychotic disorders, and social
class, 151-155
Nonwhites, infant mortality among,
115-116

Norepinephrine, 48, 50
Nursing homes, 299-300
Nurturance, family dispensers of, 67-68

Occupation: by SES, 84, 87, 89; and use of private physicians, 276
Office of Economic Opportunity, 368
Osteopaths, 287
Out-of-hospital care: need for, 351-353; types of, 353; list of organizations for, 354-356; problems and achievements, 381-388
Outpatient departments, 353, 360-363; use of by urban poor, 284; history of, 360; features of, 361; changing status of, 361-362; deficiencies of, 362-363; quality control in, 387-388
Owen, Robert, 12

Pain, and the seeking of help, 229
Parsons, Talcott, 54
Participatory democracy, 38-39
Pasteur, Louis, 41-42
Patent medicines, 239, 287
Patient care: the poor as clinical material, 336-337; crusade against disease vs. healing, 338-339; by physicians-in-training, 340-344; performance of physicians on, 344—349; auditing of, 350. *See also* Poor patient
Patient satisfaction, feature of quality control, 388
Paying for hospitalization, 326-330; length of stay related to source of, 326. *See also* Financing
Peckham Experiment, 230
Pediatric inpatient care, 346
Peer review, in quality control, 387-388
Perinatal mortality, 395
Permanente Medical Groups, 365
Perrot, George S., 366-367
Perry, Stuart, 154
Pertussis, 102

Peter Bent Brigham Hospital, community participation in, 387
Philanthropy, 14
Physical health: social differences in, 80-134; and socioeconomic strata, 83-90, 90-104, 186; and differentials in mortality, 104-115; and infant mortality, 115-121; and differentials in morbidity, 121-131; trends in, 131-134
Physician-patient relationship, 236-237; and solution of personal problems, 344—347; lay complaints concerning, 348-349
Physicians-in-training: patient care by, 341-342; personal aspects neglected by, 342-344, 349
Plague, 94
Pneumonia, and infant mortality, 118, 121
Polgar, S., 256
Pond, M. Allen, 93-94
Poor Laws, 11
Poor, the: definitions of, 1-5; attitudes toward, 5-10; help-seeking behavior of, 224-273; use of medical facilities by, 250-273; deserving vs. undeserving, 300-302; medical care system, and rehabilitation of, 321-326; as clinical material, 336-337; treatment of in medical centers, 339-344; reorganization of services for, 351-3; in Outpatient departments, 360; and neighborhood health centers, 368; special health needs of, 384; equitable distribution of services for, 389-392; health status of, 392-396
Poor patient, the, 283-287; personal problems of, 344
Portland Kaiser Study, 218-221
Post-neonatal mortality rate, 117
Posthospital performance: and family reactions, 330-331; new support systems needed for, 333. *See also* Out-of-hospital care
Poverty: institutionalized, 6-7; and social structure, 8; social response

to, 8-10; discovery of, 10-15; factors producing, 15-29; types of, 29-32; war on, 33-39; stresses of, and disease, 51-52; and infant mortality, 115-119; and mental illness, 155-172; and powerlessness, 172-179; as subculture, 255-256; medical intervention for reduction of, 392-396

Poverty class, 86; life style of, 86-90; level of living, 87-88; medical care, 88; occupations, 89; social milieu, 90; mortality in, 90-95; severe illnesses of, 103; psychiatric disorders of, 135; psychosis among, 142-151; unpsychotic disorders among, 151-155; mediatory factors in search for health care, 233-238; utilization of health services by, 264-265. *See also* Blue-collar working class; Middle class; White-collar middle class

Poverty-producing factors: geographical, 16-19; social, 19-24; psychological, 24-29

Power politics, threat to war on poverty, 37-38

Powerlessness, and poverty, 172-179, 189

Pratt, L., 225-226

Prenatal care, and income, 217

Prepaid group practice. *See* Health maintenance organizations

Prescriptions, uses of, 344-345

Preventive behavior: and income, 193-199, 222; general considerations, 221-223

Preventive service, 262; class utilization of, 264-265; buyers' market in, 266-267; studied in Aberdeen, 267-269

Primary care: importance of, 382-383; attitude of medical schools on, 383-384

Private physicians: basic in American medicine, 274; use of, 275-278, 283-284; referrals of the poor by, 336-337; treatment of personal

problems by, 344; performance of, 344-350. *See also* Family doctor

Private practice: in network of professional health care, 71-72; and SES, 88; and the poor, 300-301. *See also* Solo service

Privileges of life, 2; availability of, 7

Professional health care: and morbid episodes, 69; place of diagnosis in, 70-71; networks of, 71-72; and poverty, 72-78; and different types of disordered functioning, 182-186. *See also* Health services

Prognosis, poor, decisions concerning patients with, 347-348

Protestant ethic, 13

Psychiatry, professionalization of, 138

Psychogenic theory of illness, 45-48; weakness of, 46

Psychological factors in poverty, 16, 24-29; difficulty in removing, 37

Psychosis: changing ideology of, 140; and social class, 142-151

Psychotherapy, as means of emotional re-education, 394-395

Public clinics: in network of professional health care, 71-72; use of, 278-283

Puerto Ricans, 281; minority status of, 22-24; in poverty stratum, 86

Puritanism, American, 13

Quality control, 387-388

Race: and minority status, 22-24; and mortality, 109; and infant mortality, 115; and mental illness, 155-160; and migration, 160-161; and use of private physician, 276-277

Redlich, Frederick C., 181, 307

Regional Medical Program for heart and kidney disease, cancer and stroke, 384

Rehabilitation of patients, 303-334; bars to studying, 303-305; and length of hospital stay, 306; effect

of socioeconomic level on, 307-314; reduced potential of, 314-317; performance and social class, 317-321; medical care system and, 321-326; paying for hospitalization, 326-330; and posthospital performance, 330-334
Rein, M., 253
Residents, in outpatient clinics, 285-286
Richards, Dickinson W., 338
Robertson, Leon S., 40-79
Rochester, N. Y., health center in, 371
Role-demands, 190-191
Romans, response to poverty by, 10
Rosenblatt, D., 239
Rosenstock, Irwin M., 193-223
Roth, Julius A., 274-302, 308, 359
Rowe, D. S., 342
Rural America: poverty in, 18; accessibility of physicians in, 277-278
Rural poverty, 18, 114

Sainsbury, Peter, 153
Saint-Simon, Claude Henri, 12
Saward, Ernest W., 365-366
Scarlet fever, 103
Schachter, Stanley, 50
Schizophrenia: and social class, 144, 148; and geographical drift, 160; and minority status, 162; and social mobility, 170-172; home vs. hospital treatment of, 306-307; length of hospital stay for, 307; definition of, 312
Schneiderman, L., 257
Scott, Robert A., 312
Seipp, Conrad, 339
Self-medication, 238-250
Selye, Hans, 45
Service wards, 292-293
Sex, and the nurturant role, 67
Shepard, William P., 89
Sheps, Cecil G., 339
Sick, the: treatment of, 274-302; use of private physicians by, 275-278; use of public clinics by, 278-283; the poor patient, 283-287; and

emergency clinics, 287-291; inpatient care of, 291-294; chronic patients, 294-300; the undeserving poor, 300-302
Sick-role behavior, defined, 194
Sigerist, Henry E., 53-54, 60
Simmons, Harold E., 46, 47
Smallpox, 94, 102
Smith, Adam, 11-12
Social class: and treatment of anxiety, 62; and disruption by morbid episode, 69; and choice of network of health care, 72; and psychosis, 140, 142-151; and nonpsychotic disorders, 151-155; and suicide, 152-154; and mental retardation, 154-155; and migration, 164; and unemployment, 165-166; and social mobility, 168-172; and powerlessness, 175-179; and phenomenology of psychiatric disorder, 179-182; and disordered functioning, 185; and attitudes toward the body, 239-240; and utilization of services, 259-261; and admission to hospital, 292; and duration of hospitalization, 307-308; and rehabilitation performance, 317-321; and perinatal mortality, 395. *See also* Socioeconomic strata
Social factors of poverty, 16, 19-24; employment status, 19; age, 19-20; family structure, 20-21; race and minority status, 22-24
Social interaction pattern, place of morbid episodes in, 75-78
Social mobility, and mental illness, 168-172. *See also* Migration
Social networks, as agencies of control, 244-247
Social structure: elasticity of, 8; as human construct, 11; and war on poverty, 36-39
Socioeconomic strata, 80; classification of, 83; middle class, 84-85; blue-collar working class, 85-86; poverty class, 86; life styles of, 86-90; and health, 90-104; and

dental morbidity, 130; and lay referral, 249; and use of private physician, 276-277; and public chronic-disease institutions, 295-300; and rehabilitative hospitalization, 305; and treatment for mental disorder, 307-314. *See also* Income; Social class

Solo practice, 353, 357-360; availability of, 359-360; persistence of, 391. *See also* Private physicians; Private practice

South Dakota, poverty in, 17

South End Medical Club (Boston), 359

Southern Appalachia, poverty in, 17, 18

Spanish-Americans, and minority status, 22-24

Status, and suicide, 153-154

Stoeckle, John D., 351-396

Strauss, Anselm L., 88

Streeter, George A., 325

Stress: as factor in illness, 44-47; illnesses related to, 48-52; cumulative, 188-189

Stroke, rise in, 96

Subculture: emergence of, 255-256; concept of poverty as, 255

Suchman, Edward A., 55, 239, 241, 334

Suicide, 142, 151; and social class, 152-154, 185; Dublin on, 153; and employment, 166

Sumner, William Graham, 1

Surgery, rates of, 345-346

Survival (emergency) service, 262; class utilization of, 264; in Aberdeen study, 268-269

Sussman, Marvin B., 261, 303-334

Symptoms: assessment of, 57-58; role of in help-seeking, 228-233; changing nature of, 237-238

Syphilis, 94

Szasz, Thomas S., 56

Tannenbaum, F., 255

Tennessee, poverty in, 17

Texas, poverty in, 17

Thompson, Gerald E., 339

Tuberculosis, 94; in urban poverty areas, 111; and SES, 295-297; AMA and rehospitalization for, 318-319; isolation caused by, 324-325; tax grants for, 385

Turner, R. Jay, 170

Typhoid fever, 94

Typhus, 94

Underutilization of health services: related to functional life styles, 257; and bureaucratization, 322-323; and value orientation, 322, 323; and assessment of desirability of clients, 322, 324; potential outcome of treatment, 322; economic costs, 322, 324; family responses to discharge, 322

Undulant fever, 103

Unemployment: and suicide, 153; and mental illness, 164-168

United Kingdom, health care in, 197

United Mine Workers Health and Retirement Fund, 365

United States: attitude toward poverty in, 13-15; organized philanthropy in, 14; immigration to, 15; inaccessibility of medical care in, 240

United States National Health Survey, 100, 102

Upper respiratory conditions, 102

Urban poverty, 18, 19; and mortality rates, 95, 98

Utilizers of health services: characteristics of, 244-245; and social networks, 245-247

Vaisey, John, 353

Valentine, C. A., 256

Venereal diseases, 385

Vocational Rehabilitation, 384

Waitzkin, Howard, 367

War on poverty, 33-39

Weil, R. J., 231

Welfare benefits, differences in, 18

Welfare patients: in emergency

clinics, 289-291, 294; tuberculosis patients as, 295-297; and Medicare, 300-301
White-collar middle class, mortality in, 96-98
Whites, infant mortality among, 115-116
Whyte, William H., Jr., 89
Wilson, D. J., 345
Woodbury, Robert M., 97-98
Work satisfaction, and mental health, 167-168

World Health Organization, health defined by, 41, 53, 82
Wortis, J., 154

Yerby, Alonzo S., 216
Young Patriots Organization, Chicago, 376
Yorkville study, 225

Zola, I. K., 226, 230-231, 241